Reproduction and Its Discontents in Mexico

Reproduction and Its Discontents in Mexico

Childbirth and Contraception
from 1750 to 1905

· ·

NORA E. JAFFARY

The University of North Carolina Press   Chapel Hill

This volume was published with the assistance of the Greensboro Women's
Fund of the University of North Carolina.
Founding Contributors: Linda Arnold Carlisle, Sally Schindel Cone,
Anne Faircloth, Bonnie McElveen Hunter, Linda Bullard Jennings, Janice J.
Kerley (in honor of Margaret Supplee Smith), Nancy Rouzer May, and
Betty Hughes Nichols.

The University of North Carolina Press has been a member of the
Green Press Initiative since 2003.

Library of Congress Cataloging-in-Publication Data
Names: Jaffary, Nora E., 1968– author.
Title: Reproduction and its discontents in Mexico : childbirth and
    contraception from 1750 to 1905 / Nora E. Jaffary.
Description: Chapel Hill : University of North Carolina Press, [2016] |
    Includes bibliographical references and index.
Identifiers: LCCN 2015049993 | ISBN 9781469629391 (cloth : alk. paper) |
    ISBN 9781469629407 (pbk : alk. paper) | ISBN 9781469629414 (ebook)
Subjects: LCSH: Childbirth–Mexico–History. |
    Contraception–Mexico–History.
Classification: LCC RG67.M6 J34 2016 | DDC 618.200972–dc23
    LC record available at http://lccn.loc.gov/2015049993

Cover illustration: Fetus in the womb, Plate 4 from José Ventura Pastor,
Preceptos generales sobre las operaciones del parto (1789–90). Courtesy of
Wellcome Library, London.

Portions of chapters 2 and 3 were previously published as "Reconceiving
Motherhood: Infanticide and Abortion in Colonial Mexico," *Journal
of Family History* 37, no. 1 (2012): 3–22. Portions of chapter 5 were
previously published as "Monstrous Births and Creole Patriotism in Late
Colonial Mexico," *The Americas: A Quarterly Review of Inter-American
Cultural History* 68, no. 2 (2011): 179–207. This material is reprinted
with permission.

For Ed

Contents

Abbreviations for Archival Sources in the Notes, Appendixes, and Tables, xi

Preface, xiii

Acknowledgments, xvii

Introduction, 1
Midwifery, Monstrosity, and Motherhood

Part I
Purity and Productivity: Understanding Virginity, Conception, and Pregnancy

1   The Evolution of Virginity, 19

2   Conception and Pregnancy, 42

Part II
The Hidden History of Contraception, Abortion, and Infanticide

3   Contraception and Abortion, 77

4   Infanticide, 104

Part III
Populating the *Patria*

5   Monstrous Births, 141

6   Obstetrics, Gynecology, and Birth, 174

Conclusion, 209
Change and Constancy in Mexico's Reproductive History

Appendix I. Abortion Cases, 1823–1884, 217

Appendix II. Infanticide Cases, 1823–1897, 221

Glossary, 233

Notes, 235

Bibliography, 275

Index, 297

Figures and Tables

Figures

1 Legal abortion advertisement, Mexico City, 2011, xiv

2 Cristóbal de Villalpando, *La anunciación*, 22

3 Vaginal examination in vertical position, 1825, 70

4 A woman in labor, in bed, 1789, 71

5 María de los Santos de Pérez, 1889, 136

6 Monstrous birth: girl with two heads, 1741, 153

7 Monstrous birth: bicorporal infants, 1793, 155

8 Monstrous birth: infant with four buttocks and legs, 1789, 158

9 Monstrous birth: infant born without skull, 1893, 166

10 Midwife in naming ceremony in the *Codex Mendoza*, 180

11 Birth chamber, ca. 1830, 182

12 Birth instruments, 1789, 191

Tables

1 Midwives by ethnicity and civil status in Mexico, 1566–1888, 50

2 Abortion cases, Mexican Archives, 1652–1793, 93

3 Infanticide cases, Mexican Archives, 1699–1819, 106

4 Denunciations and convictions for infanticide in Mexico by decade, 1820s–1890s, 107

Abbreviations for Archival Sources in the Notes, Appendixes, and Tables

ACSCJ   Archivo Central de la Suprema Corte de Justicia de la Nación, Mexico City

AGI   Archivo General de Indias, Seville, Spain

AGN   Archivo General de la Nación, Mexico City

AHET   Archivo Histórico del Estado de Tlaxcala, Tlaxcala City

AHFM   Archivo Histórico de la Facultad de Medicina, Mexico City

AHJO   Archivo Histórico Judicial del Estado de Oaxaca, Oaxaca City

AHMO   Archivo Histórico Municipal de la Ciudad de Oaxaca

AHSS   Archivo Histórico de la Secretaría de Salud, Mexico City

TSJDF   Tribunal Superior de Justicia del Distrito Federal

exp.   expediente

Preface

The primary reason I wanted to write a history of childbirth and contraception was that I wanted to work on a topic that mattered to women—Mexican women, but also women outside of Mexico, women in the past, and also women today, women I know. Reproduction and its regulation is that topic. Attitudes toward female virginity and sexual activity, access to contraception and abortion, and medical decisions surrounding childbirth matter because they inform broad social practices about women's health and empowerment and because they shape intimate decisions women make at pivotal moments in their lives.

In the past century and a half, debates about abortion and contraception have riveted both the feminist movement and the political Right in Mexico and elsewhere. Such conversations have intensified in Mexico in the past decade. A woman traversing Mexico City's congested thoroughfares today might catch a glimpse of a billboard inviting her to consider undertaking a "legal interruption of pregnancy" (see fig. 1). In April 2007, Mexico's federal district passed legislation decriminalizing first-trimester abortion, and in response clinics such as Profem that provide such services have sprung up in the capital city. In response to this legislation, seventeen states in the republic passed constitutional amendments enshrining abortion's illegality except under exceptional circumstances. Other states simply maintained preexisting legislation. First-trimester abortion when pregnancy is the result of rape is currently considered criminal but not punishable in twenty-nine states in Mexico; eight states consider abortion both criminal and punishable, even in cases in which the pregnant woman faces a grave risk of dying without the procedure; a further twenty-one states currently interpret abortion as criminal and punishable even when the product of conception suffers from life-threatening congenital conditions; twenty-three view it as criminal and punishable even when the pregnancy is the result of artificial insemination practiced without the woman's consent.[1] In such a context, women who currently attempt to access abortion face heightened criminal and health risks. Women's rights advocacy groups have recently

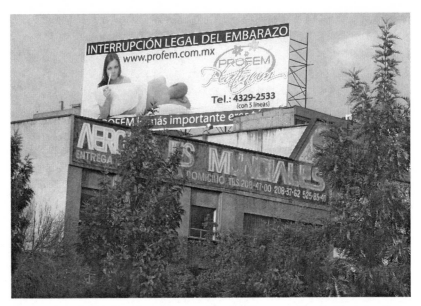

FIGURE 1 Legal abortion advertisement, Mexico City, 2011. Credit: Photo by the author.

uncovered over seven hundred cases of women prosecuted for abortion, some who have been convicted with imprisonment for twenty-five to thirty years.[2]

As such details emphasize, childbirth and its prevention are emotionally and politically charged subjects. They are subjects we care about in our personal lives and in our public forums. In the right setting, many women like to tell the stories about the birth of their children, especially when these involve heroic endurance. And pregnancy and childbirth are topics about which many people aside from pregnant women themselves feel entitled to offer advice and expertise. (I will never forget the chastisement I received a decade ago by a well-dressed stranger who followed me to the bathroom after spying me red wine–handed in a Quebec City bistro when visibly pregnant, late in my third trimester.) Decisions about the medicalization of birth are also fraught and are becoming increasingly so in Mexico, where recent figures reflect a historic transformation in birth procedures. Despite the World Health Organization's 1985 recommendation that caesarean births should only be used in high risk pregnancies and should not exceed 15 percent of a country's total births per year, in 1996 caesarean births constituted 29.3 percent of public sector hospital births and 46.8 percent of private clinic births in Mexico. By

2009, 85 percent of private clinic births resulted in caesarean rather than vaginal deliveries.[3]

Public attitudes toward virginity and private experiences of sexuality, contraception and reproduction, abortion and the medicalization of birth: all women confront one or more of these issues at some point in their lives. Current perceptions commonly formulate sexuality and reproduction, childbirth and motherhood not as matters created by agents of historical specificity but as a set of immutable, natural forces that exist outside of history. Such perceptions include, but are not limited to, the notion that women possess a biological imperative to reproduce and that when they do so nurturing comes naturally to them. Part of my objective in writing this book has been to historicize the topic of reproduction in the particular setting of eighteenth- and nineteenth-century Mexico.[4] In the very act of acknowledging that attitudes toward sexuality and practices surrounding contraception and childbirth have a changing history, we tug away at the protective cloak in which discourses of "time immemorial" and "natural and inherent" enshroud such ideas, often to the detriment of women—current, past, and future.

Acknowledgments

This book has had a long gestational period during which numerous institutions and individuals enriched its development. I acknowledge funding support from the Fonds de Recherche du Québec-Société et Culture program, the Wellcome Trust, and Concordia University. I am grateful for the important contributions that six research assistants provided to me between 2005 and 2015: Rosario Cruz Taracena, Selene del Carmen García Jiménez, Tanya Rowell Katzemba, Meg Leitold, Frida Osorio Gonsen, and Iliana Marcela Qintanar Zárate. The excellent work of the staff at various archives and libraries I used, particularly those at Mexico City's Archivo General de la Nación, the Archivo Histórico de la Ciudad de Oaxaca, and the Wellcome Library in London, was essential to the researching of this book. The efficient editorial expertise of Elaine Maisner and Allison Shay at The University of North Carolina Press and the superb copy editing of Brian Bendlin were crucial to its final formulation.

Various scholars—Linda Arnold, Ryan Amir Kashanipour, Sonya Lipsett-Rivera, Eddie Wright-Rios, and Zeb Tortorici—generously shared references, source materials, finding aids, or expert advice on particular questions. Many others, including several of those already named, along with Christian Berco, Joan Bristol, Sarah Chambers, Jacqueline Holler, Nancie Jirků, Ted McCormick, Shannon McSheffrey, Cynthia Milton, Edward Osowski, Lee Penyak, Bianca Premo, Laura Shelton, Daviken Studnicki-Gizbert, Nancy van Deusen, Yanna Yannakakis, and Anya Zilberstein, as well as The University of North Carolina Press's two anonymous readers, all provided me with various forms of valuable feedback on sections of the manuscript. Myla Junge and Maryjo Osowski both clarified aspects of medical care for me. Dear friends Julie Crawford, Aeyliya Husain, Jennifer Harvie, Erin Hurley, Monika Napier, and Joshua Rosenthal—all engaged in their own intellectual, pedagogical, and artistic pursuits—are always a source of inspiration.

My parents and my brother, Karl, Ann, and Eric Jaffary continue to show me the ongoing importance of understanding and honoring the past, while Sherrill Cheda, who is not here to see the outcome of this research, taught me the value of feminism long before I ever dreamed of becoming a Latin Americanist. My children, Luc and Simon, not yet conceived when I began work on this book, are now fine boys precocious in (among other things) their knowledge of the history of reproductive medicine and birth monstrosities. They often provided me with the first and definitely the most vocal reactions to the ideas and personages that (along with their own boisterous selves) captivated me for the past decade. Speaking of captives, the most significant assistance I received in producing this book came from my exceptional partner Ed Osowski, who as well providing me with valuable intellectual feedback on everything from central arguments to minute denotations, systematically assumes more than his fair share of our domestic commitments. If not for Ed, this book would never have been researched, written, or published. And without him, our household, our children, and my work would be less engaged, less balanced, and less musical in every sense.

Reproduction and Its Discontents in Mexico

Introduction

Midwifery, Monstrosity, and Motherhood

· ·

In mid-nineteenth-century Mexico, women's reproductive practices became a matter of intense public concern. In this period, two decades after Mexico had severed political ties with imperial Spain and embarked upon the foundation of its own legal and medical institutions, residents of small rural communities and large cities alike began to scrutinize when and if women of all classes became pregnant and how their pregnancies ended. In a small community in Coixtlahuaca, Oaxaca, in 1845, for example, sixty-one-year-old Fernando Mendoza, who described himself as both a laborer and a "fiscal actual del pueblo" (a lay assistant to the parish priest), began publicly confronting a young woman, Thomasa Maldonado, about her recent pregnancy. Mendoza declared that the local curate had engaged him "to keep vigil over [velar y ver]" women in his community and so he had repeatedly demanded that Maldonado explain to him if she was or had been pregnant, and by whom. He informed his town's chief constable, and eventually a justice of the peace, that he had known Maldonado was pregnant because he had observed it "with his own eyes since they were very immediate neighbors." Both Maldonado and her parents initially denied the pregnancy but upon Mendoza's insistence, Maldonado eventually conceded that she had been pregnant but had secretly buried the stillborn child. Mendoza and some other witnesses suspected, however, that she had in fact killed her newborn. An overseeing judge in the district of Teposcolula conducted a short investigation into her alleged crime of infanticide, but eventually absolved Maldonado, citing insufficient evidence.[1]

Thomasa Maldonado's experiences, like those of the hundreds of women whose stories are traced across the colonial period and through the nineteenth century in the chapters that follow, exemplify several issues central to the history of conception and contraception in the modernizing Mexican republic. First, Maldonado's example illustrates one of this book's primary arguments: that the emergence of a changing discourse of sexual honor and public virtue became more imperative for an increased sector of the country's female population in the later nineteenth century than it had in earlier periods. I argue that colonial populations projected their preoccupations with controlling reproduction primarily upon Spanish women of the elite and restricted their concerns primarily to the idea of their physical reproduction of suitable heirs. Understandings of virginity, the medical care available to pregnant and birthing women, and the surprisingly small numbers of infanticide and abortion cases that community members initiated all suggest that conception and childbirth did not centrally concern colonial populations. Legislation and criminal trials treating infanticide and abortion from both the colonial period and the nineteenth century reveal that the sector of women whose reproductive practices communities monitored expanded in the mid-nineteenth century. This observation substantiates the analytic conclusions Elizabeth Dore has formulated with respect to women's economic, legal, and social status in nineteenth-century Latin America more broadly. Rather than understanding the nineteenth century as representing an era of positive social change for women, Dore reads the era of political liberalism as it applied to women's experiences as innovation in a retrogressive direction.[2]

Along with examining transformations in ideas about female virtue, this book's second central argument traces the changing connections Mexicans crafted in the eighteenth and nineteenth centuries between reproduction and nation. Numerous scholars have established that after independence, reproduction and motherhood became a central concern in Mexico, as was the case for other new republics across Latin America because, as Charles Briggs expresses, "the mother-child bond was constructed as the most natural social relation *and* as the key site for reproducing religion, politics, and (with Independence) the State."[3] In Mexico—as in other parts of Latin America—after independence, state makers, legislators, physicians, lawyers, and justices all understood reproduction as central to their project of developing, in Anne-Emanuelle Birn and Raúl Necochea López's terms, "a healthy yet docile citizenry."[4]

Political control over reproduction in Mexico is most evident in the justice system's approach to treating the crimes of abortion and infanticide and in the state's increased regulation of health care providers over the time period examined here, beginning with the Spanish Royal Protomedicato's 1750 call for the licensing and regulation of midwifery in all its domains, and ending in 1905 with the closing of Mexico's first maternity hospital, the Casa de Maternidad and its incorporation into Mexico City's newly founded Hospital General.[5] Along the course of this period, as chapters 2, 3, 4, and 6 all discuss, the state incrementally expanded its medical and legal control over reproduction. In the period in which Fernando Mendoza was scrutinizing the reproductive practices of young women in his community in Coixtlahuaca, for example, contemporary physicians instructing midwives and physicians in obstetrical medicine in Republican Mexico's newly established medical institutes were also issuing directives against women's established practices of controlling reproduction by ingesting abortifacients.

In Mexico, the forging of connections between reproduction and nation predated independence. In the late eighteenth century, the rise of creole patriotism in New Spain engendered a surprising attitude toward exceptional offspring produced in the colonial setting. In response to the European Enlightenment discourse of New World climactic and biological degeneration, news editors, municipal officials and members of the public welcomed such phenomena as prodigious, as chapter 5 discusses. Novel attitudes toward motherhood, reproduction and its termination, obstetrical care, and aberrant births developed in the independent republic.

Nineteenth-century newspaper articles, medical journals, and museums all began reflecting popular attitudes of revulsion and horror toward birth monstrosities. Obstetricians, most particularly doctor Juan María Rodríguez, who became important representatives of the development of nationalist scientific achievements, generated distinctive interpretations of aberrant births. Whereas late colonial notices had restricted speculation about the causes of physical exceptionalism at birth to "the rare effects of nature" by the late nineteenth century, scientists and physicians turned their focus directly onto (and into) the bodies of the mothers who had produced such creatures. Eager to defend Mexico's status in the field of international opinion, Rodríguez advocated for the idea of Mexican monstrosity as an acquired rather than inherent trait; such a view not only allowed for the possibility of the biological redemption of monstrous productions but, as chapter 6 explores, also contributed to the pathological perception of Mexican women's reproductive anatomy that became increasingly prevalent in the institutional medicine of this period. In this same period, the Mexican state also initiated various measures involving the scientific control of reproduction and sexuality informed by contemporary eugenicist thought which sought to ensure optimal conditions for the production of a healthy national citizenry.[6] Nancy Leys

Stepan has illuminated how Mexico's eugenics movement in its early twentieth-century apex focused on eliminating "undesirable" reproducers of the national population: poor, laboring, and mixed-race women, those whose sexual and reproductive practices came under increased popular and state scrutiny in the era of the Porfiriato.[7]

The third broad argument I present here, developed particularly in chapters 2, 5, and 6, modifies the predominant and polarizing historical narrative about the development of modern obstetrical medicine by situating it within the particular circumstances in which childbirth and contraception developed in Mexico. Scholars have framed this history, in Mexico as elsewhere, according to two divergent positions. One, a positivist interpretation originating in the late nineteenth century and culminating in the 1960s, celebrated the development of modern obstetrics as the triumph of modern science.[8] According to this view, from the seventeenth to the twentieth centuries, a masculine corps of formally educated and licensed medical professionals increasingly encroached upon the previously female domain of child delivery. In the process, they introduced such innovations as the caesarean section, forceps, and anesthesia, and in so doing dramatically reduced female and child mortality in childbirth. The pioneering historian of medicine, Mexican medical student Francisco de Asis Flores y Troncoso, who published his monumental *Historia de la medicina en México* in 1886–1888, celebrated modern men of science's intervention into the realm of obstetrics, for they ostensibly rid the nation of midwives' pernicious practices.[9] More recently, and following the tradition of 1960s historian-practitioner Theodore Cianfranci's Whiggish view of the "progress points" obstetrics underwent beginning in 1700, Mexican historian and medical practitioner Roberto Uribe Elías's celebratory work, *La invención de la mujer: Nacimento de una escuela médica* continues to endorse this understanding of obstetrical developments in our own time.[10]

Since the 1960s, feminist scholars have challenged this interpretation, portraying the incursion of male physicians into the birth chamber as a process that had negative repercussions for women. For them, this process—which entailed the licensing and regulation of professional midwives—involved the obliteration of the labor and expertise of the "traditional" midwife. Thus, practitioner Phyllis L. Brodsky writes that obstetrical history illustrates "what women lost when they traded in their midwives and their female network for male practitioners"[11]—that is, autonomy, confidence, and a practice of avoiding potentially risky medical interventions. For Ana María Carillo, a historian of Mexican midwifery, the mid-eighteenth-century initiative of licensing midwives was "created by the medical profession as both a means to eliminate traditional midwives and to gain access to pregnant and puerperal women."[12] Luz María Hernández Sáenz writes in her history of the professionalization of medicine in Mexico that the rise of institutionally regulated obstetrics was achieved by the late nineteenth century, "when women were finally excluded from recognized obstetrical practice and replaced by qualified male practitioners."[13] Others stress that this process involved the displacement of midwives' expertise, which was derived from empirical knowledge, with the authority of male midwives and medical men who acquired their knowledge through formal educational institutions.[14]

Feminist critics see this process as having had disastrous consequences in terms of both women's loss of control over their own bodies and broader conceptions of women's status. European scientific developments in the seventeenth century overturned the predominant view of conception developed in the ancient world that understood human creation as the mingling of the seeds of both the mother and the father and consequently that women, like men, had similar sexual functions and needs. Antonie Philips van Leeuwenhoek's 1678 discovery of spermatozoa supported the view that "encapsulation" of humans occurred in men and that women served as little more than incubators.[15] Jo Murphy-Lawless, Lucie Jordonova, and Barbara Duden all see evidence in the era of the Enlightenment of a transformation in the depiction of the nature of women and their bodies in European physicians' medical treatises.[16] This period witnessed a new conceptualization of women's bodies as soft, passive, and natural, which contrasted with the scientific "hardness" of masculine medicine. Physicians treating obstetrics in the eighteenth century created the image of a natural maternal body, while childbirth, according to Murphy-Lawless, became "fraught with danger."[17] Medical science, in the face of such peril, needed to rescue women's weak bodies from the capriciousness of nature. Phyllis Brodsky observes, for instance, that the famous seventeenth-century *accoucheur* François Mauriceau initiated the concept that all pregnancies, even those advancing normally, were pathological.[18] Rather than seen as a process that women themselves determined, the medicalization of pregnancy and childbirth left women passive beings who experienced a process over which they had little control. Mary Daly refers to this program embedded in the rise of modern obstetrics as a "patriarchal program . . . of gynocide."[19]

In the context of colonial Mexico, this scholarly dispute takes on another layer of significance. In this setting, the rise of the modern male medical establishment was intrinsically associated with the domination of European culture over both preexistent indigenous traditions and imported African ones. In the context of medical history, the positivist position is associated, in work by such scholars as Richard Harrison Shryock and Francisco Guerra, with European science's wholehearted obliteration of preexistent indigenous practices.[20] But here, too, other writers challenge positivistic celebrations of the obliteration of "traditional" and "popular" indigenous practice, which they see as naturalistic, organic, and often, in current fashion, superior to European medical belief and practice.[21] Even such circumspect a writer as John Tate Lanning observed in his assessment of the impact of European medical practices on preexistent obstetrical knowledge that "no branch of medicine suffered more between the fall of Tenochtitlán in 1521 and the fall of Mexico City in 1821 than did that of midwifery."[22]

As the following chapters demonstrate, however, neither champions nor critics of the ascension of European medical arts and obstetrical practices accurately describe the development of childbirth and contraception in the setting of Mexico. Both positions contain some measure of accuracy, while neither is entirely correct. Various historians have successfully demonstrated that in Europe, beginning in the mid-seventeenth century, male medical professionals did intrude into the traditional domain of female midwives. By the nineteenth century, the former had largely eclipsed earlier practitioners.[23] In the case of Mexico, however, a different picture emerged. In describing this unique context, and the roles that local conditions had in forming it, this book contributes to scholarship seeking to understand the experiences of Latin America's medical and scientific history in its own terms rather than as derivatives of European creation.[24]

Although physicians began attending women at childbirth more frequently in New Spain in the late eighteenth century, unlicensed midwives still delivered the vast majority of Mexican children throughout the nineteenth century and into the twentieth.[25] Recent research has demonstrated, for instance, that even in late twentieth-century Oaxaca, midwives continued to attend the great majority of births—especially those occurring in peasant and indigenous areas.[26] In their earlier histories, both Francisco de Asis Flores y Troncoso and Nicolás León describe *parteras* (midwives) as continuing to constitute the most widespread force assisting women in childbirth. An 1874 newspaper column published in *El Siglo Diez y Nueve* described the ongoing popularity of treating pregnant and postparturient women in *temazcales* (Mesoamerican "houses of heat") in the republic.[27] In his 1910 description of the three birth positions (kneeling on all fours, sitting, or lying down) that Mexican women adopted at the time of his writing, Nícolás León observed that women who gave birth *hincadas* (on their knees)—that is, according to indigenous practice—"were the most numerous, and among those who adopt it are the women of artisans, workers, servants, and the whole poor classes of our society."[28] He later noted that *comadres* (midwives) and *parteras* continued to attend women of the proletarian class at childbirth.[29]

Despite its muted effect, the growing presence of male practitioners in the domain of obstetrical care in Mexico beginning in the late eighteenth century did have repercussions for some women, and these repercussions were neither exclusively horrific nor miraculously beneficent. While obstetricians' overzealous use of chloroform precipitated some women's deaths, for example, physicians' use of such instruments as "tenazas en cuchara" (spoon-shaped tongs) to extract fetuses intractably lodged in women's pelvises saved other lives.[30] Women in the Mexico City maternity hospital, subjected to increasing incidence of surgical intervention at birth, also underwent higher rates of puerperal infection beginning in the late 1860s. Nonetheless, the fact that beds in this institution remained in high demand throughout its existence indicates that many women sought out the medical services offered there. Further, while imported European medicine had a powerful role in determining institutional obstetrical practice up to the late nineteenth century, it did not obliterate preexistent indigenous practice and belief; nor did it prevent the female practice of midwifery, whether licensed or not. In the late colonial period and throughout the nineteenth century, midwives maintained traditional medical practices and developed new ones despite—and in some cases because of—the presence of the modernizing medical profession and the developing interventionist state.[31]

In viceregal Mexico, two medical systems functioned simultaneously: first, institutional medicine, practiced by state-sanctioned physicians, published in state-sanctioned medical texts and taught in the Royal Pontifical University's School of Medicine and, after 1768, in the Royal College of Surgery; and second, popular medicine, practiced by *curanderas* (healers), herbalists, *boticarios* (pharmacists), phlebotomists, barbers, and midwives of all ethnic backgrounds. In practice, however, few boundaries existed between these two medical systems. Given the small numbers of licensed practitioners in New Spain, most of the population sought medical treatment from any whose experience demonstrated they could provide it. Furthermore, as research on medical history in New Spain and other parts of Latin America has shown, the medical knowledge and procedures that both licensed and unlicensed healers possessed and practiced influenced one another.[32]

Martha Few contrasts her approach to obstetrical history in colonial Guatemala to earlier models of medical history in New Spain that viewed it through a prism of indigenous adaptation to European domination. Few writes instead that in Guatemala, the development of colonial medicine can be understood as a process of "medical *mestizaje*" understood as a "conflictive process that unfolded as new equilibriums of changing definitions of health and healing were continuously reworked over three hundred-plus years of Spanish colonial rule in Guatemala."[33] She also describes how in the broader realm of colonial Guatemalan health care, "Mesoamerican medical cultures interpellated the theory and practice of medicine in Enlightenment Guatemala."[34] Colonial and nineteenth-century obstetrical practices in Mexico—those advocated by licensed practitioners as well as those employed by the unlicensed—reflected interests, practices, and tensions derived from local circumstances and medical practices of diverse origins. As Jacqueline Holler has observed in her treatment of what she calls the "hybrid" medical practices of colonial Mexican midwives, since colonial physicians' obstetrical practices might include prescribing the inducement of labor through the application of enemas, a sweat pad soaked in mule's urine, or a sliced-open chicken, clients might have had a hard time distinguishing between the "magical" and "herbalistic" remedies associated with *curanderos* and the "rational" practices associated with European science.[35] As chapter 5 illustrates, even channels of institutional medicine, such as the state-endorsed late colonial periodical *Gazeta de México*, reflected the development of a creole medical practice that diverged from embodying a mere reproduction of European medicine.

In their work as *curanderas*, many midwives provided such services as divining the future, locating lost items, creating wealth, and using love magic. Although they were frequently engaged to perform such services, when their spells did not work—when love magic failed, when fortunes remained grim, or when infants or their mothers were harmed during childbirth—their clients turned against such women, denouncing them to the Inquisition or to the viceroyalty's criminal courts. As Martha Few observes, in the colonial era people feared and suspected midwives, like other medical providers, because of the apparent power they possessed over the giving and taking of human life.[36] However, more often than not, neither the Holy Office of the Inquisition nor New Spain's criminal courts judged midwives denounced for spell making threatening enough to pursue such cases beyond their initial denunciations.[37]

Suspicion of midwives' practices had a long history in Mexico. As early as a few decades after conquest, historian Francisco López de Gómara and Franciscan missionary Bernardino de Sahagún both commented on the ominous presence in sixteenth-century society of female healers who, according to Sahagún, "gave women substances they used to abort."[38] During the seventeenth century, condemnation of midwives, especially by the Holy Office of the Inquisition, more often involved their alleged practices of sorcery and superstition.[39] Doctors and medical bureaucrats in the late eighteenth-century era of the modernizing colonial state's attempted professionalization of obstetrics disdained midwives for their ignorance and poor training. Until the postindependence period, since these women often worked as *curanderas* who treated a variety of medical and spiritual ailments, midwives' conflicts with the state most often occurred in the venue of witchcraft accusations brought before the Holy Office of the Inquisition. Medical professionals' disdain for the ignorance of midwives endured—indeed, blossomed—in the nineteenth century, when such writers as Flores frequently criticized them in their work. Writing in 1888, Flores decried "the vulgar practices, sometimes absurd, sometimes ridiculous, sometimes pernicious, that have been introduced by these amateurs, practices that are still maintained with blind obedience among our people."[40]

Perhaps inadvertently, some contemporary scholars have perpetuated the assumptions of their forebears. They write that fundamental distinctions existed between midwives' "traditional" practices and those of male professionals introduced in the late eighteenth century, that the latter usurped control of childbirth from the former and that this transition implied a loss of female autonomy and a diminishment in the quality of medical care women received.[41] Taking this perspective of midwives and the work they performed one step further, some scholars imply that these early medical practitioners used "authority and power to overtly challenge gender, racial, and colonial hierarchies."[42] Laura Catalina Díaz Robles and Luciano Oropeza Sandoval describe an implicit connection between the "resistance" of nineteenth-century Guadalajaran midwives' empirical knowledge and the imperialism associated with European theoretical authority. "Doctors," they write, "tried to institutionalize the profession of the midwife through the constant opening of midwifery training courses; midwives responded with indifference and/or rebellion."[43]

The evidence gathered in *Reproduction and Its Discontents* challenges both disparaging and romanticizing views of Mexican midwives. As is most evident in the nature of evidence midwives provided to criminal courts in cases of alleged rape, these women were not predisposed to challenging the gendered, racialized, or economic inequalities that characterized their society. Neither is it accurate to say that midwives were obliterated from the field of obstetrics in late colonial and nineteenth-century Mexico. The medical establishment and members of the Mexican state may have derided the knowledge and skills of *parteras*, but such women continued to provide the majority of obstetrical services to women in Mexico throughout the period under examination here. Midwives counseled women during pregnancy, delivered their babies, and as Lee Penyak has shown, provided respected medical opinions on women's sexual and physical states to criminal courts well into the late nineteenth century. Various forms of evidence document that many aspects of pre-Columbian obstetrical practice endured into the late nineteenth century, not only circulating among indigenous practitioners but also adopted by midwives of other ethnicities and even by male physicians. In this way, the development of obstetrical medicine in Mexico exemplified the idea of "medical pluralism" that Marcos Cueto and Steven Palmer have identified as a defining feature of Latin American healing across history.[44]

Sources and Organization

Despite the centrality of childbirth and contraception to the project of nation building in Mexico and elsewhere, this is the first book-length study of the subject that traces this history through Mexico's transition from colony to developing republic and examines it by interweaving the legal, cultural, and medical history that shaped its development.[45] It tells this story by framing it, wherever possible, not only from the perspective of elite projects of state control but also from the point of view of the wider population—that of the midwives, mothers, and the networks of family members, lovers, neighbors, clients, and employers, who surrounded them.

My original intent in this project was to examine the history of "regular" birth and contraception that most women experienced during Mexico's transition from colony to nation. In practice, however, readers will see that I often discuss much earlier periods in Mexican colonial and precolonial history because many of them were preserved in the period of focus here. Readers will also note that I focus more frequently on women's extraordinary or irregular birth experiences because regular birth practices most often passed unremarked and unrecorded. The available sources—criminal and Inquisition trial records, medical records and treatises, legislation, and newspaper reporting—tend to document various types of exceptional birth and birth control practices: monstrosities, medically problematic births, instances of infanticide or abortion, or cases in which midwives acted unlawfully in one way or another. The archival record has meant, then, that this history directs perhaps undue attention to the history of birth irregularities rather than birth normalities, but in the chapters that follow I have made as much of an effort as my sources have allowed to address ordinary as well as exceptional experiences.

One way in which historians working on other contexts have understood broad patterns of change and constancy in childbirth and contraception is by studying them through quantitative analysis, using broad data treating the demographics of birth, maternal death, and infant mortality.[46] In the Mexican context, existent records indicate that birthrates in both the late colonial period and in the nineteenth century were high and were consistent with European rates. Before 1830, birthrates stood at 43 births per thousand people in Spain, and 40 per thousand in Lombardy and France, with slightly lower levels of 35 per thousand in England and Sweden.[47] Sherburne Cook and Woodrow Borah's analysis of parish records and colonial censuses in Mexico revealed a high and strikingly uniform rate of natality throughout the colonial era and into the mid-nineteenth century. They note that the most complete records existent for tracking birthrates across this period in Mexican history come from the Mixteca Alta region of Oaxaca, a region that, because of the very small demographic presence of Spaniards, would have been characterized by a strong persistence of indigenous practices—in obstetrics as in other domains—throughout the colonial era and into the nineteenth century. Viceroy Revillagigedo's 1790 census documented that the indigenous sector constituted over 88 percent of the population of the state of Oaxaca, with Spaniards representing just over 6 percent.[48] There, the mean birthrate remained almost unmoving from the mid-seventeenth century to the mid-twentieth century, fluctuating from 45 births per thousand in the seventeenth century to 44.12 per thousand in 1950, with a brief high point of 52.41 per thousand in the immediate postindependence period from 1820 to 1855.[49]

For Mexico more broadly, figures from Revillagigedo's census, as well as later records, show higher late colonial birthrates for Mexico as a whole (64.9 per thousand) than those traced in the Mixteca Alta, followed by a decline to between 50 and 55 per thousand for all of Mexico in the first half of the nineteenth century, and a further decline in the second half to 34–35 per thousand.[50] Robert McCaa largely concurs with Cook and Borah's demographic portrait of colonial and postindependent Mexico as one characterized by high and relatively uniform fertility, writing that such was also the case in pre-Columbian Mesoamerica, although he is rather more skeptical of the reliability of Revillagigedo's statistics. On both sides of the Atlantic, birthrates were kept below what would have been biologically possible through a combination of infant and fetal mortality, wide birth spacing, and some use of contraception. In Europe, late marriage age and low illegitimacy rates (at least until the late eighteenth century, when increased urbanization caused the latter to climb dramatically) were also significant factors.[51]

In terms of infant and maternal mortality, national statistics on maternal, fetal, or infant death rates in Europe do not exist before 1838, but various sources allow us to conclude that both maternal and infant death rates were high before the nineteenth century. Estimates from various districts in England indicate that in the late seventeenth century, maternal death rates at childbirth ranged from 14 to 59 deaths per thousand total births. In a northern English parish, in the first half of the eighteenth century, they averaged 57 per thousand total births.[52] According to Edward Shorter, among the ruling families of Europe in the seventeenth and eighteenth centuries, one-fourth of female deaths between ages fifteen and fifty occurred in childbirth.[53] Reliable statistics for Mexico are even scarcer, but available sources suggest consistently high rates for neonatal and infant death in Mexico as in Europe up until at least 1850. In the eighteenth century, one-fourth of the population did not live beyond their first year of life, and a another one-fourth died before the age of ten.[54] Similarly, Mexican maternal mortality remained high throughout this period, with approximately 21 percent of women between the ages of fifteen and forty-five dying at childbirth or in the postpartum period.[55] In Mexico, a significant reduction of infant and fetal mortality would not occur until well into the twentieth century.

This statistical portrait documents the persistence of high natality in Mexico from the late colonial era, persisting into the first half of the nineteenth century and then declining. But in the chapters that follow, I refrain from making too much of these trends because linking changes in obstetrical care directly to existent demographic data is a dodgy proposition given the unreliability or incompleteness of the existent data.[56] In the colonial era, for example, we must rely on a few local censuses, pseudo-censuses, and birth records from parish books. None of these sources account for stillborn infants or those who died before baptism, so while they may give us some sense of Mexican birthrates, they provide little indication of the frequency of infant mortality and say nothing about maternal death rates. While Viceroy Revillagigedo did conduct a comprehensive census of New Spain, such an exercise, on a national scale, was not repeated for over a century, until 1895. As McCaa has observed, historians and contemporary observers have drawn divergent conclusions about changes in natural growth and mortality in New Spain from even the most reliable and widely used of the colonial demographic sources.[57] McCaa notes that for the nineteenth century, "determining levels, fluctuations or trends is almost impossible because the degree of error is always greater than any likely differences."[58] Most crucially, as high as one-third of Mexico's childbirths continued to be unrecorded in any official documentation as late as at the beginning of the twentieth century.[59]

Spatially, this work concentrates on the history of south central Mexico. I base my analysis heavily on material I collected in archival repositories in Mexico City and, to a lesser extent, the city of Oaxaca.[60] My choices here are both intellectually and practically informed. In focusing on central Mexico and Oaxaca, I am following the trajectories established by earlier scholars of both women's history and the history of crime who also examined the comparative history of these regions.[61] One reason for their selection—and mine—of these collections is that they are the best organized and most easily accessible in the country.[62] I have also chosen to continue focusing on the history of south central Mexico because it was the area I had become most familiar with in performing the archival research for my first monograph.[63] Finally, I learned while conducting my research that historian Laura Shelton is in the midst of writing a history of midwifery and obstetrics in the nineteenth-century northern borderland region, and I am glad to cede the discussion of the particular dimensions of this history's development in that particular geographic context to her expert treatment.

Readers may also notice the scarce presence of religious concerns in much of the discussion of the history of childbirth and contraception in Mexico that I present here, an absence that has surprised many people with whom I have discussed this project. The minimal presence of the Catholic Church in several of the chapters that follow reflects the absence of the church from the archival record of childbirth and contraception in Mexico. When I began collecting archival data about obstetrical history, including the history of abortion and infanticide, one of my first stops was the Archivo Histórico del Arzobispado de México (AHAM), located in the Roma district of Mexico City. I hesitantly explained to the archival assistant who greeted me what I was looking for in the collection, but she did not hesitate to help me search their finding aids for any trace of materials that I would find useful. We found none. The electronic finding aid for the AHAM that bibliophile Linda Arnold generously shared with me, as she did with so many other pertinent collections, lists precisely one three-page document of interest.[64] Neither did Catholic concerns, somewhat to my surprise, feature prominently in one of the other databases I consulted for my research here, the massive Latin American Newspapers database, which makes it possible to easily search major news publications in Mexico by keyword for the period between 1805 and 1922.[65]

Certainly Catholic ideology informed some of the broad attitudes examined in this book—not least of all in terms of changing expectations about virginity in Mexican women. At particular moments—for instance, in the mid-eighteenth century formulation of the state-endorsed requirement of caesarian sections in cases of maternal death—the Catholic Church and its officers also contributed forcefully to shaping obstetrical developments in Mexico. Contrary, however, to North America's current context, in which the Christian church is one of the foremost voices in debates about control over reproduction, the church is notably mute on these topics in colonial and nineteenth-century Mexico. The state, rather than the church, most actively vociferated on the subject of reproduction and contraception, and thus the state has a much more visible presence than does the church in the organization of the chapters that follow.

When I first began writing *Reproduction and Its Discontents*, I organized the text around the different actors involved, first relegating separate chapters to mothers, midwives, doctors, and monsters. But as I wrote, I realized that such a structure imposed an artificial separation—and even an antagonism—among these parties that did not accurately reflect reality; neither did it serve me well as a means of tracing change and its absence across time. I therefore reorganized the chapters to trace the various stages and outcomes of conception and contraception across time, in most cases outlining practices and beliefs back from preconquest Mexico through salient moments in the colonial period, and then focusing on developments from the last half of the eighteenth and through the nineteenth centuries. Thus, chapter 1 treats the evolution of ideas about virginity, chapter 2 examines conception and pregnancy, and chapter 3 studies contraception and abortion. In chapter 4 and 5, I look at the history of two kinds of exceptional births: those that resulted in infanticide, and those that resulted in "monstrosities." Finally, in chapter 6, I turn to the subject of the evolution of birth itself, and to the medical practices designed to facilitate its occurrence.

By way of closing, I should explain my reasoning behind the wording of my book's title, and its echo of Sigmund Freud's classic text, originally published in 1930 as *Das Unbehagen in der Kultur*. Writing in the pessimistic shadow cast by World War I, the psychoanalyst reflected on the central conflict he believed existed between humanity and civilization. Civilization's duty was to limit human suffering, but its effect, he concluded, was to create suffering though the various mechanisms—laws, institutions, and traditions—by which it restricted human access to pleasure: gratification through sexuality and though violence.

As a historian, of course, I look for different kinds of explanations than did Freud. Uncomfortable with notions of universal laws that timelessly explain the human condition, I am more interested in the specific conditions that create humanity's varied experiences. Here, then, I am more interested in understanding instances of how and why women in Mexico in a particular time period sought to limit reproduction than I am in demonstrating their universal desire to participate in it. However, the following chapters echo Freud's thinking in two ways. First, this book does examine the ways that "civilization"—law, learning, institutions, and traditions—intervenes to shape sexuality, reproduction, and their outcomes, often in conflicted contexts. Second, if civilization in the form of laws, institutions and traditions generated what Freud saw as the essential conflicts the West endured at the start of the twentieth century, one might argue that conflicts over the legality, politics, and cultural traditions surrounding reproduction have created the most divisive conflicts of our own time.

Part I **Purity and Productivity**

Understanding Virginity, Conception, and Pregnancy

· ·

1   The Evolution of Virginity

· ·

The history of virginity is intertwined with the history of childbirth and contraception. Changes in virginity's real or perceived prevalence, the values with which colonial and nineteenth-century Mexicans associated virginity (and its loss), and the means by which they established its presence (or absence) all tell part of the story of the development of Mexico's obstetrical history. As this chapter discusses, many aspects of Mexicans' ideas about virginity remained stable from the colonial period through the nineteenth century, but others underwent transformation. In terms of stability, the importance of female virginity and its role in establishing ideas about women's value and their honor (in contrast to male virginity, and its loss, which was never the subject of energetic social scrutiny) remained constant throughout this period. Despite the growth in the late nineteenth century of a scientific discourse that posited an impartial and empirical means of determining virginity—what we might call "biological virginity"—in practice, subsequent chapters demonstrate that such factors as honor, class, and Christianity played a determinative role in establishing the state of what we might call women's "social" virginity throughout the period under consideration here. In other words, although physicians and jurists introduced new empirical discourses of virginity in the late nineteenth century, across time, female virginity was in fact always socially constructed.

Despite these facets of immobility, however, Mexicans did alter some aspects of their understandings of virginity from the mid-eighteenth to the late nineteenth century. First, it is apparent that the primary associations of virginity that Mexicans held shifted across time. In the colonial period, virginity was represented in medical texts and examined in legal contexts, but its most prevalent association was religious; it held a moral connotation even when it appeared in other—principally medical—discussions. The religious connotations of virginity persisted. However, as the nineteenth century developed, medical and criminal preoccupations with virginal status became more prevalent than in earlier periods. Second, this chapter and later ones reveal that whereas in the late colonial period the possibility of establishing "social virginity" was an option that was largely available and important only to elite families, by the late nineteenth century, plebeian women were able—and indeed, were often compelled—to advance claims of "social virginity." However much we may witness the preservation of virginity as a preoccupation for Catholic-infused eighteenth-century Mexico, the rise of the era of liberalism in the late nineteenth century saw the enshrinement of the importance of maintaining sexual purity among an ever-increasing sector of the country's female population. This chapter begins by examining colonial attitudes toward virginity and its loss and then proceeds chronologically to examine how these changed—or did not—during Mexico's passage into a modernizing liberal republic.

Sacred and Social Virginity

Historians and anthropologists have reached differing conclusions about attitudes toward female virginity in pre-Columbian and early postcontact indigenous societies in Mexico. Karen Powers observes that the Aztecs, like the Inca, endorsed the idea of premarital sex and did not place a high value on female virginity.[1] Similarly, Susan Kellogg discusses the rural Nahua practice of *montequitl*, recorded in the early colonial period, in which bridegrooms lived with their future brides' families before marriage, and suggests that, excepting elites, these communities did not fetishize female virginity before marriage.[2] Several other scholars, however, argue that pre-Columbian Mesoamerican culture did place a high value on women's virginity and policed female sexuality in a way that did not differ significantly from contemporary western Europe in the early modern era.[3]

Despite these differences, there is considerable consensus that by the mature colonial period, when Catholic ideology became increasingly prevalent among large portions of the population, Mexicans from a broad range of class and ethnic backgrounds espoused the ideal of premarital female virginity. It is also clear that the importance of publicly maintaining a reputation for virginity rose in direct proportion to a woman's position in New Spain's social hierarchy.[4] Reverence for female virginity is evident in historical documentation recording women's legal, spiritual, and social experiences in colonial and nineteenth-century Mexico. Particularly in the colonial period, the primary association Mexicans made with virginity in women was religious. Catholicism—the foundational ideology of New Spain—reinforced the estimation of female virginity in religious iconography, prayer, and music. Both women and men worshipped popular incarnations of the Virgin Mary that the Counter-Reformation Catholic Church so successfully promoted in Mexico. Moralistic and spiritual tracts addressing the religious education of elite women, such as Juan Luis Vives's influential *Instrucción de la mujer cristiana*, reinforced the cult of virginity.[5] Vives counseled that mothers in general (and Catherine of Aragon in particular) should take the example of Saint Anne, who raised the Virgin Mary, as their role model.

The Virgin Mary's impossible example was the most widely reproduced image of womanhood available to colonial Mexicans. Her embodiment of virginal conception, gestation, and birth was explicitly reiterated in the Catholic catechism that all dutiful Christians memorized, for this text reminded the faithful that Mary "was herself a virgin, before the birth, during the birth, and after the birth."[6] Colonial Mexicans who studied their catechisms on the topic of Mary's perpetual virginity at the moment of Christ's conception would have also read that he was created "from the purest blood of the Virgin Mary found in the natural place of conception, which is called the uterus." There, "without any contact whatsoever with a man, with miraculous supplication to the Holy Spirit, [Christ] was formed instantaneously into a human body and a rational soul."[7] Elsewhere, the catechism taught that the devout could understand Mary's perpetual virginity by considering "with what greater perfection than the sun which penetrates a crystal without breaking it, did Christ penetrate the womb of the Virgin Mary without staining her virginity."[8] Colonial artists frequently depicted this moment in their rendering of the Annunciation, when the archangel Gabriel announced Christ's miraculous conception to Mary, as shown in Mexican painter Cristóbal de Villalpando's late seventeenth-century work (see fig. 2), which pictured Mary listening to Gabriel's message while the Holy Spirit, represented as a dove hovered above their heads, radiated a white light that shone down toward Mary's head.

Women and men of all classes celebrated Mary in her ubiquitous localized forms—in miraculous appearances in the devotions practiced by confraternities and in the altarpieces, paintings, and sculptures before which Mexicans prayed in colonial churches and private homes throughout the viceroyalty. Such depictions no doubt inspired colonial women who sought to create blessed associations for themselves when they became expectant mothers, for they entrusted themselves in prayers, icons, and engravings to Mary's protection throughout pregnancy, labor,

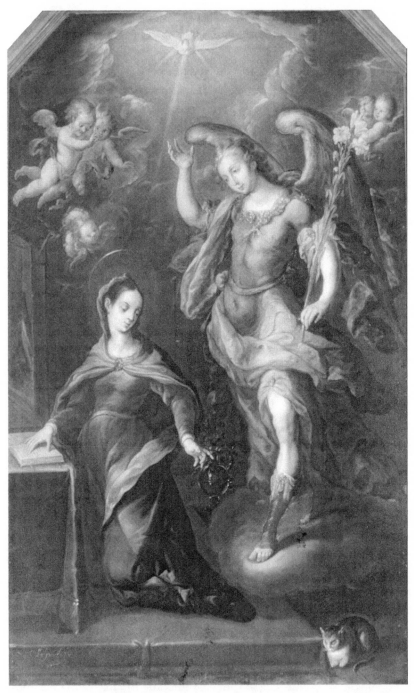

FIGURE 2 Cristóbal de Villalpando, *La anunciación*. Credit: Used with permission of the Instituto Nacional de Bellas Artes y Literatura, 2015.

and delivery. When nearing or entering labor, some consumed holy wafers upon which were inscribed a text, known as the "words of the Virgin" that read, "In your conception, oh Virgin Mary, you were immaculate: Pray for us to the father to whose son you gave birth."[9] Others carried these words, inscribed on special papers, in small linen sacks they wore around their necks or fastened to the heads of their beds.

Such practices sparked some controversy within both the church hierarchy and the pious laity of New Spain, but apparently grew in popularity in the closing decades of the colonial era. In 1777, a curate, ecclesiastical judge, and *comisario* (local agent) for the Holy Office of the Inquisition in Pachuca wrote his superiors in Mexico's central tribunal to inform them of the "general custom that existed in his region of writing on a wafer the words from the verses *in conceptione* and giving them to parturient women to drink."[10] The central tribunal advised him to teach his parish that "there is no power in material words to obtain the goal and favor that they purport to bring if those who recite them lack the confidence they must have in God and in the intercession of the Virgin, for in the absence of this faith, the Tribunal will find the abuse of superstition."[11]

Thirty years later, the Inquisition heard a second denunciation about the practice of writing the words to the prayer "In your *Conception o Purest Virgin*" on paper, burning them, and mixing the ashes into a drink for pregnant women's consumption.[12] According to Carlos Pérez de León, a layman who denounced the practice as superstitious, by 1809 the words to the prayer to the Virgin were found posted "in nearly all the doors of the churches of Mexico." As well as studying the popular practice, the court's theological qualifiers examined the Archbishopric of Mexico's 1807 decision to regularize the recitation of the prayers into sanctioned indulgences worth eighty days' concession to all the faithful who devoutly recited them.[13] In their 1809 ruling, the qualifiers of the Holy Office upheld the court's earlier assessment of the practice, judging that the practice consisted of "a false devotion and a use of total superstition contrary to the decrees of the Church and inductive to false confidence."[14] The tribunal prohibited subsequent printing of the prayers and indicated the prohibition should be included in the subsequent Edicts of the Faith that instructed the populace on the upholding of orthodox Christianity.

Although this ruling would have signified the end of the exchange of indulgences for the recitation of the prayers, it is much less likely that it secured an end to the prayers' recitation. Pregnant and laboring women appealed to Mary, and many other saints, with various other sacred rituals to facilitate pregnancy and birth through the close of the colonial era and into the next century.[15] Some placed black leather belts, such as were worn by members of the Augustine order and by members of the Confraternity of Nuestra Señora de Consolación, upon their wombs and recited a prayer for unbaptized children and pregnant women beginning, "Oh blessed Belt! In mystical regalia you girded and adorned the chaste body of Holy Mary. Belt, that tightly embraced, in purest cloister, that joyful abode which could not be housed in heaven."[16] The opening lines of the text show reverence for the divine, but also hint at the pride that worshippers might have felt in the acknowledgment of the importance Mary's flesh, which "could not be housed in heaven," had played in producing the miracle of Christ.

Just as Mary's marvelous womb had been necessary to the production of Christ, virginal brides were essential to the functioning of colonial Mexican society in more prosaic terms. The arrangement of elite marriages in New Spain, with its thoroughly racialized social organization, required virginal brides. Colonial society, at least at the elite level, policed female sexuality and reproduction because claims to both blood purity and civil legitimacy could only be absolutely established through the maternal line, while paternity could never be proven.[17] Responsibility for child care in cases of the production of "deviant" offspring—products of extramarital or incestuous unions, for example—always rested with mothers, according to Juan Sala, one of the foundational jurists of the early republican period, because "maternity is always certain but paternity never is."[18]

Throughout the colonial period, wealthy families promoted the maintenance of their social positions by encouraging (and, whenever possible, requiring) their children to ascend in social status by marrying spouses of equal or higher *calidad* (quality), a term encompassing a person's racial lineage, economic status, and public reputation. The church, as Patricia Seed's extensive research has demonstrated, long championed children's rights to the free selection of their partners in the face of parental and—especially after the Royal Pragmatic of 1776—state-based objections to such matches.[19] However, the church had also long been sympathetic to petitioners' arguments that they should obtain dispensation from ecclesiastical impediments to marriage in the face of otherwise sanctioned socially unequal marital unions. In granting nearly every impediment dispensation made to it in the late eighteenth century, the office of the Mexican vicar general demonstrated that it viewed the marriage of close blood relatives, including first cousins and uncles and nieces, as a preferable option to the possibility that unequal unions might take place in the absence of these matches.[20] Petitioners in such cases successfully argued to the court that they be granted dispensation to marry their close relatives because "the *cortedad* (smallness) of [their] towns [made] it difficult for those of *sangre limpia* (clean blood) to marry equally."[21]

Beyond the particular context of the creation of marital unions, the maintenance of virginity had significant ramifications on a woman's social value in colonial society.[22] In this era, civil and ecclesiastical records carefully identified most single women by their status as *doncellas* (virgins) or *solteras* (single women who were not virgins); the distinction, as Asunción Lavrin describes, attributed moral superiority and upgraded social status to the former while deriding the latter.[23] Virginity's key role in determining a woman's social reputation in the setting of colonial Latin America is perhaps most famously illustrated by the example of Catalina de Erauso, the "lieutenant nun." Erauso's memoir described how, in 1599, she had managed to escape a Basque convent dressed in men's clothing and journeyed to the New World, where she lived as a clerk, a gambler, and eventually a soldier for the Spanish crown, killing and maiming dozens of men in personal and professional ventures. At last arrested for murder, Erauso managed to win the approbation of Pope Urban VIII, who absolved her of all her crimes and granted her permission to resume her practice of dressing in men's clothing after a physical examination confirmed that Erauso's virginity had survived her many adventures intact.[24] Her all-important preservation of her virginity secured her considerable liberty. After some years, Erauso returned to New Spain to spend the rest of her life working as a muleteer, using the name Antonio de Erauso. When questioned about his decision, Pope Urban VIII affirmed, "Give me another Lieutenant nun and I will do the same."[25]

Medical and Legal Virginity

Although more documentation survives from the colonial period attesting to elite women's need to establish the public record of their virginity—and hence their honor—in such contexts as *palabra de casamiento* (promise of matrimony) legal cases, colonial sources—such as Richard Boyer's exposition of the documents treating a deflowerment suit initiated by a late seventeenth-century indigenous woman, Catarina María, in Malinalco—also indicate that plebeian women also sought to publicly establish their virginity through such means.[26] Here Catarina and her brothers, who eventually petitioned the *juzgado general de los naturales* (general Indian court) on her behalf, sought material compensation for the loss of her virginity. Her brothers declared that they would also be satisfied if the accused married their sister.[27] Catarina María's case differed from the majority of those processed by colonial magistrates in that, in this instance, she initiated the suit on her own behalf. In the vast majority of rape and breach of marriage trials, instead, women's male guardians initiated legal suits since it was their lost honor, rather than that of the alleged female victims, that courts sought to restore. The sentences they issued often mandated the payment of fines to victim's families or the requirement, in cases of unmarried assailants and victims, that the former marry the latter.[28] This was why the rape of a virgin was always considered more heinous than the rape of a married woman; the crime carried a greater potential loss to her family's future marital prospects regardless of the ramifications of the experience on the woman herself. The one instance in which magistrates passed severe sentences against assailants involved cases of child rape when the victims were under age fifteen.[29]

Although such did not occur in Catarina María's case, in criminal accusations of deflowerment and rape in the colonial era, magistrates often required medical examinations for female plaintiffs to establish whether sexual intercourse had occurred, whether there was evidence demonstrated the act had been forced, and whether the plaintiff appeared to have recently lost her virginity. In the colonial period and for much of the nineteenth century, courts most often requested that midwives perform such examinations. As Antonio Medina's 1806 text for the instruction of Mexican midwives asserted, midwives needed to be familiar with the anatomy of women's genitalia as a foundation for "the declarations they are instructed to give before judges in questions involving suspicions of virginity, rape, or impotency."[30] Medina informed his readers that in making such assessments, an evaluation of the hymen was critical, describing this anatomical element as "a thin rounded tissue comprising the orifice of the vagina, having a tiny opening that in the first act of coitus or carnal act was ruptured with some effusion of blood, which left it divided in three or four masses, similar to the leaves of the Myrtle plant."[31]

Here, Medina's text, first published in Spain in 1750 but in circulation in Mexico until at least the mid-nineteenth century, stated decisively that a ruptured hymen normally occurred with first coitus and was a sign that this act had transpired, but his position was exceptional.[32] Other early modern European writers whose works circulated in late colonial Mexico were more equivocal. In eighteenth-century Mexico, among the most prominent obstetrical works physicians consulted were those by French obstetricians Jean-Louis Baudelocque, André Levret, and François Mauriceau. Doctors also studied the texts of various Spanish physicians including Jaime Alcalá Martínez, José Ventura Pastor, Pedro Vidart, and Pedro Virgili, along with writings by the Mexican professor of medicine Juan Manuel Venegas, whose work appeared frequently in the *Gazeta de México* in the 1780s.[33] Many of these writers reported multiple findings about the implications of the hymen's presence or absence.

Seventeenth-century physician François Mauriceau wrote in his *Traité des maladies des femmes grosses,* for example, that the notion that female virginity could be determined by the state of a woman's hymen "was a potent error . . . for if this membrane is found in some women, it is very clear that this goes against the design of nature since it is not found even in the female fetus . . . nor in all girls or women of any age among whom there is no other sign by which we may conjecture their virginity."[34] Baudelocque observed in his *Principes sur l'art des accouchements,* first published in 1775 and frequently republished thereafter, that while the presence of the hymen was normally recognized as the physical sign of virginity, in fact, "this sign is not at all a certain one; neither do tears in this membrane any more certainly indicate the opposite." He continued, "The hymen can exist even after a woman has undergone the approaches of a man, and even when she is pregnant; and this membrane can be destroyed by causes that have no bearing on the achievement of this moral virtue that alone merits the name of *virginity.*"[35] Even within the context of this medical tract, Baudelocque portrays virginity as a moral virtue rather than a biological state and notes that physical signs should not be relied upon to judge it.[36]

Some midcentury medical tracts published in Mexico maintained this more nuanced appraisal of the implications of the state of the hymen. The *Cartilla de partos* (1863), the formally adopted text for use in midwives' training at Oaxaca's medical institute, maintained the perspective that such writers as Baudelocque and Levret had earlier advocated: "Much has been said about the existence and importance of the hymen: the most common interpretation is that in those cases where it exists, it is easily torn and destroyed—by menstruation, vaginal discharge, by the stimulating substances contained in urine, by a long and forced bowel movement, by illicit touching and by a multitude of illnesses, such that it is not prudent to qualify virginity by the presence or absence of the hymen."[37] Similarly, prominent Mexican obstetrician Ignacio Torres's 1858 *Manual de partos* proffered the view that the implications of the hymen's physical state were necessarily inconclusive, for it might persist intact in pregnant women: "Some midwives say they have encountered hymens so resistant that they obstruct the termination of birth; and they say that to facilitate it, it has been necessary for them to cut the hymen."[38]

Another text contemporary to Torres's work, however, offered an interpretation that resembled the more definitive assessment of the implications of the hymen's presence or absence that Antonio Medina had earlier voiced. As the *Tratado práctico de partos* (1857) that the state of Michoacán's medical faculty adopted for midwives' instruction declared more simply, "In nonvirgins, with very few exceptions, the hymen is broken, leaving between two and five scars evident on the sides of the opening."[39] From the late colonial period to the mid-nineteenth century, then, some discrepancies existed within Mexican medical texts over the question of whether physical examinations—particularly of the hymen— could conclusively establish virginity, but a majority of authors asserted that the biological evidence was inconclusive. These texts themselves indicated that those assessing the state of women's virginity would necessarily have to use other criterion to make such assessments.

In the expert testimony they provided to courts, midwives rather than doctors most often performed such services in criminal suits in Mexico beginning as early as the late sixteenth century and continuing through the late nineteenth century.[40] Courts most often requested such examinations in the most serious rape cases they investigated—those in which the victims were minors, under the age of fifteen. In their testimony, midwives normally restricted their judgments to assessments of the physical evidence they observed on the bodies of women and girls they examined. As well as examining their genital areas, midwives recorded signs of physical struggle anywhere on the bodies of alleged victims, for, as Lee Penyak reminds us, "contemporaries assumed that [those] who did not physically struggle with their attackers must have willingly participated."[41] Midwives who provided expert testimony to criminal courts in rape trials in Mexico were less prone to subtle interpretations of the hymen's presence or absence than were the various medical texts referred to above, perhaps because these women were normally examining bodies that showed various other physical signs of rape and defloration: blood and inflammation in the genital region, or wounds or signs of struggle on other parts of the body. The types of assessments they provided in such cases did not vary greatly over time.

In 1684, for example, the *teniente* (deputy of a municipal council officer) of the community of Yanhuitlán, Oaxaca, called upon two midwives to assess a young girl's virginity. In this case, an indigenous man had denounced an acquaintance for having violently raped his daughter, a girl younger than eight years old.[42] After interviewing both of her parents, the victim, and another community member, the *teniente* listened to the testimony of Úrsula Hernández, a mestiza *partera*. Hernández testified that her examination of the girl revealed that "all her membranes were open and torn and that her hips were damaged and that liquids were flowing from the opening of her uterus."[43] A second midwife, Agnes Dias, a free mulata, found the girl's "parts defective and open and apparently broken open by a man, with the membranes torn and open and with some materials flowing from the mouth of the vagina."[44] The midwives' testimony, along with the assailant's own confession of his crime, led to the tribunal's unusual condemnation that he should be condemned to death by hanging.[45] In a much later case, in 1870, two midwives in Ejutla, Oaxaca, examined a girl of twelve; after detailing the wounds she carried on all of her limbs, they described the bloody flux and inflammation found on her genitals, but said there was little of the latter because the "tearing was recent."[46]

During the late colonial era and through the nineteenth century, magistrates most often respected the judgments midwives provided. Luz María Hernández found that in thirteen out of fourteen expert testimony cases she examined from between 1756 and 1831, "the outcome of the trial not only agreed with, but depended to a large extent on the partera's opinion." In the one exceptional case, the judge decided "without detriment" to the *matronas* (midwives) that the accused was innocent.[47] Penyak has observed that between 1740 and 1846, both "prosecutors and defense attorneys frequently relied on the findings of midwives to buttress their arguments."[48] Occasionally, court officials selectively dismissed midwives' testimony. For example, in one eighteenth-century suit originating in Tenango del Valle, Toluca, and involving the accusation of the "violent deflowering" of a ten-year-old indigenous girl, two midwives examined the alleged victim. The first, a Spanish widow, declared on November 4, 1763, that the girl had been "deflowered, and injured beyond what would be natural."[49] But a second midwife, Antonia de Zalasar, an Indian who conducted her examination over a month later, found the girl had "no sign of having been with a man; rather it is clear that she is a virgin."[50] Despite the fact that Zalasar's examination occurred after so much time had passed, the judge ignored the testimony of the first midwife. He wrote that the only evidence supporting the rape charge was the declaration of the alleged victim, and concluded that "this is not to be believed because the testimonies of the two midwives who examined her found her without injury or damage at all." He dismissed the case.[51]

Penyak discovered that in the Mexican capital, male physicians had replaced female midwives as expert witnesses in such cases after the mid-eighteenth century.[52] Yet in outlying districts, Mexican criminal courts apparently relied on them much later. In the community of Ejutla, Oaxaca, for instance, in seventeen *estupro* (deflowering) trials occurring between 1863 and 1888 the local magistrate requested that midwives rather than physicians provide such evidence. As late as 1863, Ejutla's *alcalde* (first instance judge and municipal official) still consulted with *curanderas* in such cases as well as midwives, but in the 1870s also occasionally began calling upon male physicians to provide expert evidence.[53] When presented with conflicting testimony from midwives and doctors, such courts tended to assume the latter provided more reliable evidence. In 1879 Romualda Pacheco, a widow living in the small community of San Agustín Amatengo, denounced one Andrés Mendoza for having raped her thirteen-year-old daughter, Dominga Gonzáles.[54] Two *matronas* examined Gonzáles; one of these, Felipa Pacheco, possibly a relative, assessed that the state of the girl's genitals indicated she had been raped one or two days earlier.[55] Three days later, after her aggressor had denied the act, the court ordered Gonzáles examined again, this time by a surgeon. He declared her genitals revealed "no sign of violence."[56]

This assessment likely weighed in the court's decision to acquit Mendoza of the crime. Perhaps motivated by this incident, the victim's mother, Romualda Pacheco, decided herself to become a midwife, and eight years after initiating her daughter's case, Pacheco appeared as the expert witness in the rape trial of a six-year-old girl whose father denounced a man for having "forced" his daughter.[57] Having been a mother who unsuccessfully pressed rape charges against a man whom she claimed had violated her own daughter, it seems reasonable to expect that Pacheco might have been particularly sensitive to the issue of producing assessments supporting the claims of alleged rape victims, particularly when these were young girls. When called upon to assess the physical state of the child in the 1887 trial, Romualda Pacheco and the other examining midwife both testified—like the surgeon who had examined Pacheco's own daughter eight years earlier—that the girl had not been raped, for they saw evidence only that a "light material" was exiting the urinary tract, which they judged had "originated in some blow that the patient had received."[58] The court subsequently investigated the aggressor for the lesser charge of "attempted rape." As in this instance, midwives remained neutral in the testimony they provided to courts in rape cases. When they saw physical evidence that girls had been raped, they reported it.[59] But in many other cases, even when the alleged victims were children, they refrained from judging that rape had occurred if they saw no indication that it had.

Throughout the time period treated here, in their appearances before criminal tribunals midwives provided assessments about female virginity based on their empirical examinations of female bodies. No doubt they were also aware of the social implications of these judgments. The social value and honor of unmarried females of any age was dramatically diminished when they lost their virginity, whether or not this loss occurred in the context of a rape, as is illustrated in one 1756 trial from the city of Taxco. There, mulata *soltera* Josepha de la Cruz denounced a man for raping her seven-year-old daughter, Luiza Francisca, over whom she possessed *patria potestad* (parental rights).[60] One of the midwives, Josepha de Ocampo, whom the court called to examine the girl, declared that the man "had certainly deflowered [Luiza Francisca] and left her wounded, not on the labia of her pudenda, but rather inside, on the top and on one side, and she is still bleeding from this, for she was scraped, as when a fingernail scrapes a delicate body part; since she is being treated, she will recuperate, but she will always remain a fallen woman [siempre quedará perdida mujer del mundo]."[61] These and similar cases illustrate that in the late colonial era, the loss of virginity for even for the nonelite population had grave potential implications for a girl's future social status, signaling the dividing line between honor and dishonor. This trajectory continued to develop even more strongly in the course of the nineteenth century, as chapters 3 and 4 further explore.

Elites and "Social" Virginity

Beyond this medicojuridical context, other mechanisms and other discourses helped determine the state of women's virginity and hence their honor. At the most basic level, there is the fact of the astonishingly high illegitimacy rates characterizing New Spain and the rest of Spanish

America in the colonial era. In Spanish colonies, illegitimacy rates rose to quadruple that of European and Anglo-American societies; in Mexico, these rates ranged geographically, between 7 and 50 percent in the seventeenth century, declining to between 7 and 35 percent in the eighteenth.[62] These high indications of sexual activity outside of the confines of marriage suggest that for some substantial portion of the population, at least, reverence for virginity occurred at a more abstract than actualized level.[63]

Marital documentation also provides further evidence about attitudes toward female virginity that nonelites espoused. *Palabra de casamiento* suits document that plebeian families and sometimes individual women themselves pursued honorable marriages or suitable compensation for virginity lost under its promise. But other types of suits, particularly applications for dispensation of marriage impediments, illustrate various ways that members of colonial society, from a range of economic positions and ethnicities, in practice ignored the church's mandates on various forms of sexual and marital propriety, including the desirability of premarital virginity. In one 1772 application for the dispensation of consanguineous ties, two indigenous applicants demonstrated that the question of the preservation of premarital virginity was of no concern to either party. Sebastián Fabian de Lara, the applicant for the dispensation, was a candle vendor who testified that he was "a poor official" who earned a daily wage of three or four reales.[64] Fabian de Lara declared to the archbishop's office that, without force or violence, he had violated the virginity of his first cousin without having given her any promise to marry. When his paramour had become pregnant, they had pledged to marry and had subsequently had three children before applying for marriage dispensation.[65] In another trial initiated the same year, two black slaves similarly applied for dispensation of consanguineous ties based on their claim of wishing to regularize their relations, having previously engaged in "illicit copulation."[66] In such cases, parishioners' curates normally counseled them to apply for dispensation to marry and formalize their unions.

Regardless of their sexual histories, the determination of women's virginity and honor depended on factors other than medical assessments made by midwives and doctors. First, the voice of public opinion formed by acquaintances, family members, and servants could help determine the status of women's virginity in the colonial era. As Asunción Lavrin, Ann Twinam, and Sonya Lipsett-Rivera have demonstrated, such determination was really only possible for women who possessed economic means, lofty *calidad*, and the protection of reputable male family members.[67] The mechanisms by which communal discourses regarding a woman's virtue could determine her state of virginity is apparent in the mid-seventeenth-century Inquisition trial of a mestiza *partera* and *curandera*. Among the charges leveled against Isabel Hernández was her alleged provision of an abortion to a woman believed publicly to be a virgin.[68] This woman's family, Hernández testified, had publicized her condition simply as "the detention of the menses."

This was a condition well known in the colony's medical literature. Jesuit cleric Juan de Esteyneffer's important *Florilegio medicinal*, first published in 1712, described that the "detention of the menses," as well as being possibly caused by pregnancy, might also originate in various illnesses and diverse causes. Esteyneffer said the menses might be detained because of "cold, dry winds, because of bathing in cold water . . . [or ingesting] hot foods, excessive salt, too much activity . . . or great sorrow, jealousy, or anger, or from eating unseasonal fruits, particularly limes and oranges."[69] According to physician Juan Manuel Venegas, who published the *Compendio de la medicina práctica* in Mexico in 1788, detention of the menses was understood to have such morally innocent (and self-contradictory) origins as "the good or bad disposition of the organs, health or sickness, robust and weak complexions, [or] hot or cold climates,"[70] He also posited that menstrual suppression could be caused by humoral imbalances, fright, weakness, hysteria, and age.[71] Medical works circulating in New Spain provided various remedies for inducing the resumption of the menses when these had been "suppressed." These works suggest that in this context, as John Riddle discovered was the case in Europe before the late nineteenth century, "most authorities did not consider the taking of a menstrual regulator, regardless of whether there was a pregnancy, as an abortifacient. Unless a woman was demonstrably and visibly pregnant, she was not pregnant until she so declared."[72] Similarly, in late colonial Mexico, institutional medical authorities believed women's menses could become legitimately suppressed for various reasons other than impregnation; hence the ingestion of a menstrual "regulator" did not imply the ingestion of an abortifacient.[73]

In the case of the seventeenth-century Inquisition trial of *partera* Isabel Hernández, the father of a woman whose menses had ostensibly been "detained" called Hernández to her side when his daughter went into labor. Hernández had given her some powders, and the woman had given birth that same night. In the aftermath of the night, however, the midwife testified that "talk ran in Tlaxcala of this confessant, and how she had cured the woman with some powders, and while many friends asked her what powders she had used, she responded that they were some powders that she knew and did not want to say, when the truth was that she had said this because she had not wanted people to know about the moral laxity of this woman because of her good reputation."[74] Hernández clearly helped this woman—whose family she described as *gente honrada* (honorable people)—dispatch her fetus, allowing the public to believe that she had merely cured the woman of her "menstrual detention."

Elites often succeeded in altering the official public record about the state of virginity of young female family members. Ann Twinam and Muriel Nazzari have both demonstrated that women of the Latin American elite successfully avoided having premarital pregnancies damage their reputations of virginity by using various strategies, including immediate or post hoc matrimony or concealing pregnancies.[75] Often they were later able to integrate the resultant offspring into their families as *agregados* (dependents), and occasionally succeeded in eventually legitimizing them.[76]

Successful applications for the dispensation of marriage banns represent another example of elites' use of one such strategy. In such cases, families sought secret marriages that could transpire without public banns—announcements made from the pulpit on three successive holy days—to avoid calling attention to the date upon which a marriage and its consummation might have taken place. In one such case dating from 1772, Francisco Ignacio Para, a Spaniard who originated from Cadiz and served as the *alcalde mayor* (magistrate and district administrator) in the province of Apan,[77] applied to the vicar general of the archdiocese of Mexico to dispense with the requirement of publicizing his betrothal to Margarita Sotomayor, a woman whom, Para confessed, "in my fragility and misery I knew carnally and from which incontinence, she has found herself several months' pregnant."[78] Para pleaded that because Sotomayor was from a "distinguished family of great honor" it would be "gravely inconvenient" that the timing of their marriage be public, for Sotomayor's father, if he learned of his daughter's state before she was safely married to Para, would likely be so enraged that he would kill his daughter and the fetus she carried. Furthermore, declared Para, for the sake of his own profession and honor it was not convenient that news of the timing of his marriage should be made public, for if it were, he would suffer in the estimation of "subjects of high character." The archbishop's office, in this and several similar petitions, granted dispensation of the banns, thus allowing for secret marriages to occur, and through them, the official preservation of elite women's premarital virginity.[79]

Plebeian Virginity

Over the course of the nineteenth century, as the new republic of Mexico developed its liberal and capitalist institutions, its citizens' attitudes toward virginity began shifting. Various forms of evidence from early and mid-nineteenth-century criminal cases support the idea that in this later period, the importance of publicly establishing a reputation of premarital virginity, honor, and respectability became increasingly prevalent among women who belonged to lower social groups. Lipsett-Rivera's research into popular attitudes toward sexual honor and space in this period reveals the extent to which the populace associated female respectability and virginity; these values were cemented into the very designs of Mexican domestic architecture, and into the attitudes women displayed in their occupation of it. Female enclosure within the home signified respectability, whereas moving beyond it—into the street, and even into doorways, windows, thresholds and breezeways (*zaguáns*)— could signify moral laxity and sexual licentiousness.[80]

Lipsett-Rivera describes various criminal denunciations by women who were assaulted or raped when they allegedly indicated their sexual availability to their assailants by stepping from a doorway and into a *zaguán*. One Mexico City trial from 1849 involved a woman's description of sexual assault she had suffered one evening when her mother had sent her out to buy meat. (We may presume that the family was not wealthy, since a family member rather than a servant was dispatched for the task.) A male acquaintance invited her to join him in a *zaguán* near the butcher shop, and she "entered the zaguán only a little to avoid scandal."[81] Lipsett-Rivera comments that "surely she understood the implications of her acceptance of [the man's] invitation."[82] He dragged her further into the space, then into an adjoining street, and at the entryway to the Alameda park, had sexual intercourse with her, taking her virginity. Lipsett-Rivera describes several similar episodes, and characterizes all parties as cognizant that a female's presence in the *zaguán*, which was "not the moral space of the courtyard in which all was observed," often signified sexual availability. Whereas colonial era documentation suggests that the concern with preserving virginity in women was a most particular concern with Mexican elites, Lipsett-Rivera's research conveys a sense that this preoccupation permeated all sectors of Mexican society by midcentury, when women stationed themselves in particular architectural features of their homes to convey the correct message of "morality and honorable behavior that women tried to convey to their neighbors."[83]

Kathryn Sloan's work on nineteenth-century *rapto* cases seems at first to contradict my claim of the degree to which the cult of virginity had permeated the value systems of plebeian Mexicans by the mid-nineteenth century.[84] *Rapto*, as defined by the 1871 Mexican Penal Code, was the forced abduction of a woman for sexual or conjugal purposes through violence, deception, or seduction, or a female under age sixteen's voluntary accompaniment with a man. Sloan studied over two hundred *rapto* trials between 1841 and 1919 in the city of Oaxaca, most of them dealing with working class subjects, many of whom were indigenous. One of Sloan's startling findings is that "in more than 90 percent of the 212 cases . . . the girls voluntarily ran away with their suitors, and some even engineered the entire escapade."[85] If Mexicans of all classes and ethnicities espoused the value of premarital female virginity so deeply, how and why could these girls and women have acted as they did?

Sloan herself presents the answer: this group of young working class Mexicans in effect used their society's preoccupation with their own virginity in order to achieve their desired ends. Most often, Sloan found, couples resorted to *rapto* as a way of contravening parental opposition to their personal choices in marital partners. Repeating a pattern of behavior that Seed uncovered in Bourbon Mexico with respect to more elite households, these Oaxacan couples successfully challenged familial opposition by willfully and publicly flouting the injunction against women's loss of virginity. Once this had occurred, women and men successfully petitioned municipal criminal courts in the Oaxacan capital to allow them to regularize their unions through lawful civil marriage. "Both officials and youngsters supported virginity as a normative value," writes Sloan. "Yet the young women also knew that virginity could be wielded as a bargaining chip not only with their suitors but also with parents and the state in order to achieve their aims of independence and the desire to forge a new family."[86] She asserts that the attitude toward virginity these couples espoused demonstrates their adherence to "an alternative code of honor and sexuality" in which girls and women could have sexual relations before marriage and retain their honor as long as they had received betrothal promises beforehand.[87] In fact, this attitude does not appear "alternative" to that which Mexican elites had displayed since New Spain's foundation. What may be novel about it was its greater pervasiveness by this era among members of the less affluent ranks of Mexican society.

It would be impossible to prove that plebeian Mexicans in the late nineteenth century engaged in premarital or extramarital sex either less or more frequently than in earlier periods, although we do see evidence of ongoing high rates of extramarital reproduction in this era. Federal government statistics recorded ongoing high rates of illegitimacy for both the capital city and the country as a whole at the close of the nineteenth century. Of roughly 372,000 births recorded by federal agencies in Mexico in 1895, for example, roughly 218,000 (under 59 percent) were legitimate. In Mexico City, the same sources report that in 1900, of nearly 30,000 recorded births, just under one-third were legitimate.[88] My argument, however, is not that behavior changed per se, but rather that attitudes toward illegitimacy shifted. Ann Blum observes that "a continued weakening of the stigma attached to bearing children outside marriage" characterized the later nineteenth century.[89] My contrasting interpretation is that in this era the pressure for plebeian women to adhere to the mores of sexual purity that had earlier been more strongly represented in elite classes increased.[90]

While at the time of its creation in 1806, administrators of the Mexico City Poor House's Department of Secret Births restricted its usage "uniquely and exclusively to Spanish women of all states" by the mid-nineteenth century, Mexican newspapers called for the foundation of a similar institution for a broader segment of the female population in order the avoid the "infamy, humiliation, and tears of shame" that public births would bring to them.[91] After the establishment of Mexico City's Casa de Maternidad in 1866 in the same location that had housed its colonial predecessor (by then in disrepair), the institution's director, doctor Ramón Pacheco, ensured that public announcements were posted "on the street corners and public spaces" that "all pregnant women, by deed of being in the eighth month of pregnancy will be admitted without any other requirement to the Casa."[92] Those who wished to be admitted in secrecy did not have to reveal any element of their identity or qualify in any way for the service.

A Scientific Look at Virginity

In the era of the Porfiriato (1876–1911), societal preoccupations with the need to defend Mexican women's premarital virginity on a national scale emerged within the positivistic and internationalist *científico* climate of the era. In this period with intellectual support from the emergent eugenics movement and the growth of studies of hygiene and criminology, prominent physicians and criminologists examined a series of physiological and sociological problems they understood to be threatening the potential of the Mexican nation: crime, disease, alcoholism, and drug addiction. The Mexican state directed many initiatives at what many understood to be the source of such ills: the female body. It embraced initiatives to penalize syphilitics and police prostitution. Celebrated criminologists Carlos Rougmanac and Julio Guerrero argued that abnormal sexual behavior lay at the root of Mexico's crime problems, the latter asserting that poor women were prone to promiscuity and consequently to illegal abortions.[93]

Within this context, Francisco de Asis Flores y Troncoso, pharmacy professor at the Mexican School of Medicine, produced his 1885 study *El hímen en México*, contributing to the blossoming late nineteenth-century scientific field of "hymenology." Flores's text on the Mexican hymen, along with a host of materials dealing with public sanitation, policing and incarceration, and health, was included in the works Mexico chose to represent its national scientific achievements at the 1889 Exposition Universelle in Paris.[94] Flores declared that his aim in creating his tract was to produce a reliable work that could be used in medicojuridical proceedings when it was necessary to determine the state of female virginity and assess the possibility of rape and deflowerment.[95] He sought to undertake a scientific classification of the hymen in Mexico in order to catalog its varying physical attributes (subdividing it into five "regular" and six "anomalous" forms) and, most explicitly, to generate a scientific formula by which to measure the force of the resistance characteristic of various forms of the hymen. He wished to produce a formula through which different types of hymens could be measured in terms of the likelihood they possessed to resist penetration whether by "the penis (in ravishment or rape), the finger, the mouth of a bottle, a plug (*tapon*), etc. (in lesbian lovemaking.)"[96] He elaborated on several declinations of his basic equation appropriate to each form of hymen studied, but at the most basic level, his formula articulated that $T_m = P \times t$, where T_m represented mechanical force, P represented the sum of all forces, and t the time involved "to overcome the resistance of the labial hymen,"[97] subsequently describing the decomposition of the hymen upon its contact with the force of "the foreign body."

El hímen en México, apparently celebrated in its own time, jars the modern reader. Flores's mathematical answer to the problem of assessing whether rape or intercourse had occurred reads like a parody of positivism. It is hard not to recoil from imagining the professor, perhaps aided by assistants, moving about his laboratory, conducting resistance experiments on the hymens of female bodies—presumably corpses—including those belonging to infants. Flores was not explicit in his text about the subjects he used to generate his findings, but he did comment that the data he used "were presented in the department of Legal Medicine in the Escuela de México in 1882."[98] Another faculty member of that institution, doctor Adrián de Garay, later charged Flores with plagiarism, declaring that his data was "not the property of Sr. Francisco Flores, but rather that of the students of legal medicine of the year 1884."[99] (Flores later successfully contested this charge in a defamation suit.) Flores provided information about the staging of the experiments themselves in only one passage of *El hímen* when he commented that he had detected the existence of a hymen in every one of the 181 females he had examined for his study except one. In this instance, "an examination practiced on the cadaver of a 9-day-old girl . . . observation of the hymen, perhaps in a rudimentary state, escaped the observer."[100]

Flores's text most explicitly aimed to be a resource for physicians and jurists in their assessments of females involved in criminal proceedings for, he observed, if he could demonstrate that the "mechanical force used to overcome (*vencer*) [the hymen] was different in each of its forms, it is probable that my theory approaches the truth and that this data could have some value in expert testimonies treating the crimes of sexual incontinence."[101] Knowledge of the type of hymen a young woman possessed, and its level of "resistance" and flexibility, could help substantiate young women's claims to virginity and grooms' perhaps unjustified accusations of their brides' obvious prior sexual experience.[102] While a majority of medical texts dating from the colonial era and the mid-nineteenth century that physicians and midwives consulted in Mexico endorsed the view that examinations of the hymen could only ever be an inexact science because its (torn or intact) state need not necessarily and definitely imply virginity or its loss, by the late nineteenth century physicians of Flores's cohort sought to create a scientifically exacting science of virginity.

Besides seeking to make this contribution to medicojuridical proceedings, Flores also sought to chart the unique biological qualities of

Mexican women in a framework of nationalistic claims of their physiological—and specifically gynecological—features. He repeatedly asserted in *El hímen en México* that one particular formation of hymen— the *herradura*—was manifest more frequently in Mexican females than in those of any other nation that had examined the topic.[103] A few years earlier in his career, Flores had produced a tract attempting to chart the particularly national characteristics of Mexican women's pelvises—a position, as chapter 6 will further elaborate, that the most celebrated Mexican obstetrician of his day, Juan María Rodriguez, also championed.[104]

Finally, Flores also used this work to voice support for his era's new perspective of the importance of widespread premartial female virginity. In the sixteenth and seventeenth centuries, many Mexicans abstractly associated female virginity with the supreme religious virtue of the Virgin Mary's example, but they also managed to accept the contradiction between the idea of reverence for virginal purity and practices that embraced a reality of women's participation in sexual acts. Elite Mexican society, whose concern with maintaining the viceroyalty's racial and class-based social hierarchies, augmented its need to police premartial female virginity, but even among this group, the possibility of "social virginity" correctly deployed might trump the taint of the loss of biological virginity.

By the late nineteenth century, however, female virginity had become—for Flores, as for his contemporaries—a crucial indicator of a measure of a nation's civilization, and a reliable mechanism was therefore necessary to scientifically account for its presence.[105] "Today," he exclaimed, "virginity is one of the most precious jewels for which man searches. Civilized nations all scrutinize its maintenance, establishing rigorous punishments against all acts committed against it."[106] Flores described societies in Peru, Arabia, Petrea, and Asia that so esteemed female virginity that they sutured virginal lips together at birth, preventing their later unsealing except by a surgical operation, while characterizing societies that did not value virginity as "remaining forever in primitive infancy."[107] The stakes for virginity, it would seem, had been raised; no longer a requirement only for the preservation of the racial purity of elite dynasties, the preservation of virginity before marriage had become a requirement for all Mexican women, since they were all implicated in the work of producing and reproducing a civilized and prosperous nation.

Developing Virginity

Mexican society from the late colonial era through the nineteenth century esteemed female virginity. However, why and how society esteemed it changed over time. In the colonial era, residents of New Spain principally associated female virginity with the Holy Mother and the traits of female honor that Catholicism upheld. This status-obsessed society policed elite Spanish women's virginity particularly, since women were the only genetic receptacles through which claims to family lineage and racial purity could be traced. But although they were under greater scrutiny, women who formed part of the colonial elite also had the greatest chances of restoring their virginity through social means—law suits, marriages, and other domestic arrangements—when doubts about their sexual purity arose.

Over the course of the nineteenth century, new preoccupations regarding female virginity in the developing nation of Mexico arose. First, we can see that notions of virginity underwent a transformation in this era in terms of the discourses with which it was most associated, from its sacred connotations in the colonial era to the predomination of medico-juridical associations in the late nineteenth century. Second, it is apparent that as the nineteenth century progressed, larger numbers of women from a broader demographic in the nation's socioeconomic scale, families, neighborhoods, and sometimes individual women themselves began articulating a greater concern with preserving female virginity. It became possible, or more frequently imperative, that these larger sectors of women defend and pursue public recognition of female sexual virtue. Larger sectors of Mexican women came under scrutiny in terms of the preservation of their virginity because what was at stake was no longer only the impeccable reproduction of a small elite's security over undisputed racial and social legitimacy, but the purity and productivity of the entire nation. When women failed to safeguard their sexual virtue, as contemporary criminologists contended, they opened the door to all manner of disorder, social decay, and crime.

2 Conception and Pregnancy

Of all the aspects of childbirth and contraception in colonial and nineteenth-century Mexico, ideas and practices surrounding conception and pregnancy remained the most stable across time. Societal expectations about female virginity shifted, as did practices surrounding abortion and child delivery, but beliefs about conception and notions about the health regimes women should follow during pregnancy remained relatively unchanged. Midwives, who had been charged with pregnant women's medical care in precontact Europe and Mexico, persisted as the most important sector attending women during pregnancy and at birth through the nineteenth century and into the twentieth. This chapter details the knowledge midwives possessed and the services they provided concerning conception and pregnancy to Mexican women, courts, and medical institutions in colonial and nineteenth-century Mexico.

Despite the relative stability of conception and pregnancy across time, some transformations did alter women's experiences. In our own era, certainty about conception's occurrence is assumed; we joke that women cannot be "a *little* pregnant." In colonial and early nineteenth-century Mexico, biological certainty of the state of pregnancy was much rarer. As Cathy McClive has argued was the case in early modern Europe, ambiguity and uncertainty characterized many women's experiences of conception and pregnancy.[1] Throughout the colonial period, pregnant women, midwives, and judicial authorities alike acknowledged the uncertainty of their understanding of conception's occurrence; by the close of the nineteenth century, they had developed greater certainty about detecting pregnancy. This increased certainty coincided with the rise of more aggressive penalization of the crimes of infanticide and abortion.

Criminal trials, Inquisition cases, obstetrical guides, medical histories, and Mexican newspapers document that beginning in the second half of the eighteenth century, a new group of medical professionals—licensed physicians—began to study obstetrics, assist women at childbirth, and produce new medical literature about these experiences. The numbers of women they treated remained small at the end of the colonial period, but grew over the course of the nineteenth century. The most dramatic obstetrical changes this group introduced did not involve conception and pregnancy but instead shaped practices relating to abortion and birth. However, physicians' entrance into the field of obstetrical medicine, and specifically their introduction of the performance of internal gynecological exams during pregnancy initiated some conflicts between them and expectant mothers and their families and midwives while all of these parties readjusted themselves to the new circumstances of childbearing in the era of modernization.

Pre-Colombian Obstetrical Knowledge

Throughout the colonial period and beyond, indigenous women were the most popular choice for expectant Mexican mothers seeking birth attendants. Indigenous health care providers had developed a sophisticated knowledge of obstetrics and gynecology in the pre-Columbian era, much of which survived throughout the colonial era. Although pre-Columbian and early modern European ideas about conception diverged in significant ways, medical knowledge in New Spain tended to build upon, rather than bury, developments from the pre-Hispanic era. As Noemí Quezada observes, Spain's conquest society, while rejecting the spiritual elements of indigenous medical practice, accepted and assimilated many aspects of pre-Columbian medical therapy, which it recognized as further evolved in experimental terms than existent European botanical knowledge.[2]

Aztec civilization, in particular, had accorded midwives a prominent social role in the rituals surrounding childbirth and in the reinforcement of that society's entrenched gender roles. Franciscan missionary Bernardino de Sahagún's 1569 tract *Historia general de las cosas de Nueva España*, a work treating a broad spectrum of Nahua social practices and historical narratives based on the testimonies of indigenous informants, details various aspects of pre-Columbian obstetrics. Despite ongoing questions over the extent to which a Europeanized filter mediates this source's presentation of pre-Columbian history, Sahagún's text remains paramount in historians' understanding of midwives' work in pre-Columbian Mexico.[3]

Sahagún's informants told him that the most prominent Nahua healers were *ticitl*. Beyond dealing with bodily complaints, as Sherry Fields observes, their knowledge involved coordinating the material with the supernatural world; they "combined sacerdotal functions with hands-on, empirically based therapy."[4] Their realm of expertise included bone setting, bleeding, purging, closing wounds, and knowledge of herbs, roots, and minerals. They knew how to counteract the ill effects of witchcraft and how to recognize the symptoms of numerous diseases. The *Florentine Codex* recorded that such figures understood, among other things, "the properties of herbs, and roots, trees, and stones . . . how to bleed, administer purges, give medicine, apply ointments, palpitate what is hard in the body to make it soft, set bones, to cup and cure sores and gout, and diseases of the eyes, and to cut small tumors from them."[5] Both men and women worked as *ticitl* in Nahua communities, but the healers who worked exclusively as midwives—*tepalehuiani* (the one that helps)—were female, as were those figures who, according to Sahagún, "provided herbs to cause abortions."[6]

In the early sixteenth century—and likely before that—the Nahuas had a sacred, rather than a physiological, understanding of the moment of conception.[7] Sahagún's informants described how they believed that the creative duality of the gods formed new creatures in the heavens and, from there, placed them in the wombs of women. The Nahuas called these newly formed beings "precious stones" and "rich feathers," and wrote that our "god wished to complete and bring them to perfection in the womb of the young woman."[8] Here, his informants likely referred to Cihuacoatl, the first woman to give birth on the earth. The Nahuas also honored many other gods whose domain touched obstetrics, including Tzinteutl, goddess and advocate of pregnant women, and Xoalteuctli, god of the night and patron of recently born children. Pre-Hispanic society also revered women who died in their first birth as goddesses, henceforth called *mocihuaquetzque*.[9]

Nahua society accorded great reverence to both pregnant women and to the *ticitl* who supplied women with medicines that encouraged fertility, guided them through pregnancy, and aided them in childbirth. Sixteenth-century naturalists recorded that the Nahuas supplied women with various plants, including *cozolmécatl* (which, according to naturalist Francisco Hernández, "restored energy to those who are drained by sexual excesses"[10]) and *talapayatzin*, which encouraged conception. They also frequently prescribed the root *iztacpactli* and the herb *chichilpiltic*, mixed with the plant *yolopatli* to encourage fertility.[11] The Nahuas commemorated recently married noble women's announcements of pregnancy with elaborate public ceremonies, and according to Sahagún, developed an extensive body of beliefs about the practices in which pregnant women should engage in order to ensure the health of their fetuses. They were to avoid heavy lifting, bathing too frequently, excessive intercourse, looking upon frightful sights, or fighting with their spouses. Most important, they were to remain respectful to the gods throughout pregnancy.[12] *Ticitl* became active participants in impending births beginning in the seventh or eighth month of a pregnancy, when women were ceremoniously entrusted to their care. On this occasion, *ticitl* provided expectant women with further counsel in order to ensure safe deliveries: they were not to overheat their wombs, their backs, nor the ground upon which they slept in order to avoid harming their fetuses. They were not to sleep during the day, view the color red, or eat earth because of the deformities these acts would provoke in their newborns.[13] Midwives advised women to ensure they ate sufficiently and avoided both overtaxing themselves and encountering grave frights. During the first three months of pregnancy, women were to "have temperate congress with their husbands, for if they abstained completely from the carnal act, their children would be born sick and lacking strength." In the later months of pregnancy, however, they advised women to abstain completely from intercourse.[14]

Nahua midwives also prepared a *temazcalli*, a Mesoamerican "house of heat" into which they accompanied pregnant women to palpitate their wombs to ensure fetuses had assumed correct positions. Midwives continued the practice of these external manipulations of the fetus throughout pregnancy and often during labor as well. Repositioning fetuses through both external and internal manipulation was, as Francisco de Asis Flores y Troncoso remarked in 1886, "one of the least serious tocological operations most popularly practiced in Mexico today."[15] He noted that it was ancient practice in both the Old World and the New, "where, at least from the era of the conquest we know it existed among the Indians, and where it remained relegated to the common people, who applied it especially in cases of [buttocks-forward] presentations." Pre-Columbian midwives were also skilled in the practice of breaking the amniotic sac to provoke labor.[16]

Pre-Columbian midwives possessed extensive botanical knowledge, which they used to address sterility and to assist women throughout pregnancy, labor, and postpartum recovery. Prominent sixteenth-century Spaniards accumulated painstaking encyclopedias of the qualities and uses of Mexican flora and fauna. Martha Eugenia Rodríguez contends that all medical texts produced in New Spain, beginning with Francisco Bravo's 1570 *Opera medicinalia*, the first medical work published in the New

World, "borrowed from traditional Mexican medicine in their discussions of indigenous therapeutic remedies."[17] Along with Bravo and Sahagún, these writers included Francisco Hernández de Toledo, naturalist and court physician to Phillip II, and the venerable hermit Gregorio López.

The range of treatments available to assist women from conception to the postparturient period that these writers recorded is astonishing. They listed hundreds of remedies to provide contraception, encourage fertility, counteract the side effects of pregnancy, assist in complicated deliveries, and remedy postpartum complaints. Treatments existed for labor pain, stalled labor, facilitating the placenta's expulsion, encouraging lactation, and soothing postpartum hemorrhoids.[18] For amenorrhea (the absence of the menstrual period), Nahua midwives prescribed several plants including *xiuhtotonqui*, the juice of the herb *tlalquequetzal*, the pepper *xocoxochitl*, and the flower of the *cempoalxochitl* (prescribing the latter for urinary retention as well). For uterine-related afflictions they recommended *tepitzin*, *patlahoac*, and *xoxoparucina*.[19] Early postconquest sources recorded that the Aztecs also used the powdered herbs *malinali* and *tlahotil* as antiabortives, and Francisco Hernández discovered that indigenous midwives used the roots of *apancholoa* and *atehuapatli* to arrest undesired miscarriages.[20]

A Portrait of Mexican Midwives

Colonial and nineteenth-century sources document that various obstetrical practices of pre-Columbian origin endured throughout the colonial era and persisted in postindependence Mexico. José Ignacio Bartolache, the eminent eighteenth-century physician and publisher of *Mercurio Volante*, deplored Mexican women's ongoing reliance on such practices and the personnel who provided them, lamenting that so many of his contemporaries chose midwives who prescribed temazcal baths and performed external manipulations of the fetus to attend them at childbirth.[21]

Through the colonial period and much of the nineteenth century, few Mexican women delivered their children with the assistance of doctors. As physician Juan Bautista Arechederreta, future rector of the college of San Juan de Letrán, wrote in his 1802 appeal to the Mexican Protomedicato (medical board) requesting the establishment of a faculty of medicine, obstetrics, and nursing, "In America . . . only some of the most well-off women seek to use surgeons at childbirth."[22] Up until the end of the colonial period, licensed physicians were in short supply in New Spain.

In the first century of colonization, most accredited doctors practicing in the viceroyalty were *peninsulares* (Spaniards born in Iberia). They were a rarity throughout the viceroyalty in large part because of the rigid social codes and the requirement of demonstrating *limpieza de sangre* and legitimacy excluded the vast majority of the population from studying medicine. In the colonial era, *médicos* (physicians) had to fulfill a four-year course of university training and spend two years apprenticed to a licensed physician. Their studies dealt exclusively with the realms of "internal medicine"—fevers, epidemics, and the like. "External medicine"—wounds, broken bones, and amputations—were the domain of surgeons, either "Latin," those who followed a formal course of medical studies (although the rigorousness of this program varied considerably) or "romance," who acquired their knowledge purely through five years of practical experience and proof of clean blood. Romance surgeons, responsible for bleedings, amputations, and bone setting, occupied the lowest position in medicine's professional hierarchy.

Nicolás León notes that only one Latin surgeon was accredited by the University of Mexico in the seventeenth century, suggesting that romance surgeons formed the vast majority of practitioners.[23] By the second half of the seventeenth century, forty-seven *médicos* and only one surgeon worked in all of New Spain.[24] At the start of the eighteenth century in Mexico City and the surrounding area, there were 27 *facultativos* (accredited physicians) who had trained a total of 359 doctors, 16 Latin surgeons, and 542 romance surgeons to service a population of well over 100,000 people. By 1790, the census of New Spain's capital recorded an urban population of nearly 105,000 ministered by 94 doctors, 51 surgeons, and 227 *sangradores* (bloodletters) and barbers.[25] By 1822, Mexico City's Ayuntamiento recorded that 27 *médicos*, 46 *cirujanos* (surgeons), 29 *boticarios* and 25 bloodletters practiced in the capital. The inventory noted that "midwives were not included because it is not known who they are and where they live; the only one who has been licensed is Doña Angela Leiti, on the calle del Factor en el Molino."[26]

Along with the explanation of the scarcity of doctors, midwives remained active in Mexico because, until the late eighteenth century, physicians considered obstetrics a debased area of medicine, unworthy of their attention.[27] Until the late eighteenth century, obstetrics was not part of the medical curricula taught at the University of Mexico. Even such medical officers as the "physician to the city" (the Mexico City council's name for the jail doctor) who treated such illnesses as cataracts, urinary stoppages, and hernias in prison inmates never assisted women in childbirth. Neither did the town council ever appoint a midwife or surgeon to handle the difficult deliveries of inmates.[28] Only the Hospital de San Pedro in Puebla included such material in its standard curricula, likely modeled on the *cátredra de partos* (formal curriculum of obstetrics) taught in Spanish surgical colleges after 1787.[29] Consequently, male professionals did not actually attend women giving birth on either side of the Atlantic before the seventeenth century, though male physicians as far back ancient Greece had theorized about conception and birth. As French physician Jean Astruc declared in the preface to his 1767 tract *The Art of Midwifery*, which circulated widely in Europe and Spanish America alike, "I have never practiced midwifery: though I undertake, nevertheless, to teach the art of delivery."[30]

Until the end of the colonial period, European medical tracts influential in Mexico derived much of their wisdom from ancient writers—Aristotle, Galen of Pergmon, and Hippocrates.[31] Elaine Hobby observes that early modern midwifery manuals as a whole were largely dependent on these earlier writings: "The endlessly repeated descriptions of the qualities of a good midwife—she must be healthy and strong, of middle years, discreet, clean and cheerful, have small hands and short nails—come ultimately from Galen and Hippocrates."[32] Such direct continuity is certainly represented in a late colonial midwifery tract published in Mexico, Antonio Medina's *Cartilla nueva util y necesaria para instruirse las matronas*, which advised—in a near direct citation from Hippocrates—that midwives must be neither too old nor too young and must be healthy, strong, and with medium-sized hands. In an early modern innovation, however, Medina further observed that midwives should have sufficient literacy and intelligence to be able to learn from their instructors and to benefit from the reading of books. Finally, he noted they needed to possess a "docile humor and be predisposed to submit to the judgment of those of superior competence, requesting help and consultation at the opportune moment from doctors and surgeons in cases in which any complications occur."[33]

The majority of the midwives who attended women in pregnancy and childbirth in the colonial era and through the nineteenth century would likely have been illiterate and so would not have consumed such texts. There were exceptions, however. One fascinating 1721 Inquisition trial originating in the city of Veracruz details the tribunal's investigation, under charges of superstition, heretical witchcraft, and pact making with the devil, of Josefa "la madre" Chepa, a midwife other witnesses identified as a mulata but who referred to herself as a mestiza. The bailiff's inventory of Chepa's belongings, seized upon her imprisonment, included "two books, one that deals with surgery and the other entitled pastoral letter."[34]

Chepa's apparent literacy and her practice of consulting surgical tracts was likely unusual. Her racial classification, however, may have been more representative of women who practiced midwifery in urban centers of New Spain in the midcolonial period. A sampling of fifty-three civil, criminal, and Inquisition documents involving Mexican midwives in the period between 1566 and 1888 (see table 1) revealed the largest numbers of midwives whose ethnicity is declared in contemporary documentation were mulata or Afro-Mexican (eleven), followed by Spaniards (nine), and mestizas (six). Indigenous women, who numbered only three, were the smallest group represented in this sample. After independence, courts did not normally identify parties according to racial labels, so tracking their identity along these lines becomes virtually impossible.

Mulata midwives were likely more prevalent in urban capitals and in the Caribbean coastal region, where the Afro-Mexican population as a whole was most strongly represented in the seventeenth and eighteenth centuries. Lee Penyak's analysis of thirty-seven midwives who served as expert witnesses in rape trials to criminal tribunals in Mexico City between 1740 and 1846 revealed higher numbers of indigenous women. In his pool, 41 percent were Spanish, 36 percent were indigenous, and 7 percent were *castiza* (women with one mestizo and one Spanish parent).[35]

The differing ethnic composition of members of these two data sets reflects the types of sources consulted. Criminal courts relied on indigenous women's testimony as expert witnesses in rape trials, but indigenous women, who feature more prominently in Penyak's sample, did not appear as defendants in Inquisition trials, which accounted for nearly two-thirds of the types of cases in my data, since they were jurisdictionally exempted from trial by the Holy Office. Disgruntled former clients and members of the piously minded public, on the other hand, frequently denounced Afro-Mexican midwives to criminal courts and to the Inquisition on charges of sorcery or charlatanism. Because both data sets document only particular types of anomalous cases—when foul play of one kind or another was suspected—they cannot be understood to necessarily represent the typical demographics of the pool of women who worked as midwives in the colonial era. We only know definitively that women of all castes worked as midwives in New Spain.

TABLE 1 Midwives by ethnicity and civil status in Mexico, 1566–1888

Date	Name	Age	Place	Ethnicity	Civil Status
1566	Francisca Díaz		Spain	Spanish	Widowed
1627	Isabel Arias		Culiacán	Mulata	Widowed
1627	Luisa de Trujillo		Culiacán	Mestiza	
1627	Ana de Valencia		Cuilacán	Mulata	Widowed
1627	Catalina Gonzáles		Cuuilacán	Mulata	Widowed
1652	Isabel Hernández		Tlaxcala	Mestiza	Widowed
1664	Estefanía de los Reyes		Mexico City	Mulata	
1665	Francisca		Zacatecas	Mulata	
1684	Úrsula Hernández		Yancuitlan	Mestiza	
1684	Agnes Díaz		Yancuitlan	Mulata	
1705	Juana		Mexico City	Mestiza	Soltera
1708	Petrona Fuentes		Mexico City	Spanish	Widowed
1709	Agustina de Lara		Mexico City	Spanish/ Mestiza	Married
1713				Mulata	
1713	María Calvillo		Acámbaro	Mestiza	
1721	Josefa de Zárate	40	San Juan de Ulúa	Mulata/ Mestiza	Widowed
1736	Teresa García		Iraputo	Mulata	
1743	Lucia Berrueta		Zultepec		Widowed
1753	Marcela		Merida		Married
1754	Pascuala de los Reyes		Tenancingo	India/ Castiza	
1754	Juana Hernández	64		Loba	Married
1756	Josepha de Ocampo				
1756	Agustina de Valera		Taxco		Widowed
1763	Juana Gomes	80	Tenango	Spanish	
1763	Antonia de Zalasan	70	Tenango	India	
1766	Petra de Torres		Tlayacapa	Spanish	Widowed
1774	María Guadalupe Sánchez	38	Mexico City	Mestiza	Married
1792	Agustina Carrasco		Tuxpan	Mulata	
1798	Lorenza		Zacatecas		
1805	Isabel Guadalupe García	55	Mapantlan	Spanish	Married
1806	Barbara Localilla	70	Mexico City	Spanish	Widowed
1806	Lorenza Abalos	53	Mexico City	Spanish	Married
1819	Rosa María Villeras	40	San Cristobal y Ecatepec	Spanish	Married

TABLE 1 (continued)

Date	Name	Age	Place	Ethnicity	Civil Status
1819	Valentina Marta	55	San Cristobal y Ecatepec	Indian	Married
1837	Felipa Romero	40	Oaxaca City		Widowed
1837	María Barbara	50	Tamazulapa		Widowed
1837	Francisca Estolana	30	Tamazulapa		Widowed
1837	Ignacia Medina	30	Tamazulapa		Married
1844	María Diego de Paz	63	Teposcolula		Widowed
1844	Dominga de la Cruz	45	Teposcolula		Married
1855	María Luz Gonzáles	69	Ejutla		Widowed
1857	María Dominga de las Nieves	59	Tepscolula		Widowed
1870	Marcela Gonzáles		Ejutla		Widowed
1870	Paula Ortiz		Ejutla		Widowed
1870	Agustina Sánchez		Oaxaca City		
1879	Isabel Atlamirano		Ejutla		Married
1879	Getrudis Ramírez	58	Ejutla		
1880	Dolores García	50	Mexico City		Widowed
1880	Romula Bravo	42	Mexico City		Widowed
1880	Dolores Ortiz	44	Mexico City		Widowed
1884	Felipa Sánchez	50	Oaxaca City		Soltera
1885	Josefa Vázquez	40	Mexico City		
1888	Margarita Mesinas	40	Oaxaca City		

Sources: AGI, Indiferente; AGN, Criminal, Inquisición, Indiferente Virreinal, TSJDF; AHJO, Ejutla, Criminal; AHJO, Tepscolula, Criminal; AHMO, Justicia.

In the earliest part of the colonial era, midwives might have had a tendency to work only with clients who shared their ethnic background, as is suggested by the biographical details of one mid-sixteenth-century peninsular midwife who established a business in Mexico City in the 1550s. In 1566, the Spaniard Francisca Díaz applied to the Casa de Contratacíon in Seville for permission to return to New Spain.[36] Elderly and avowedly ill at the time of her application, Díaz had first traveled to Mexico to work as a midwife six years earlier. She declared that she had found "very great fortune" in Mexico. Having earned enough capital to purchase a black slave, Ana, Díaz had returned to Seville, according to one witness "to resume married life with her husband."[37] However, by the time of her arrival there, Díaz had discovered that her husband had died, so she elected to return to Mexico accompanied by Ana, personal goods valued at five hundred pesos, and her fifteen-year-old son. Although "very ancient" and ailing, Díaz had apparently been so impressed by the opportunities that life in Mexico had offered her that she desired to undertake the overseas passage a second time, seeking also to establish her son, whom she hoped soon would marry, in the colonial capital.[38]

Díaz declared that one of the reasons why she had so quickly amassed substantial capital in Mexico City was "due to her ability and also because of the lack of midwives who have scientific training and experience in this said office."[39] Given what we know of pre-Columbian obstetrics, however, it is unlikely there would have been a shortage of indigenous women with expertise and experience in the art of childbirth operating in Díaz's milieu. Her statement thus implies that in the early postconquest era, Spanish and perhaps also mestiza women living in the urban capital sought out Spanish *parteras* instead of indigenous midwives, thus creating a lucrative market for Spanish women like Díaz. However, the ethnic classifications of midwives and their clients in the cases discussed below reveals that, by at least the early seventeenth century, *parteras* of all racial backgrounds attended the births of women who, in turn, came from all ranks and ethnicities of colonial society. Perhaps we see in Díaz's declaration, nevertheless, some indication of the class of women, who by the era of Mexican independence would form the clientele for the male medical professionals who emerged in that period's burgeoning field of obstetrical medicine.

The few records that reveal information about the economic status of Mexican midwives suggest that their class positions also varied. Researchers often characterize them as poor and uneducated.[40] Colonial records do not indicate how much pay midwives normally received for delivering children. It is likely that there was no fixed wage for their work, but that they accepted whatever families were able to offer them. When clients were too poor to pay, as one woman testified to the criminal court of Ejutla, Oaxaca, in 1881 was her situation, midwives charitably donated their services.[41] The inventories of their possessions that the Inquisition produced when it imprisoned defendants reveals many of the women lived in fairly humble economic circumstances. In 1652, for instance, goods belonging to the *partera* Isabel Hernández that the Holy Office seized included several items of clothing, a number of cases, various powders and stones, some reliquaries, dishes, and gourds; their total value was only nine pesos.[42] Most midwives in the colonial period are described as illiterate, although starting with the formalization of the profession in the late eighteenth and early nineteenth centuries, literacy began to be a requirement of those who aspired to be licensed midwives.

Some midwives, then, were relatively poor. However, midwives might also, particularly in comparison to the vocations available to women in the colonial period, amass quite respectable incomes. Silvia Arrom indicates that by the nineteenth century, midwives were likely to earn more money than most women working for pay in urban Mexico.[43] Archival records occasionally allow us a glimpse of such wealth—as in, for example, the case of Josefa de Zárate, the literate mestiza or mulata.[44] Zárate, a woman over forty years old, was the widow of a mestizo fisherman. Besides working as a midwife, Zárate was also known as a *curandera*. She first came to the attention of sailors working in the port, and eventually to religious authorities for her alleged ability to retrieve lost items and bring good fortune to her clients. Unlike Isabel Hernández, when the Inquisition imprisoned Zárate, it seized considerable wealth from her. Among her possessions were two black slaves, worth a substantial sum of 450 pesos.[45]

Spanish women may have preferred their births overseen by midwives who shared their ethnic identities in the first decades of Spanish rule in Mexico, but documentation from later periods reveals that by the seventeenth century, women sought obstetrical care across race and class divisions. This material depicts the interethnic and interclass networks that existed in the maturing viceroyalty wherein Spanish women might be attended in childbirth by indigenous, mestiza, mulata, or Spanish midwives, and that *parteras* of various ethnicities used medical knowledge and treatments originating in different traditions and communities. Isabel Hernández, described in Inquisition records as a *casta* (a person of non-European ancestry, usually of mixed race), descended on her mother's side "from the principal Indians of the Kings of Tlaxcala" and counted among her clients the provincial governor, Don Diego de Villegas, for whom she had performed "love magic," as well as a black slave whose birthing she had assisted.[46] Another mid-seventeenth-century mulata *partera* told one witness who testified at her Inquisition trial that she often used herbs she procured from Indians in order to cure both her clients' medical and their romantic troubles.[47] A Spanish midwife, Petra de Torres, whom the Inquisition investigated in 1766 in Tlalnepantla, a community slightly northwest of Mexico City, served a mainly indigenous clientele in her work as both a *curandera* and *partera*.[48]

Despite the evidence contained in table 1, the basic demographics of colonial society render it most likely that indigenous women were those who would have most commonly acted as midwives in both colonial and nineteenth-century Mexico. Indigenous people formed the majority of the population of Mexico throughout this period, though their numbers did diminish in inverse proportion to the steady growth of Mexico's mixed-race population beginning in the mid-seventeenth century. In that period, New Spain was roughly 85 percent indigenous, 10 percent Spanish, and 5 percent *casta*.[49] In the mid-eighteenth century, the Indian population constituted nearly two-thirds of New Spain's total, while the mixed-race population had expanded to just over one-third.[50] By the turn of the nineteenth century, according to the Prussian scientist and traveler Alexander von Humboldt, half of New Spain's 5.5 million inhabitants were indigenous, while one-fourth were *casta*.[51] Over the course of the nineteenth century, and particularly during its final decades, these numbers inverted, and by the late nineteenth century, official documents listed a little over one-third of the country's population as indigenous.[52] Lower numbers of both European and African women immigrated to Mexico than did men throughout the colonial period, which also contributed to the maintenance of proportionately higher numbers of indigenous women than those of other ethnicities into the nineteenth century. Although this demographic portrait suggests that the majority of midwives working in Mexico in both the colonial and postindependence eras were likely to have been indigenous, such women do not form the majority of those who appear in many historical records. Either indigenous midwives' clients had fewer reasons to denounce these *parteras* to criminal or ecclesiastical courts, or their clients in the rural settings in which they were more likely to live had fewer opportunities to encounter the bureaucracies of colonial or republican justice.

Midwives practicing in colonial Mexico were most often women who had themselves experienced childbirth. Almost all the women included in table 1 were or had been married. Of the thirty-five midwives in table 1 whose civil status was indicated, thirty-three were or had been married, and only two were *solteras* but, tellingly, not *doncellas* (virgins). All the midwives in this group were mature, with ages ranging from thirty to eighty years; the majority were women in their forties, fifties, and sixties. Many had learned their art from their own mothers.[53] One of the first midwives that Mexico's Protomedicato licensed in 1817 declared, for example, that she had begun her education in obstetrics with her mother.[54] A common prerequisite for becoming a midwife was the personal experience of having given birth. Felipa Romero, a Oaxaqueña midwife investigated in 1837 for having injured a client and committed infanticide, articulated the importance of this desirable attribute in the defense letter she presented to the judge investigating her case. Romero declared that authorities should not be so quick to suspect midwives of infanticide, but should instead fix their attention upon new mothers. Labor and childbirth, she attested, were so devastating that simply undergoing them provided women with sufficient cause for seeking to destroy the babies they had just birthed, a fact that no male doctor could ever personally appreciate. "How many times," she asked, "has it happened that mothers are murderers of their own children?" Since at the time of birthing them, "the force of having expelled them and the pain that accompanies this, whose details and intention no doctor can clearly apprehend since not one of them, including the great Hippocrates, has ever given birth nor ever will."[55] One source indicates that among the indigenous population of Michoacán, a more specialized form of anatomical expertise than motherhood was often a prerequisite to midwifery. Writing in 1887, medical historian Nicolás León bemoaned the immorality of the young women who eventually matured into the work of midwifery, "for it is common that a woman, having been a prostitute in her youth will become a midwife in her old age."[56]

For reasons of availability, familiarity, and confidence, then, women in late colonial society normally sought out midwives rather than physicians to attend them. The thirty-nine year-old *criolla* (creole, a Spaniard born in the New World) resident of Zacatecas, Doña María Barbara Comales, sought out such assistance in 1797. As she subsequently described to an Inquisition officer, upon her arrival to the city she had asked several people to recommend a *partera* who could assist her in her approaching labor. "Most of them," she testified, "said that the best one was an old woman called Lorenza who was very well known in the whole city." Comales had contacted the midwife and the latter had had told Comales that she possessed "some good little *yervitas* [herbs] that could help women to give birth without pain and without a *tenedora* [birth assistant responsible for physically restraining laboring women] other than her own sister."[57] Lorenza had then "shown her the herbs wrapped in some ordinary papers, but she had never known their quality nor had she wanted to take them, and for this reason she had asked what kind of herbs they were and the answer was that only in the botico [pharmacy] that they were known, and with this, she had sent away the old woman."[58]

In subsequent interviews with townspeople, Comales learned that a local magistrate had previously put Lorenza in jail for not revealing the nature of the medicines she used, and that the justice had ordered both "the surgeon Moreno" and "the Boticario Espinosa" to examine them, but neither had been able to identify the substances. Comales had then interrogated both Moreno and Espinosa, but neither could provide any further information about the herbs, "but only said that just as they had their remedies, [Lorenza] also had hers." When Comales learned from another acquaintance in Zacatecas that the herbs that Lorenza administered "had taken the lives of various expectant women," she was prompted to denounce the midwife to the Inquisition.[59]

Besides revealing information about one of the forms of service—the easing of the pain of birth—that midwives purported to provide to colonial women, the case illustrates the esteem in which townspeople apparently held Lorenza. Despite the rumors that had circulated about the ill effects of her remedies, the majority of Zacatecaños valued Lorenza's skills sufficiently to have recommended her services to the expectant mother even though a surgeon was available. Neither did the Inquisition view the denunciation against the midwife as sufficiently grave to prompt further investigation.

Even in complicated births—those, for instance, involving multiple or "monstrous" offspring, as treated below—women of means still often opted for the care of midwives rather than physicians in the late eighteenth century. This occurred in the case of a pair of conjoined twins born in the city of Guanajuato in 1785. In this instance, the *Gazeta de México* reported, "One was born foot-first, and in delivering him, the midwife discovered the knot that joined the two heads."[60] Here, the expectant mother, Doña Rafaela Cortés, had contracted a midwife rather than a doctor to assist her in the birth despite the honorific's implication of her probable high social status and the fact that her presumably larger than usual antepartum size might have indicated a potentially arduous labor. In other cases, the *Gazeta's* birth announcements recorded that either doctors alone, or both doctors and midwives, were called to aid women in labor.[61]

Colonial Beliefs and Practices

What kind of advice and what services did midwives provide to women who suspected they were pregnant in the maturing viceroyalty? It is clear that while many women suspected they could themselves determine whether conception had occurred, they often sought confirmation from midwives. Without such confirmation they remained in doubt (or ignorance) of their states throughout their pregnancies. One 1614 Inquisition denunciation detailed how a free mulata woman whose "stomach had grown large" had consulted an Indian woman to find out if she was pregnant. The latter told her that she was not pregnant but that some "creepy-crawly" (*sanbadijae*) had caused her stomach to rise. The mulata, unsatisfied with the diagnosis, had then drunk some hallucinogenic peyote to discover the truth, and "had seen that she was pregnant."[62] The friar who denounced the mulata in this case was likely concerned about her use of peyote, a substance the Inquisition would formally ban in 1620.[63] Church officials, community members, and former clients made similar denunciations against midwives who also operated as *curanderas* and whose services included providing love charms, reading the future, and locating lost objects.[64]

For some Mexican women, the question of whether conception had occurred could not be unambiguously determined by their own biological knowledge. Some women did declare in Inquisition trails and criminal cases that they knew they had conceived because of such commonly known physical indications of pregnancy as suspension of the menses and swelling of the womb. In one 1786 criminal trial, for instance, fifteen-year-old Juana Trinidad Márquez accused her cousin, Antonio Márquez, of having abandoned her after having given her his *palabra de casamiento* and impregnating her. She declared that "some days after her incontinence, she felt she was pregnant [se sintío embarazada]," without specifying how she had known.[65] In one 1857 infanticide trial, the accused confessed she had suspected she was pregnant because she had stopped menstruating.[66] In a third case, dating from 1883, a woman declared that she had known she was pregnant because her "menstrual illness had stopped and because her womb had swollen in a very apparent way."[67]

In other instances, including in instances of very advanced pregnancies, women or their close companions claimed total ignorance of their state right up to the moment of birth. In one 1802 criminal trial, a twenty-year-old mother accused of killing an infant, her second child, declared that although she had been raped repeatedly by a man, she did not realize that she was pregnant with his child right up to the instant of the infant's birth, adding that various doctors "who had assisted her in this period, and cured her for another illness" had also remained ignorant of her state right up until the very day of her labor.[68] In a second criminal case, originating in Teposcolula, Oaxaca, both parents of a seventeen-year-old declared that they had remained ignorant of their daughter's pregnancy and childbirth even though they had lived with her through both events.[69] In a third criminal trial dating from 1840, a woman from Aguascalientes accused of infanticide denied that she had ever been pregnant. Although a midwife and an acquaintance both declared they had known she was pregnant, Mexico City's Supreme Court judged that the prosecution had presented insufficient evidence that the defendant had, in fact, been pregnant since their only evidence rested on the fact that her womb was large. The court observed that women could have large bellies for reasons other than pregnancy, and upheld a lower court's decision to absolve her of the charge of infanticide.[70]

We cannot now determine whether these women and their peers spoke truthfully when they claimed ignorance of pregnancy. Nevertheless, we can conclude that up until the late nineteenth century, sufficient ambiguity existed about whether or not a woman was pregnant based on her physical appearance and such biological indications as amenorrhea that it was feasible for women and their peers to claim ignorance about whether conception had occurred. Such claims were strong enough to convince criminal courts that sufficient doubt existed about the matter to avert convictions for infanticide and abortion. A large belly, suspension of the menses, nausea, and other such established signs of pregnancy were not necessarily clear evidence of pregnancy. Rather than relying on women's own judgment, determination of conception remained ambiguous in the absence of expert confirmation.

Incipient Professional Obstetrics

Beginning in the late eighteenth century, principally under the encouragement of the modernizing Bourbon state, male physicians rather than female midwives began to attempt medical confirmation of pregnancy for a limited number of elite women in the colonial capital. In 1780, for instance, the sister of the *corregidor* (district administrator) of Coyoacán requested that surgeon Andrés Montaner y Virgili attend her during the birth of her child.[71] And in the era of Mexico's independence, physician Francisco Montes de Oca was the *partero* (male midwife) of the empress Doña Ana María Harte, wife of Agustín de Iturbide.[72]

In these cases expectant mothers could be assured of the credentials of their birth attendants, but such was infrequently the case. The problem of licensing and regulating medical practitioners, purportedly in order to eliminate fraud, but also as a means of generating revenue though the collection of licensing fees, had plagued the Spanish crown since the late fifteenth century. As early as 1538 the Mexico City municipal council enjoined medical examiners to inspect apothecary shops in the capital and to examine all those practicing midwifery, but apparently this legislation was rarely enforced.[73] Between 1567 and 1750, the Spanish crown restricted those medical positions that would be subjected to formal examination and licensing to physicians, surgeons, and druggists.[74]

In the second half of the eighteenth century, the Bourbon state increasingly formalized medical care in Iberia and abroad, seeking to modernize medicine, eradicate unregulated health providers, and generate profit through its investment in scientific exploration and research (most successfully in the form of the 1788 foundation of the Royal Botanical Gardens).[75] Doctors themselves were the most outspoken proponents of stricter state regulation of the medical profession. The celebrated physician and mathematician José Ignacio Bartolache was one of the most vocal critics of Mexican midwives; in his 1772–73 medical periodical *Mercurio Volante*, the first scientific journal published in the Americas, Bartolache admonished that the women of New Spain "abandoned themselves in their pregnancies and births to the indiscretion of these *parteras* and *comadres* whose work bears no relation to that of the licensed doctors that these people normally seek out, not without grave damage to these patients. I have noted among them infinite abuses of great consequence. People who reject a medicine prescribed by a learned doctor will still drink the most absurd and foolish drinks at the behest of their midwives."[76] Bartolache concluded that until these practitioners learned the art of midwifery from the *Arte de Partear* (likely referring to a Barcelona publication dating from 1765), written and perfected by "the most intelligent of men . . . it is nonsense to believe that midwives can be of use for anything other than to receive and bathe the newborn and bring clean clothing to the laboring mother."[77]

In 1788, the director of the medical faculty at the University of Mexico, several professors from the faculty, and representatives from the

Royal Botanical Gardens wrote a series of letters of complaint to the Count of Revillagigedo, viceroy of New Spain, bemoaning the deplorable state of professional regulation of medicine in the kingdom: "We know that the kingdom has been infiltrated by charlatans and empirical [i.e., unschooled] curanderos who do not have the authorization of the Faculty of Anatomy," they wrote. They described the poor state of *boticos*, where "a multitude of remedies are available in any store selling oil and vinegar, that are dispensed without consultation with licensed doctors."[78]

The field of obstetrics was among the many affected by the move toward heightened regulation. In the last decades of the eighteenth century, obstetrics was starting to be formally taught in medical schools in New Spain. In 1768, the Bourbons founded the Royal College of Surgery (Real Escuela de Cirugía) in the Royal Indian Hospital. Although it did not admit women, by 1804 the College had begun instructing students in obstetrics. In 1792, colonial authorities also founded an obstetrics *cátedra* in the Hospital of San Miguel de Belén in Nueva Galicia to instruct female students.[79] More extensive obstetrical instruction and research did not occur in Mexico until the 1830s. A fully fledged maternity hospital, emerging from the 1806 Department of Secret Births of the Mexico City Poor House, would not be created in Mexico until 1865.

The Bourbons also attempted to initiate the professionalization of midwifery. As early as 1742, an influential Spanish Enlightenment writer, Benito Jerónimo Feijóo y Montenegro, called for women's absolute exclusion from midwifery.[80] In 1750, King Fernando VI ordered the Protomedicato to establish a process by which midwives would be formally examined and licensed. That same year the Royal Protomedicato, avowedly responding to recent instances of women and infants dying in routine childbirth when attended by incompetent midwives, introduced requirements mandating that midwives in Castile and other realms of the Spanish Empire be required to study for four years with an approved instructor, produce documentation demonstrating their *limpieza de sangre*, attain three or four years' training under a licensed surgeon or midwife, and achieve a certificate of good conduct. They prohibited single women from becoming *parteras* and required women to pay 128 reales for their licenses.[81]

The royal decree of 1750 also engendered prohibitions on the types of medical procedures midwives were permitted to perform. Physician Antonio Medina's midwifery tract *Cartilla nueva util y necesaria para instruirse las matronas*, originally published in Madrid in 1750 at the behest of the Royal Protomedicato, specified that in cases of fetuses who had died inside the womb, midwives were not to attempt dilation of the cervix because the procedure was difficult and could provoke accidental complications that they were ill equipped to handle. Medina believed that midwives were competent to deliver babies in routine births, but that "a good surgeon" should always be called to attend women in the cases of any kind of complication. Here and in many other contemporary and later sources, medical authorities and the state warned midwives and their clients against these female practitioners' attempts at practicing interventionist medical procedures.[82] In 1798, the Mexican Protomedicato, possibly influenced by Ignacio Bartolache's earlier recommendations, decreed that midwives should be further restricted from the kinds of medical services they provided to women at childbirth. "Midwives," the board ordained, "should consider themselves purely as receivers of newborn babies." Doctors were to be called in cases of any and all complications.[83]

This was a radical effort. Throughout the early modern period, midwives in Spain (and in Mexico, long before then) had assisted women in all the complications that might be presented in childbirth. Francisco Núñez's 1580 *Libro del parto humano*, a Spanish tract directed at midwives and written in the vernacular, observed, for instance, that midwives knew "how to carry out a caesarean postmortem."[84] But the Bourbon and eventually the early republican Mexican states attempted to dramatically reduce the complexity of the cases midwives would be licensed to treat. In 1804, the Ordenanzas, regulations governing the Royal College of Surgery, required that "in cases of laborious or difficult births, a licensed surgeon should be called."[85] By this point, such cases included molar pregnancies, instances in which the placenta did not emerge naturally, or in situations when laboring women had lost much blood, those with nonstandard fetal presentations, or in cases of stillborn fetuses.[86] Decrees against midwives' participation in complicated births were, however, unenforced and unenforceable. A century after the publication of the 1804 Ordenazas, the Ministro de Gobernación of president Porfirio Díaz was still attempting to mandate that licensed midwives would be permitted to assist women only in "normal" deliveries and prohibited them from practicing obstetrical operations using instruments or applying anesthesia or intrauterine injections unless prescribed by a physician.[87]

The strictness of midwives' licensing requirements meant that few women applied for such certification, even though physicians increasingly cited the deplorable absence of licensed midwives in New Spain. In 1793, several professors from the University of Mexico complained to Mexico City's council about "the swollen crowd of women who have introduced themselves into this city" to practice midwifery unlicensed.[88] According to the Mexican Protomedicato's own records, by 1831 it had licensed only two midwives: Angela María Leite in 1816 and María Francisca Ignacia Sánchez in 1818.[89] Although male midwives became more popular in Europe in the eighteenth century, they had a negligible presence in Mexico; in the second half of the eighteenth century, the Mexican Protomedicato licensed only one surgeon as a *partero*.[90]

It is possible that larger numbers of midwives were licensed than these records suggest. The crown often recruited the professional advice of midwives in criminal trials, and presumably would have been reluctant to call for evidence from unlicensed practitioners.[91] Also, a mandate Viceroy Revillagigedo issued in May 1794 and circulated to at least nineteen *subdelegados* (provincial administrators) in the valley of Mexico reminded medical care providers of all levels—doctors, surgeons, *boticarios*, and midwives—of their legal obligation to "help all patients who need their assistance," suggesting that the office of the viceroy believed a larger body of licensed midwives existed.[92] Finally, outside the capital city, local governments also established means of officially training and licensing midwives in the closing decades of the colonial era, including at the Hospital of San Miguel de Belén in Nueva Galicia.[93]

Whether licensed or not, through the close of the colonial era *parteras* continued to attend women in childbirth. The Mexico City census of 1811 listed twenty-four midwives operating in the capital that year although their ethnic or civil status should have disqualified many in this group from legally undertaking such work: five were *casta*, eleven were Indians, and four were single.[94] In his 1804 report to the director of Mexico's Royal College of Surgery, doctor Antonio Serrano bemoaned the ongoing inadequacy of the regulation of midwifery in the viceroyalty, where licensed doctors were scarce and where "a plague of curanderos, destroyers of humanity," served the public. "Even in this capital," Serrano warned, "there are women who, without principals or knowledge, exercise the art of midwifery." Their only training came from what they had learned from their mothers or sisters. Such women, Serrano continued, "in attempting to extract a baby and placenta, instead remove the intestines. And if the arm of a baby presents itself, when a doctor would insert his hand to seize the baby by the feet, instead try to yank it by the arm and seeing their efforts are in vain, cut it off! Unhappy victims of ignorance!"[95]

Despite the foundation of some venues for formal obstetrical instruction in New Spain beginning in the 1760s, Serrano complained that there were no educated midwives anywhere in the viceroyalty and there was no obstetrical *cátedra* in the kingdom. By the mid-nineteenth century, the numbers of licensed midwives had grown. Training programs for midwives were established in the capital, Guadalajara, and Mérida in the 1830s; in Morelia and Puebla in the 1840s; in Monterrey in 1853; and in Oaxaca, San Luis Potosí, Zacatecas, and several other major urban centers by century's end.[96] Mexico City's Escuela de Medicina graduated its first midwife, Carlota Romero, in 1841. By 1888, 140 women had successfully passed through the program.[97]

Medical publications and other sources suggest that while midwives continued to attend the births of the majority of Mexican women, male professionals became increasingly common—at least in urban settings for upper-class women—by 1800. After the turn of the century, new obstetrical publications appeared in Mexico that were aimed at male professionals who could perform more interventionist obstetrical operations. These included an 1821 translation of Parisian physician Jacques Pierre Maygrier's 1817 work under the title *Nuevo metodo para operar en los partos*, which instructed physicians on various techniques, including the use of the forceps and the hook (*gancho agudo*) to extract fetuses presented abnormally at delivery.[98] Forceps deliveries eventually held dramatic repercussions for women's experience of childbearing and for the broader perception of reproduction and motherhood in Mexico. By the late nineteenth century, adoption of these instruments in the republic's urban centers had become institutionalized, and practitioners viewed their use as a necessary and distinctive element of birthing in the evolving mestizo nation.

Conception and Pregnancy in Modern Obstetrics

The advent of professionalization and the development of new medicalized obstetrical procedures in Mexico thus followed a gradual rather than immediate trajectory after the Royal Protomedicato's call for professionalization in 1750. (Subsequent chapters in this book will treat how changes in both health care personnel and the medical care they offered affected women's exposure to contraception and abortion and their experiences of childbirth itself.) New medical practitioners also affected the kind of knowledge women might have of conception, and the practices and beliefs they adopted during their pregnancies. In late eighteenth-century Mexico, among the works doctors interested in women's health consulted were those of French physicians François Mauriceau (*Traité des maladies des femmes grosses*, 1668), Jean-Louis Baudelocque (*Principes sur l'art d'accoucher*, 1775), and André Levret (*Observations sur les causes et les accidents de plusieurs accouchements laborieux*, 1750). They also studied the writings of various Spanish physicians including Antonio Medina (*Cartilla nueva util y necesaria, para instruirse las matronas*, 1750), Pedro Vidart (*El discípulo instruido en el arte de partear*, 1785) and José Ventura Pastor (*Preceptos generales sobres las operaciones de los partos*, 1789), along with Mexican professor of medicine Juan Manuel Venegas (*Compendio de la medicina*, 1788), whose writings also appeared frequently in the *Gazeta de México* in the 1780s.[99]

The works of Medina and Ventura had the most pronounced impact and readership in the viceroyalty. Medical historians Nicolás León and José Joaquín Izquierdo have traced their circulation among eighteenth-century medical practitioners in New Spain, and both appeared in late colonial medical libraries.[100] A citation to Ventura's tract found its way into a list of medical texts possessed by a party apparently investigated by the Mexican Inquisition in the late eighteenth century. This unique, undated document is an inventory of medical texts, likely those in possession of someone the Inquisition had incarcerated in the late eighteenth century. Among other works, this collection included William Buchan's *Medicina doméstica*, Herman Boerhaave's *Aforismos de cirugía,* and a text listed as "Pastor, Tratado de Partos, 2 tomos."[101]

Obstetrical texts of this period clearly described the mechanics of conception, although, as Andrés Levret observed in 1778, no one had yet adequately explained how the mystery of propagation occurred.[102] Like his contemporaries, Vidart detailed the semen's passage via the fallopian tubes to the fertilization of an egg in the ovaries.[103] Drawing from Hippocratic theory, most contemporary writers also believed that for conception to occur both parties had to achieve orgasm. Ventura, citing Jean Louis Baudelocque's 1781 *L'Art des accouchements*, for instance, wrote that various explanations for sterility in women existed, including that they had not taken pleasure in intercourse.[104] Fifty years later, medical opinion in Mexico had apparently shifted on this point. A medical primer prepared for the training of midwives in Morelia in 1857 advised that conception was most probable when copulation had occurred just before or after a woman's menstrual period, but noted that "for conception to occur, pleasure is not necessary, as is often believed."[105]

In terms of the detection of conception, Antonio Medina's midwifery primer instructed that midwives could use various means to determine if women were pregnant, but cautioned that these were much more reliable later in pregnancy. Medina wrote that a *comadre* could ask her patient if, after "cohabitation," she had felt a light pain near the navel or a light trembling throughout the entire body. Pregnant women might also experience an appetite for unusual foods, and were likely to suffer bouts of nausea (especially in the morning), abundant salivation, or headaches and backaches. If they experienced all of these symptoms along with the complete absence of menstruation, it was very likely they were pregnant.[106] The same observations continued to characterize obstetrical manuals for the next century.

Nevertheless, the inconclusive nature of these symptoms also remained current throughout the era of obstetrical professionalization, for Medina observed that the absence of menstruation was not "as is commonly believed" a sure sign of pregnancy since "some poor mixing of their humors, or some other thing" could provoke this symptom. By 1863, the *Cartilla de partos* produced for midwives by the state of Oaxaca advised that conception could be detected by the suppression of the menses and expansion of the uterus, but also observed that various illnesses could also provoke both symptoms.[107]

Likewise, Medina's counsel for the good health of expectant mothers did not differ greatly from that which Nahua *ticitl* provided in the pre-Columbian era: they were to abstain from frequent cohabitation and avoid immoderate exercise. Also, "as much as possible, they should maintain a serene soul."[108] To alleviate severe nausea, Spanish surgeon Pedro Vidart counseled afflicted women to drink "a light infusion of the herbs veronica or chamomile, or a glass of orange juice or lemonade."[109] Vidart's discussion of women's unpleasant physical experiences during pregnancy was somewhat unusual, for when most texts from the eighteenth century onward discussed pregnancy, they discussed only those steps women should take to avoid miscarriage. Ventura advised that they should not be allowed to ingest "unnatural" substances, but should be able to satisfy their cravings at whatever time these might strike. They were to avoid violent exercise, great shock, fear, and the application of pressure on their wombs in the act of coitus.[110]

Juan de Esteyneffer, a Jesuit missionary who published the influential *Florilegio medicinal* in Mexico in 1712, apparently drew his knowledge about pregnancy from centuries-old humoral theory and likely the domestic remedies that European midwives had long used. He advised that women could prevent miscarriage by avoiding heavy blows or vigorous exercise, but wrote that women who were naturally sanguineous or phlegmatic were more prone to miscarry than others.[111] Esteynferrer's antiabortive remedies included the ingestion of the seed of the herb *lanten*, and that of a mixture of powdered deer antlers (*asta de venado*) cooked in broth. To "comfort and calm" the fetus, he counseled that a warm compress made of roast beef sprinkled with cloves, nutmeg, or cinnamon be applied to the womb.[112]

A handwritten pharmaceutical manual produced in the closing decades of the eighteenth century described various substances that could be proscribed for women to inhibit miscarriages. These included *pildoras contra fluxo* (pills to inhibit flux), astringents that could "detain the flow of blood or of matter from the womb," *Gotas para disentería* (dysentery drops) that could arrest "the flow of blood of any type," and a treatment made from blond sandalwood that similarly halted blood flow.[113] More explicitly, the same manual described "Palacios's Anti-Miscarriage Powders" (*Polvos de Contra Abortos de Palacios*). This remedy "prevented fetuses from being sent to limbo" by preventing miscarriage in those had suffered a fright, a fall, or other accident. The powders detained the fetus in the uterus, but were only effective when women who took them remained in bed for the six-day duration of their treatment.[114]

In the republican period, Ignacio Torres's weighty 1858 *Manual de partos*, like earlier colonial texts, concentrated on counseling women on how to prevent miscarriage rather than on how to alleviate physical discomfort during pregnancy. Torres's tract briefly discussed afflictions women might experience while pregnant, and then detailed how women in such a state should avoid all strong emotions, vigorous movement, heavy exertion, genital stimulation, tight clothing, and spicy food. He advised pregnant women to take in pure air, eat healthy food, and embrace good hygiene.[115] By the late nineteenth century, obstetrician Juan María Rodríguez's counsel retained much continuity: to prevent miscarriage, women should avoid experiencing powerful emotions, physical violence, and even moderate engagement in coitus. Rodríguez cautioned that women should also avoid dancing, wearing corsets, and horseback, carriage, or train riding.[116]

By the mid-nineteenth century, obstetrical guides did not detail the treatments pregnant women could be offered to address such side effects as nausea, constipation, hemorrhoids, and backache that had formed a part of both European and Mexican midwives' realm of medical specialization in earlier eras. In this period, however, various newspaper ads from publications in the Mexican capital reveal that druggists and doctors advertised remedies for such symptoms, often basing their legitimacy on their mixtures' European credentials. In 1863, one Dr. Corvisar, "physician to the French emperor, Maximilian II," advertised in *El Siglo Diez y Nueve* his medical tonic, the *Elixir de pensina*—a digestive remedy the Medical Academy of Paris had supported that would alleviate the nausea from which pregnant women frequently suffered.[117] Another 1870 advertisement published in *El Siglo Diez y Nueve* invited residents of the Mexican capital to try an elixir created by one Dr. Theremes, "used in the best hospitals of Paris," to treat various illnesses including consumption, anemia, and the "palpitations of pregnant women."[118] A third mixture, the *jarabe y vino de lactofosfato de Cal*, developed by the Parisian Dr. Conte, would awaken the appetite in pregnant and nursing women who were repelled by the idea of eating.[119]

In terms of knowledge about conception, and advice during pregnancy, the changes the professionalization of obstetrics initially brought to Mexico do not, thus, appear dramatic. The personnel who provided obstetrical care began shifting, but this occurred only gradually. Women who sought obstetrical care from physicians might have received less detailed information about treating the side effects of pregnancy than midwives might have provided them with, but some could seek remedies from other venues. One aspect of obstetrical care that did begin to change dramatically was the initiation of internal examination as a more conclusive means to determine if conception had occurred. Although in the early colonial period Mexican midwives had performed physical examinations of women's exterior genital region in rape cases, there is no evidence that they undertook internal examinations of women's cervixes in pregnancy or during labor. Neither does evidence of such examinations survive in most early modern midwifery tracts, including the earliest such work published in Spain, Damián Carbón's 1541 *Libro del arte de las comadres y del regimiento de las preñadas y paridas y de los niños*.[120] European midwives did, however, determine the extent of cervical dilation during labor itself.[121]

In the era of the incipient professionalization of obstetrics, however, cervical examinations became more standard. Medina's 1750 manual advised that midwives could also tell if a woman was pregnant if her breasts or womb were harder than usual, if her navel had changed color, or if the cervix, upon examination, felt totally closed, soft, and nearly flat. Similarly, Ventura wrote that early signs of pregnancy included suspension of menstruation, elevation and tenderness of the breasts, and the complete closing and hardening of the cervix. He added that the surest sign of pregnancy remained the movements of the fetus, which might be felt at four and a half or five months.[122] During their pregnancies, several other guides counseled midwives and physicians to monitor the development of the uterus through internal manual examinations of the cervix. In 1858, Torres counseled midwives to perform internal examinations of upright women in order to determine the thickness, strength, and dilation of the cervix.[123] By 1878, Juan María Rodríguez, Torres's former pupil and then director of Mexico City's birthing hospital, the Casa de Maternidad, listed all of the above-mentioned probable signs of pregnancy, and added "neurosis" and "hysteria" to the list of "probable" signs associated with the state.[124] Rodríguez also wrote that medical practitioners (whom he titled *parteros*) should conduct thorough internal examinations in the seventh or eighth month of pregnancy by "applying the tip of the index finger to the base of the uterus . . . and making a violent push upward, so that a solid body can be perceived displacing itself and falling on the tip of the finger."[125] Rodríguez noted, not surprisingly, that this method disturbed his patients excessively, so it was preferable to instead perform an abdominal exam.

The advent of more frequent and more intrusive internal examinations of pregnant and laboring women beginning in the era of obstetrics' professionalization in turn initiated a problem for the new professionals who were attempting to establish a foothold in the birthing chamber. Beginning with the detection of conception and continuing throughout pregnancy and in the final act of birth itself, pregnant women and male physicians experienced considerable discomfort maneuvering within the physical and social intimacy these moments created. Midwives' undoubtedly less formal bedside manner and their more habitual physical familiarity with women's bodies rendered them more approachable to expectant women.

Physicians' inexperience with women's bodies was at best uncomfortable and at worst fatal. As doctor Juan Bautista Arechederreta commented in his 1802 appeal to the Mexican Protomedicato on the topic of the professionalization of obstetrics, it was necessary for midwives to have formal training in obstetrics practices and in "other surgical operations that men find shameful to practice upon the other sex such as, for example, the catheter . . . sucking cups . . . and others such that their natural modesty has meant that some women cruelly suffer, and even perish from these, in order to avoid their exposure and perhaps even the insults and jeers of some doctors."[126]

Spanish physician Ventura addressed this issue explicitly in his writing because years of practical experience in birthing chambers unusually informed the obstetrical tract he produced. He commented that physicians, when called to aid women in labor, must "present themselves before their patients not with a sad, harsh, or imperious manner, which imprints terror and fear to the core of their hearts." Evidently, emotions described how laboring women received many of his professional contemporaries. Instead, Ventura advised adopting a "pleasant, agreeable, sweet, and happy countenance (in moderation)."[127]

He also instructed practitioners to avoid touching their patients unless it was absolutely necessary and, even then, counseled that this should be done "with all possible honesty and delicacy."[128] He further advised practitioners to use a "modesty blanket" during cervical examinations and in the last stages of delivery to protect the dignity of all parties. Images depicting obstetrical exams and women in labor published in the eighteenth and nineteenth centuries illustrate the extent to which concerns over modesty and physical discomfort characterized women's experiences of obstetrical care (see figs. 3 and 4).[129] José Ventura Pastor advised that it was imperative for obstetricians to embody the perfect measure of good cheer, intimacy, and authority, but these were habits about which obstetrical texts did not and could not instruct them.

Mexicans, and specifically Mexican midwives, greeted physicians' arrival at the bed chambers of late colonial birthing women with mixed reactions. While evidence of a cooperative spirit between physicians and midwives was sometimes evident, doctors' presence provoked hostility among some midwives as one Inquisition case originating in Mérida in 1753 illustrates. There, one Doña Josepha Pastrana denounced a midwife described only by the name "Marcela" for having bewitched her. Pastrana was presumably a Spaniard and a woman of some substance, for her husband was the collector of the *santos diezmos* (church tithes) for the district of Campeche. Pastrana testified to the *comisario* (local agent of the inquisition) of Mérida that the previous year she had given birth with Marcela's assistance, seemingly without incident. Seven days later, she had

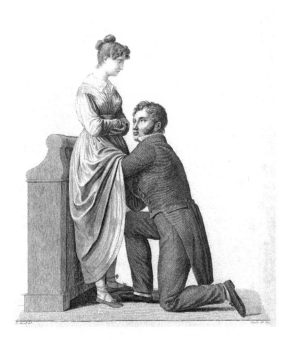

FIGURE 3 Vaginal examination in vertical position. From Jacques Pierre Maygrier, *Nouvelles demonstrations d'acchouchements* (1825). Credit: Wellcome Library, London.

had a disagreement with Marcela and afterward had begun "to suffer gravely from ailments of the stomach and womb, lacking totally the use of her head." She declared she felt oppressive "forces and airs" in the midwife's presence that prevented her from getting up without assistance and said that she had been provoked to move her head and make strange movements with her hands "like a senseless person."[130]

Her husband had called a doctor, Don Phelipe de León, to her aid. Pastrana described the remedies that León provided her with in largely supernatural terms: "The first thing he did was to order that she take the sacraments." He then pursued his unspecified "cure," which she found to be effective only when she was in his presence. "Whenever the doctor approached her bed, she found herself much relieved and did not feel anything, and when he distanced himself, she felt all her fatigue and anxiety."[131] Pastrana further declared that Marcela, the midwife, was much distressed that she had involved Dr. León in her treatment: "she continuously told her that if she wanted to get well, the said don Phelipe would not cure her, but only she [Marcela]."[132] Eventually Pastrana's husband persuaded Marcela herself to cure his wife, which she did shortly thereafter, "by placing her hand underneath the sheets of her bed, while the denouncer simultaneously felt better airs, and then, as if tearing out

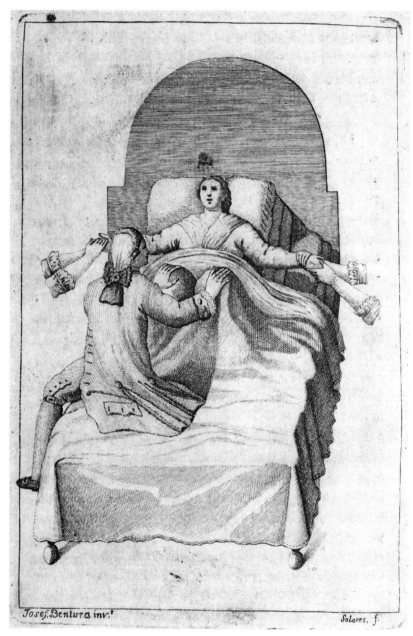

FIGURE 4 A woman in labor, in bed. From José Ventura Pastor, *Preceptos generales sobre las operaciones del parto* vol. 1 (1789), plate opposite page 191. Credit: Wellcome Library, London.

her womb inside her, she took her hand back out, which made the pain go away, and the said midwife took her hand out from the sheets and was holding on to her underclothes, and on them there were three drops of blood and when she saw this, the denouncer was already better."[133] Possibly Marcela had merely massaged Pastrana's uterus to encourage its postpartum contraction, a procedure midwives normally performed immediately following childbirth. In any case, though she seemed cured, Pastrana subsequently denounced Marcela for sorcery and secured her husband's promise that he would not permit Marcela subsequent entrance into their house.

Midwife Marcela's professional competitiveness was directed toward both her patient and the doctor whom she evidently viewed as poaching on her client base, but midwives also expressed such professional competitiveness toward one another. In one 1792 Inquisition trial from Veracruz, a man denounced the mulata midwife Agustina Carrasco to the Holy Office for having cursed his pregnant wife. He declared that his wife, suspecting herself pregnant, had engaged Carrasco to examine her belly. Carrasco had determined she was pregnant, but had also threateningly informed her: "*You are pregnant, but I must be your midwife and if this is not the case, you will give birth only when frogs grow hair.*"[134] He further declared that his wife suffered so much in the days leading up to her labor that they feared for her life. Her family then called Carrasco, and when she arrived she removed from the woman's vagina "a chile of the kind that is used in food and then remained until she delivered a dead child."[135] The child itself was born with "very strange" marks, including only one eye—on its forehead.

Individual midwives, physicians, and pregnant women had varying reactions to the changing landscape of obstetrical professionals at the end of the colonial period. In the "Observaciones" section of his late eighteenth-century tract, written from his experiences in the peninsular context, José Ventura Pastor described various incidents in which he condemned midwives' involvement with his clients. In one instance, he wrote of a birth scene in which a woman had miscarried and the fetus had remained inside her uterus. The midwife, "who lacked experience in the execution of a birth of this nature, and surrendering to the cruel vanity of not calling an educated surgeon," had pulled too hard on the trunk of the corpse and severed the body from its head, until Ventura was able to remove the latter with the use of his obstetrical spoons.[136]

In Mexico by the third quarter of the nineteenth century, Francisco de Asis Flores y Troncoso's description of a birth scene he pronounced typical of his era accords control of childbirth to midwives, even in those cases when doctors were also called to attend deliveries: "The midwife, both because she arrives before the doctor [to the house of the laboring woman] and due to her sex, gains the trust of the patient and of the family to such a degree that, when the doctor arrives, she limits herself to giving him only the data she chooses to share, and she invites him to prescribe this or that medicine." For his part, Flores was incensed: "The doctor, for dignity and for conscience, must not accept this role, and must procure to form an opinion himself on the case in question, and must recuperate the supremacy that society and the law have both assigned him."[137]

But other sources suggest cooperation was also possible. Juan Wecesalao Sánchez de la Barquera, a noted journalist and editor of *El Diario de México*, published a series of articles in 1806 addressing the question of contemporary health and social practices relating to pregnancy, birth, and neonatal care. In one piece, Sánchez criticized the persistence of the concoctions that some "old women" ignorantly continued to administer to pregnant and laboring women: boiled *zuapatle* [*cihuapatle*, the aster flower], chocolate with chiles, and "other thousands of absurdities of this type."[138] But he also wrote admiringly of the great facility with which "barbarous women"—undoubtedly rural indigenous women, who would likely have been accompanied by *parteras*—gave birth, although he judged their success was likely due to the sensible clothing they wore, the pure air they breathed, and the robust lifestyles they practiced.[139] Other evidence of cooperation and mutual learning between midwives and doctors is apparent in later periods. In nineteenth-century Oaxaca, legislation required doctors to learn the art of obstetrics from midwives rather than the other way around.[140] And writing in 1910, Nicolás León commented that he himself had decided to study at the side of a midwife because his teacher, a Dr. Pérez Gil, could not explain the mechanism of birth satisfactorily to him.[141]

Conception across Time

Most women who suspected themselves pregnant in late nineteenth-century Mexico would have experienced knowledge about conception and medical advice during pregnancy that did not differ enormously from women's experiences one or even two centuries earlier. Many of them would likely have decided for themselves whether or not they were pregnant based on a set of fairly commonly recognized symptoms. However, some would have doubted they were pregnant—or remained in total ignorance of their state—right up to the point of labor itself. Most would have had only a rough idea of their babies' due date, and most would have only have sought out medical assistance as birth became imminent, often securing midwives' commitment to assist them at birth in the last weeks, days, or hours of their pregnancies. And the advice midwives—or in rarer cases, beginning in the late eighteenth century, physicians—supplied them with as they prepared for childbirth differed little from that which was offered in earlier periods.

One difference that women increasingly experienced beginning in the era of the professionalization of obstetrics in 1750, however, was the introduction of internal obstetrical examinations—whether performed by midwives or physicians—that professionals declared should be used to confirm conception and track the course of pregnancy. These intimate procedures marked one change in the certainty by which pregnancy could be detected and also altered the dynamics of women's social and physical experiences with their health care attendants. They were also early manifestations of the more elaborate scrutiny of Mexican women's reproductive anatomy that medical professionals developed one century later with the emergence of works such as Francisco de Asis Flores y Troncoso's *El hímen en México* and Juan María Rodríguez's discovery of his female compatriots' distinctively narrow pelves. Along with physicians' adoption of the late eighteenth-century pelvic examination, more dramatic changes affected other aspects of women's obstetrical experiences in this period, particularly in the realms of anticonceptive and abortive procedures, to which we will now turn.

Part II **The Hidden History of Contraception, Abortion, and Infanticide**

· ·

3 Contraception and Abortion

· ·

While the medical counsel Mexican women received during pregnancy did not change dramatically between the colonial era and the late nineteenth century, the same was not true of women's attempts to regulate childbirth through either contraception or abortion. Over twenty years ago, Thomas Calvo remarked that while it would be foolhardy to account for Guadalajara's low seventeenth-century birthrate exclusively with women's use of contraceptives and abortion, "the issue cannot be lightly dismissed."[1] And yet the history of contraception, abortion, and infanticide have gone largely untreated in existent scholarship, particularly in English, where the most prominent history of Mexican women covering the period of transition from colony to republic dispenses with the topic in a single footnote and demographic research contends that colonial women had no knowledge or practice of contraception.[2] Rather than accepting that women in eighteenth- and nineteenth-century Mexico had no knowledge of contraception or abortion, this chapter uses ethnohistorical accounts, medical texts, legal codes, and criminal and Inquisition records to trace both practices and attitudes toward abortion and contraception in Mexico beginning in the pre-Columbian era and carrying through the nineteenth century.

In the colonial period, Mexican midwives employed a variety of medicinal substances to assist women in regulating their pregnancies. Available documentation suggests that women of all classes and ethnicities used such substances regularly and that the state and medical authorities did little to monitor their use. It is also apparent that although the law condemned abortion, Mexican communities condoned or ignored women's use of both contraception and abortion. Such was also the case, as chapter 4 will argue, for infanticide.

The era of the professionalization of obstetrics—the century following the Royal Protomedicato's (medical board's) call for midwifery's professionalization in 1750—witnessed several changes in abortive and contraceptive practices in Mexico. First, the sources and forces of institutional medicine repressed or ignored existent medicinal knowledge about both contraception and abortion. State-approved medical texts, the decrees of medical regulatory bodies, and the writings of prominent obstetricians often did not acknowledge, and sometimes actively condemned, information about contraception and abortion that midwives, *curanderas*, *boticarios*, and physicians in earlier periods, whether advertently or inadvertently, had long provided to Mexican women. At the same time, however, Mexico also experienced some liberalization in terms of the legal ramifications of abortion in the treatment of the crime in the country's first national penal code in 1871. This code decriminalized the procurement of an abortion to save the life of a pregnant woman and dramatically lessened the sentences colonial jurisprudence had dictated for the crime. Intriguingly, however, in the last decades of the nineteenth century, popular attitudes toward women who committed abortion diverged from the liberalizing tendency toward abortion the state exhibited. Significantly more Mexicans denounced women to judicial authorities for performing or procuring abortions and for committing infanticide in the closing decades of the nineteenth century than they had done in earlier periods. Despite popular and official condemnations of abortion, however, it is also clear that Mexican women continued to circulate knowledge and employ the techniques of inducing early labor to regulate their pregnancies throughout the period under examination. Given the public climate of growing opposition to abortion, they must have done so under conditions of increased secrecy.

I examine contraception and abortion together in this chapter because medical practitioners, state authorities, and women themselves did not draw as great a distinction between contraception and abortion as we do today. Throughout this period, midwives' most widely recorded practice for controlling reproduction was the prescription of substances that induced miscarriages by provoking uterine contractions in preterm pregnant women. Mexican populations and medical authorities alike comfortably accepted the idea of the legitimate use of "menstrual regulators" that might now be classified as abortifacients.

Tracking evidence of colonial and nineteenth-century abortion and contraception is difficult because documentation about the practices is scarce and because sources do not always clearly distinguish between accidental miscarriages and intentional abortions. Witnesses, judges, defendants, physicians, and bureaucrats often used the term *aborto* to describe any preterm fetuses' expulsion from the uterus, whether intentional or accidental, only exceptionally distinguishing between *abortos de voluntad* and *abortos provocados*. Thus, when staff in Mexico's first maternity hospital, the Casa de Maternidad, recorded that 21 of 911 pregnant women admitted between July 1886 and June 1888 had had *abortos*, they were presumably indicating the number of women who had miscarried rather than that this state institution had entered the business of performing abortions.[3]

Contraception and Abortion in the Pre-Columbian and Early Colonial Eras

Various sources document midwives' use of a variety of plant- and animal-based substances as both contraceptives and abortifacients in the pre-Columbian era. Nahua midwives did not understand how women might achieve periodic contraception, but they were knowledgeable about how women might induce long-term sterility. The sixteenth-century botanist and Mexican *protomédico* Francisco Hernández learned in the course of his research into New Spain's natural history that the plant *tetexquilitl* would make men infertile, while the herbs *axoxoquilitl* and *tlacoxiloxóchitl* could render both sexes "impotent to conceive."[4] The ubiquity with which pre-Colombian communities availed themselves of such plants is suggested in a passage contained in sixteenth-century missionary Bernardino de Sahagún's *Historia general de las cosas de la Nueva España*. Sahagún recorded that poor women in central Mexico were able to earn modest incomes by keeping small gardens where they grew edible plants, among which was *axoxoquilitl*.[5] In the pre-Columbian era, Sahagún further noted that those who ingested hummingbirds, creatures colonial Mexicans later associated with love magic, would be rendered infertile.[6]

Sources on early postcontact Mexico record more extensive information about indigenous women's use of abortifacients, and considerable evidence suggests that many continued to use them throughout the colonial period and in the nineteenth century. Spanish historian Gonzalo Fernández de Oviedo noted in his early postconquest *Historia general y natural de las Indias* that "there are other women so friendly with lust that if they become pregnant they take a certain herb, that later stirs up and casts out the pregnancy."[7] The early sixteenth-century Franciscan, Toribio de Benavente Motolinía, described with alarm the "witches" he had seen represented in a Corpus Christi pageant who knew of the substances that could make women miscarry.[8] Sahagún's informants also described various medicinal substances pre-Columbian midwives used to stimulate menstruation, to induce labor or, administered in higher doses earlier in pregnancies, to provoke miscarriages. These included *tlilxochitl* (vanilla bean) mixed with *mecaxochitl* (a pepper plant) in a drink of chocolate, *ancoas* (ginger root), the root of the *phehuame* plant prepared as an infusion, *nochtli* (nopal cactus), and *tlaquatzin* (the dried tail of an opossum ground into a powder and believed to have powerful expulsive properties).[9] Francisco Hernández recorded that the cooked leaves of *tlapechmecatl* or the application of *yahuatli* (marigold) "provoked abortion and expelled dead fetuses."[10] The most widely recorded, and apparently highly efficient, labor accelerator was *cihuapatli* (the aster flower). Sahagún wrote that when a pregnant woman was given this herb to drink after a *temazcal* bath, "the baby is propelled or pushed out."[11]

Mature Colonial Continuities

Throughout the late colonial period and into the nineteenth century, *parteras* continued to share their knowledge about contraception and abortion with their clients.[12] The eighteenth-century physician Ignacio Segura suggests as much in his 1775 midwifery treatise *Avisos saludables a las parteras*, in which he warned that "because parteras mingle with people of great coarseness, it is worth warning them that it is a mortal sin to do anything that can impede generation [of offspring]."[13] Medina's midwifery tract, published in Spain in 1750 and reissued in Mexico in 1806, included similar admonitions against performing or counseling abortion.[14] Confessional guides, including Fray Bartolomé de Alva's 1634 *Confessionario mayor y menor en lengua mexicana*, advised priests to routinely question women about whether they had "[taken] some potion in order to expel the baby."[15]

Other sources document that midwives continued employing various elements of pre-Columbian birth practices, particularly that of administering *cihuapatli* to pregnant or laboring women throughout the colonial period and the nineteenth century. In 1652, for instance, the Holy Office of the Inquisition investigated *partera* Isabel Hernández, a woman born of a mestiza mother and Spanish father, for *hechicería*, or spell making.[16] Several of Hernández's former clients testified against her, declaring that she had used various powders and potions to cast spells on them. The court requested that Hernández identify each of the powders, roots, and objects seized from her room. Among them were a powder that she declared was made from "the ground-up tail of a little animal said to be called tlacuache" (another rendition of *tlaquatzin*, one of the contraction-producing substances Sahagún had described midwives administering a century earlier), which she administered to laboring women in *pulque* (a fermented beverage made from maguey cactus), as well as fried onion and almond oil. Hernández also identified her possession of an herb she called *suapatle* (*cihuapatli*), the potent contraction-inducing aster flower Sahagún and others had recorded in their texts in the mid-sixteenth century.[17]

Various other Inquisition trials document *parteras'* provision of women with herbal abortifacients and with remedies to "regularize" their menses.[18] According to a tract the prolific scientific writer Antonio León y Gama composed in 1795, "all the uterine illnesses that women suffer from find efficient remedy in the multitude of herbs known by the generic name of *cihuapatli*; or medicine of women."[19] He also commented that even so ubiquitous a substance as pulque could be used "to provoke the menses in women."[20]

During the colonial period, women, midwives, and institutional medical authorities such as León y Gama referred to such substances as "menstrual regulators." Colonial Mexicans considered provoking the menses to be legally and socially acceptable, while Mexican legal and medicinal authorities viewed providing or receiving intentional abortions as both unlawful and immoral. While early modern physicians understood the cessation of the menses as one reliable indicator of pregnancy, they also believed menstruation could be "suppressed" for a variety of other reasons including the onset of many illnesses. Physicians, midwives, and *boticarios* all prescribed medicines to provoke the menses when these had been "suppressed" or "detained." It is not always apparent whether their prescriptions of such remedies—which sometimes acted as abortifacients— was self-conscious or inadvertent, but it is clear that effective herbal abortifacients circulated in colonial Mexico.

Physician Juan Manuel Venegas wrote in his 1788 *Compendio de la medicina*, for instance, that various treatments could restore a woman's menses including infusions of the plants chamomile, pennyroyal, and *altamisa* (artemisia).[21] All three are substances women long used on one or both sides of the Atlantic to induce abortions.[22] One late eighteenth-century medical text, an anonymous compilation of remedies and cures, included a recipe for an *altamisa* brew: "a tested, true, and infallible remedy to induce menstruation in women."[23] The *Gazeta de México*, one of New Spain's earliest news publications, also published a remedy for suspension of the menses; the September 18, 1795, edition announced that a daily dosage of a mixture formed by the reduction of the herb *viperina*, mixed with wine, cream of tartar, *aguardiente*, and *quina* leaves would successfully treat various chronic illnesses including menstrual detention, hysteria, hypochondria, and pulmonary disorders.[24]

In the late colonial period, *boticarios* who provided women with such often cautioned against ingesting medicines that might provoke miscarriage, suggesting that the prevention of preterm labor remained a central aspect of medical counsel given to pregnant women but also that various substances were available to women who used them to intentionally provoke miscarriage. One fascinating source, a handwritten late eighteenth-century pharmacy manual produced in Mexico City, discussed various medicines that might provoke miscarriage, including the "agua de la vida de las mugeres." The manual does not describe the composition of this elixir, but says it is used to treat hysteria and warns that it should not be given to pregnant women, "although it may be given to those in labor to facilitate the birth and fortify the newborn."[25] Similarly, a tincture made from the Cantueso flower was not recommended for women who were pregnant.[26] Another contemporary tract, a handwritten catalog of Mexican medicines compiled by Jesuit missionary Lucas Vásquez, described several medicines that could be taken "to provoke childbirth and release the afterbirth." The main ingredient of one of these was *altamisa*.[27] A third anonymous late eighteenth-century medical tract included a remedy for "difficult birth" that could serve as a cure in cases of stalled or lengthy labor. The tract instructed readers to make a plaster by mixing the cooked leaves of *altamisa* with barley flour and apply the warm plaster to the outside of the womb and the thighs.[28]

Colonial physicians and pharmacists prescribed such remedies to provoke menstruation in cases of "detention" or "suppression" of the menses. It is unclear whether they knew they could be used as abortifacients, but colonial women knowingly ingested them for such purposes. In one late eighteenth-century criminal trial originating in San Antonio Xacala, for example, a Spanish woman initiated a suit for breach of promise to marry, along with accusations of incest and forced abortion against her cousin, whom she said had given her word of marriage and then violated her virginity. He had then counseled her to abort her fetus, which she claimed to have done successfully by having "drunk a little altamisa."[29]

The fact women in Mexican colonial society actively controlled reproduction more widely than hitherto acknowledged is also suggested by an examination of birthrates in this context. Late colonial and early republican demographic records document that women in the Mexican capital gave birth unexpectedly infrequently. The Prussian naturalist Alexander von Humboldt, who traveled to New Spain at the turn of the nineteenth century, remarked upon the "very small number of births in the capital."[30] Historian Silvia Arrom, who drew her findings from a sample of Mexico City wills dating from 1802 to 1855, substantiates Humboldt's observation. Contrary to misconceptions of the timelessly enormous size of Latin American families and scholarship documenting rapid eighteenth-century population increase in the Mexican capital, it is striking that of the women Arrom studied from the last years of the colony through the first half of the nineteenth century, over 14 percent had given birth to no children at all by age forty-five; a further 17 percent had borne only one child, while another 15 percent had only had two children.[31] It seems unlikely that nearly half of the female population of urban Mexico had managed to limit family size so dramatically without recourse to either contraception or abortion.

Humboldt believed that celibacy, indigenous poverty, and the scarcity of medical services provided the principal explanations for the capital's low birthrates. Arrom, in contrast, saw low birthrates as the result of the large numbers of women who remained single or were widowed early. Her conclusion implies that reproduction could only occur within matrimony, however—a reading belied by the staggering rates of illegitimacy characteristic of this setting. In some cities, including San Luis Potosí, illegitimacy reached 51 percent in the mid-eighteenth century. Throughout the eighteenth century, in one affluent Mexico City parish, over one-fourth of those born were illegitimate.[32] The combined instance of high rates of extramarital sexual activity and low birthrates in particular contexts in colonial Mexico suggest that women's practices of contraception, abortion, and infanticide were more common than historians have hitherto acknowledged.

Abortion and Contraception in the Era of Professionalization

Beginning in the second half of the eighteenth century, medical professionals publicly condemned the practices women on both sides of the Atlantic had long used to provoke miscarriages and regulate reproduction. Spanish physician Cristóbal Nieto de Piña published an exhortation in 1783, for instance, in which he treated the means by which dead fetuses could be extracted from women's wombs. He opened his tract by vilifying those women who actively sought out abortions by feigning illnesses in order that the remedies physicians prescribed for them, including bleedings, might induce abortions.[33]

The medical texts that Mexican physicians consulted in the late colonial period generally omitted all discussion of contraception and abortion. In his *Preceptos generales sobre las operaciones de los partos*, for example, José Ventura Pastor exhaustively cataloged women's reproductive anatomy and minutely detailed the acts of conception, pregnancy, and birth, but avoided nearly all mention of contraception. He did, however, acknowledge that women in his milieu occasionally induced abortions. Condemning the practice, he described it as the "depraved and pernicious use of repeated bleedings, and other medicinal abortifacients that women use with the explicit goal of provoking abortion to cover their honor . . . without considering that they put their lives in danger with the violence of the strong oral emmenagogues [agents provoking menstrual flow] that they take."[34]

In the mid-nineteenth century, abortion appeared more frequently in medical texts than it had in the late colonial era, though always as a subject of condemnation rather than of instruction. María Magdalena de Flores's 1854 transcription of physician José Ferrer Espejo y Cienfuegos's second-year obstetrical course taught in Mexico City contains detailed information about contemporary medical understandings of abortion. In his lectures, Espejo distinguished between accidental (those caused by illness), spontaneous (those produced by physical or emotional violence to the mother), and intentional causes of abortion.[35] Intentional abortions, he lectured, were provoked by "those criminal maneuvers that women execute to make themselves abort, even with danger to their own lives either through violent exercise, taking harmful drinks, or attempting any means possible to abort."[36] The physician also discussed the question of whether, by examining their patients' symptoms, medical practitioners could distinguish between the simple "restoration of the menses" after they had been suspended due to disease and the occurrence of a "true abortion," although without indicating here if he referred to accidental or intentional abortions or both. He observed that the distinction between an actual abortion and the simple "restoration of the menses" had long confounded medical practitioners because the external signs—principally the onset of heavy vaginal bleeding—were the same in both cases. Citing the French midwife Marie LaChapelle's observations about the question, however, Espejo declared that practitioners could distinguish between the two. Only in the case of abortions, he noted, would the cervix be extremely dilated. Second, only in abortions would labor pains always precede hemorrhaging.[37] Espejo's attention to this matter suggests that medical practitioners of his day had begun to question Mexican women's practice of intentionally consuming medicines to provoke abortions, representing such acts as merely the routine medicinal restoration of the menses.

Physicians in this period actively and openly decried women's ongoing use of such herbal labor accelerators as *cihuapatli* and *altamisa*. In 1857, a midwifery manual the medical faculty of Michoacán produced commented that substances stimulating uterine contractions "like Altamisa and Zihuapatzli [an alternative spelling of *cihuapatli*] and others . . . are very dangerous and should only be used in very particular cases."[38] Instead, this text recommended the use of *cuernecillo de centeno*, or ergot, a drug derived from a fungus grown on rye that provoked uterine contractions and had long been used in European midwifery.[39] In his 1888 treatise on nineteenth-century medical practices, Francisco de Asis Flores y Troncoso also commented on the contemporary use of *cihuapatli*. Although Flores cautioned that the plant was "abused" in current obstetrical practice and caused many "unfortunate accidents," he also observed that its effect in stimulating labor contractions was the same as *cuernecillo de centeno*, and stated "its extract is recommended and the solution of its active ingredient at the same dose as the analogues prepared with centeno, especially as a hemostatic."[40] An 1892 investigation into a possible abortion that a woman had received prior to her admission to Mexico City's Casa de Maternidad also indicated she may have consumed *cihuapatli*. The Casa's head midwife reported to the hospital's director that she had been unable to "extract the product of birth" that remained in the woman's uterus after the *zipualpatle* (*cihuapatli*) she had taken had produced an infection in her womb.[41] Public health officials investigating high rates of maternal mortality at the Casa in the 1880s also disparaged Mexican women's ongoing practices of endangering their health by taking either "Zinapatle" or *cuernecillo de centeno* before arriving at the hospital.[42]

Despite broad condemnation of such medicines, individual physicians were sometimes more accepting of their value. Aniceto Ortega, a candidate for the professorship of obstetrics at the Escuela de Medicina in 1867, published a thesis describing various treatments for postpartum complications. He commented that *zoapatle*, "a plant that had abortive capabilities," could be used to great effect in encouraging the desired uterine contractions after birth.[43] And in his field observations of the obstetrical practices of Tarascan communities in Michoacán published in 1887, Nicolas León remarked, "I have had the opportunity to observe an intentional abortion that was brought about by the ingestion of a powerful infusion of the seeds of strong *Phurénchequa* (Eritrina coralloides *Sess* et *Moc*. Leguminosas). . . . I have also been informed that the plant called in Mexican *Chihuapatli* is used for this end as well as mechanical manipulations with the hands."[44]

Nineteenth-century judicial and medical records reveal little about practices involving surgical abortions, although limited evidence (including the 1871 penal code that provided specific punishments for medical professionals who helped women to abort) suggests some physicians and other practitioners provided surgical abortions. One newspaper story originating in a Matamoros newspaper and reprinted in Mexico City's *El Siglo Diez y Nueve* in 1844 recounted that two women had given a third woman a mixture of aguardiente and some kind of narcotic and had then "opened her belly with a well-sharpened barber's blade to take from her the fetus that was inside her."[45] They had failed to extract the fetus, which perished, along with the woman, one month later. The internal records of Mexico City's Casa de Maternidad describe one case of a possibly surgical abortion in 1876. In recording deaths that occurred in the institution in August of that year, a Casa administrator, likely the head doctor, observed that a woman who had arrived at the Casa after having lost much blood from an "abortion that an ignorant midwife had brutally performed on her, who, having failed to extract the afterbirth had administered a strong dose of zoapatle."[46] The following month, the administrator noted that two women had aborted in the Casa. One had miscarried "a dead baby whose death was caused by some blow she had received to her belly." Three months later, the administrator noted that two other women had arrived at the Casa "with indications of abortion."[47]

The only criminal case uncovered in this research that touched on surgical abortion was the criminal investigation of doctor Federico Abrego initiated in 1896.[48] Mexico City police suspected that Abrego had performed an abortion on his lover and nurse, María Barrera, whose body was discovered on an operating table in Abrego's house. Several witnesses informed investigating detectives that Berrera had been suffering inordinate vaginal blood loss in the days leading up to her death. Abrego himself declared that he and his colleague, one Dr. Alvira, had attempted to treat Berrera for blood loss that she had been suffering for a week prior to her death. They had sedated her in order to apply a surgical "plug" to terminate her menstrual bleeding.[49] Detectives ordered Berrera's corpse exhumed and medical experts who examined her remains concluded that "she had been four or five months pregnant at the time of her death and that she had died from internal bleeding as a result of an abortion."[50] Abrego eventually confessed that an abortion had been the cause of Berrera's hemorrhaging, but claimed that she had performed the procedure upon herself. Despite the various forms of circumstantial evidence linking Abrego to the crime, neither the Third Criminal Court nor the federal Supreme Court convicted Abrego of abortion and he was released in the spring of 1899. In Abrego's case, as in all criminal investigations of abortion examined in colonial and nineteenth-century Mexico, magistrates exercised extreme caution in convicting defendants for the crime of abortion, which by nature a secretive and private act unlikely to involve eyewitnesses.

Prohibitions on Abortion

Over time, state authorities condemned Mexican women's ongoing usage of various methods to provoke miscarriages abortions, many of which dated to the pre-Columbian and early colonial eras. Sahagún recorded that in pre-Columbian Mexico, the Nahuas viewed abortion as a crime punishable by death.[51] New Spain's systems of criminal and canonical law likewise dictated that abortion, like infanticide, be judged severely. The administration of law in the Spanish Empire rested largely in the hands of the provincial magistry, *alcaldes mayores* (who also acted as municipal authorities in nonjudicial matters) and their inferiors, *tenientes de justicia*. These officials approached the resolution of disputes in the empire through the application *derecho indiano* (the law of the Indies). *Derecho indiano* derived both from peninsular and New World sources. It was founded upon medieval and early modern Castilian legal codes, including the Ordenamiento de Alcalá (1348), the Laws of Toro (1505), the Nueva Recopilación de Castilla (1569), *fueros* (municipal charters), the Fuero Real (1255) and, most important, the Siete Partidas (1265).[52] Distinctive American contexts also influenced the formation of Spanish imperial law, particularly after 1614 when Philip III ordered that only laws formulated specifically for the Americas would govern the region.[53] The collection of royal decrees pertaining to the governance of the Indies was first collected in the 1680 *Recopilación de leyes de los reynos de las Indias*. The

Recopilación did not explicitly address the crimes of either infanticide or abortion, but the older peninsular legal codes treated both crimes severely. Infanticide carried the penalty of death by burning in medieval Spain.[54] The Siete Partidas considered abortion as homicide, generally punishable by death for both the mother and the abortionist, and did not follow the ancient distinction between "quickened" or "ensouled" fetuses and unanimated ones.[55]

Midwives in colonial Mexico were instructed that their involvement in abortion would incur the death penalty. One midwifery manual published in Mexico in 1775 warned, "Midwives, and any other person, who counsel or cooperate in any way with abortion, sin mortally, even if the creature is not animated, even if they do this to protect the honor, or life, of the pregnant woman. And if the creature is animated, they incur excommunication . . . and they will receive the death penalty for this act."[56] Canonical law also condemned abortion. Starting in 1588 with Pope Sixtus V's bull Ad Effraenatum (Without Restraint), abortion carried with it the penalty of excommunication.[57] In 1679, Pope Innocent XI condemned two propositions regarding abortion: the claim that abortion was not homicide, and that "it was lawful to procure abortion before ensoulment of the fetus lest a girl, detected as pregnant, be killed or defamed."[58] The Mexican tribunal of the Holy Office endorsed Sixtus V's bull in 1684, and the Diocese of Mexico did the same in the eighteenth century.[59] Martha Eugenia Rodríguez observes that midwives were threatened, on pain of capital punishment, to keep their knowledge of abortion in total secrecy; neither was it licit for them to kill any newborn, even if it was "too ugly or monstrous."[60]

As the discussion below reveals, although colonial criminal codes treated abortion—like infanticide—with great severity on paper, in practice colonial magistrates judged those accused of both crimes with far greater leniency. Justices were able to do this because they exercised considerable flexibility in interpreting the law according to their own discretion. Elisa Speckman Guerra observes that despite the centralist and standardizing initiatives of the Bourbons, throughout the colonial era judges interpreted the law with reference to formal legal codes but also according to "ideas and shared practices (common law) and particularly according to the customs of the place and the particular circumstances of the accused."[61] Over the course of the nineteenth century, the maturing republic revised the letter of the law, rendering it consistent with the more liberal judgments that Mexican magistrates had long pronounced even in those cases when they found defendants guilty of these crimes. Near the start of the century, Joaquín Escriche's canonical *Diccionario razonado de legislación y jurisprudencia*, first published in 1837 and then reissued repeatedly throughout the century set out the medieval and early modern precedents of criminal law in its definitions of crimes and their appropriate punishments. Escriche declared that both infanticide and intentional abortion of a fetus should carry the death penalty.[62] Ramón Francisco Valdés's *Diccionario de jurisprudencia criminal Mexicana*, published in 1850, concurred. Valdes observed that pregnant women who sought to miscarry "voluntarily take herbs or other concoctions, or give themselves blows in the stomach."[63] He indicated that those who voluntarily procured or induced abortions after the fetus was animated should be sentenced with capital punishment. In other cases, they should incur the penalty of five years' exile or imprisonment.[64]

By the time Mexico enacted its first national penal code in 1871, however, the state introduced a number of innovations to how both abortion and infanticide should be judged. In 1870, a federal commission headed by Antonio Martínez de Castro, minister of justice and public instruction under President Benito Juárez, completed the framing of Mexico's first national criminal code, initiated eight years earlier. The Mexican Congress ratified the text the following year.[65] This ideologically liberal code, along with the first national civil code of 1870, was severed from its political association with the Liberal Constitution of 1857 by the War of Reform (1857–61) and the resurrection of imperial rule under Maximilian Habsburg (1863–67). Martínez de Castro, like earlier liberal theorists José Luis Mora and Manuel Otero, sought with the code to create a politically liberal structure that would reform convoluted colonial law, penal institutions unfashionably designed for punitive rather than reformative outcomes, and judicial personnel he characterized as corrupt, arbitrary, and inefficient.[66] One of the code's salient characteristics was its exhaustive classification of the exact penalties—derived from exhaustive examinations of aggravating or attenuating circumstances that judges who applied the code were to administer in their sentences.[67]

Martínez de Castro also privileged the notion of popular participation in the reformed criminal legal system. In theory, he and his fellow commissioners sought the public's involvement in the implementation of justice. As he observed, "in publishing a good Penal Code that even the poorest can acquire at little cost, so that they might learn their duties, know the deformity of the crime, and advise themselves of the punishments they might incur, one will doubtless see a rapid decline in the number of delinquents."[68] Martínez de Castro and his team sought to design a code that would attract popular support and secure national participation in a project of governance that would assist the state in guaranteeing public security and prosperity for Mexico.[69]

One of the central features of the 1871 code was its heightened articulation of the importance of public honor in Mexican society. While colonial historians have long recognized the centrality of honor in the social operation of gender, the novelty of honor's articulation in the late nineteenth century lay in both its legal codification and its explicit connections to the notion of public order.[70] Pablo Piccato has described this as late nineteenth-century state makers' desires to craft a "stable notion of honor" that would legitimize their claim "to embody the virtues of the nation and to speak in its name."[71] Mexico's 1871 penal code detailed the primacy of honor and its relationship to the public sphere in several ways. First, a sizable section of the code was dedicated to regulation crimes "against reputation" and another section "against the order of families, public morality, and *buenas costumbres* [moral habits]"; these dealt with instances in which private legal matters normally contained within the sphere of domestic regulation became linked to offenses against public morality.[72] Such crimes included suppressing the existence of offspring by failing to record them in the civil registry, circulating obscenity, or committing adultery. The commission considered such acts as pederasty, statutory rape, and bestiality crimes against the public order when they were committed "with scandal, obscenity or violence."[73]

Honor featured prominently in the 1871 code in other ways. The code's second chapter, which dealt with circumstances that removed criminal responsibility from defendants, mandated that a defendant should be absolved of responsibility for criminal infractions "when the accused worked in defense of his or her person, honor, or goods, or the person, honor or goods of another."[74] Elisa Speckman Guerra has also observed that the 1871 code's treatment of the crime of infanticide in particular demonstrated the centrality of public honor.[75] The code defined infanticide as the killing of an infant in the first seventy-two hours of its life, precisely because there was a greater possibility of hiding the crime during this period of high newborn mortality.

Finally, in its attempted elimination of the arbitrariness of judicial sentencing, the 1871 code painstakingly enumerated all mitigating circumstances that might apply to the commission of particular crimes and their associated reductions in criminal sentences. For the crimes of both abortion and infanticide, the defense of honor was one of several possible mitigating circumstances. The 1871 penal code specified that abortion was permissible in cases when, if it were not performed, the pregnant woman ran the risk of death.[76] It also distinguished between accidental and intentional abortions, declaring that the former, when "caused only by the pregnant mother is not punishable," and when caused by doctors or midwives would be punishable with suspension from the exercise of their professions for one year.[77] A pregnant woman, on the other hand, would be punished with two years' imprisonment when she sought out an intentional abortion as long as she met the following criteria: "I. That she did not have a bad reputation [Que no tenga mala fama]; II. That she had successfully hidden her pregnancy; III. That the pregnancy was the fruit of an illegitimate union."[78] In cases of the absence of either the first or second circumstances, her sentence was to be increased by one more year of imprisonment. If the pregnancy resulted from the union of a married couple, the penalty rose to five years' imprisonment. Medical practitioners of intentional abortions could be sentenced anywhere from four years' imprisonment up to the death penalty in cases of their patients' demise.

The 1871 code signified two important reforms in how the law declared the judiciary should view abortion and infanticide. First, it dramatically reduced the severity by which judges were to sentence the accused, changing the standard (theoretical) sentence from capital punishment as dictated by Escriche, and elsewhere, to several years' imprisonment. Secondly, it mandated that accused parties' efforts to preserve their honor from public spectacle should further mitigate the severity with which judges should treat them. The killing of children from legitimate unions was to be treated more severely than the same actions in cases of illegitimate offspring, presumably because illegitimate children could bring dishonor to women's reputations while legitimate offspring could not. Protection from the dishonor implied by illegitimacy mitigated the severity of abortion and provided a partially justifiable, motive for its commission.

The Commission of Abortion in the Colonial Period

The medical knowledge circulating in Mexico about abortion, and the theoretical if not actual condemnation of its practice, remained remarkably consistent from the colonial era through much of the nineteenth century. We know that women obtained abortifacients throughout the period under examination, but given the limitations on the kinds of source materials that survive, it is difficult to assess with any certainty changes in the frequency with which women procured or induced abortions. We can detect with much more certainty the changing frequency with which family members, community members, and judicial authorities denounced women for having committed or procured abortions. In this regard, a notable transformation is evident: As also occurred with regard to infanticide in the seventeenth and eighteenth centuries, an astonishingly small number of residents of Mexico denounced women to local authorities under suspicion of abortion. Also, colonial authorities treated such cases with notable leniency, almost always dismissing the charges against defendants or occasionally sentencing them with punishments far more mild than the death penalty that colonial law dictated the crime should carry. Over the course of the nineteenth century, however, Mexico witnessed a marked increase in the numbers of women denounced to criminal courts for committing or procuring abortions. Particularly during the era of the Porfiriato, increased numbers of neighbors, patrons, policemen, and municipal administrators denounced women they suspected of having aborted. Increased denunciation rates suggest that toward century's close, Mexicans were shifting their expectations about the gendered behavior they understood as socially acceptable—especially for the unmarried, working-class women who formed the vast majority of those denounced.

Judicial authorities pursued few criminal or Inquisition cases involving abortion in the colonial era. To date, my search of the most thoroughly cataloged archival holdings for New Spain has uncovered only eleven cases featuring criminal or Inquisition investigations of abortion across the entire colonial period (see table 2).[79] Beyond the low frequency with which members of the public and state officials denounced women for procuring abortions, such trials are also intriguing because of the remarkable degree of leniency with which both criminal and ecclesiastical courts in New Spain treated both infanticide and abortion cases. Seven of the eleven abortion trials examined here were cases brought before the Holy Office of the Inquisition, and in all of these trials the court either did not pursue the cases beyond the initial denunciation or did not focus on the crime of abortion in either its formal accusation or its sentence.[80] In a trial dating from 1731, priest Gregorio de Jesús María denounced himself to the Holy Office for soliciting and impregnating two women and—citing Innocent XI's condemnation of the deed—for attempting to procure

TABLE 2 Abortion cases, Mexican Archives, 1652–1793

#	Date	Accused	Outcome	Reference
1	1652	*Partera* Isabel Hernández	Convicted of *hechizería*; abortion not featured centrally in her sentence.	AGN, Inquisición, vol. 561, exp. 6
2	1717	María Marta de la Encarnación	Convicted for being an *ilusa*; abortion not featured centrally in her sentence.	AGN, Inquisición, vol. 788, exp. 24
3	1731	Fr. Gregorio Jesus María	Self-denounced for counseling abortion. Not pursued.	AGN, Inquisición, vol. 757, exp. 5
4	1743	*Partera* Lucia Berrueta	Not pursued.	AGN, Inquisición, vol. 826, exp. 54
5	1783	María Manuela	Escaped from prison during trial.	AGN, Indiferente Virreinal, caja 6473, exp. 29
6	1784	Matiana María	Put in *depósito*; not convicted of abortion.	AGN, Bienes Nacionales, vol. 731, exp. 4
7	1785	Barbara de Echagaray	Convicted of *heregía mixta*; abortion not featured centrally in her sentence.	AGN, Inquisición, vol. 1231, exp. 1
8	1786	Juana Trinidad Márquez	Convicted of abortion. One year banishment; spiritual penance.	AGN, Indiferente Virreinal, caja 6271, exp. 26
9	1788	Sor Ana María La Cal	Not pursued.	AGN, Inquisición, vol. 1246, exp. 5
10	1793	María Manuela Sanabria	Investigated for being an *embustera*; three alleged abortions; not pursued.	AGN, Inquisición vol. 1364, exp. 3.
11	nd	Don Gregorio Balde Olibar	Not pursued.	AGN, Indiferente Virreinal, caja 5969, exp. 19

Source: AGN, Bienes Nacionales, Indiferente Virreinal, Inquisición.

abortions for them. On one occasion he had attempted to arrange for a *partera* to abort the fetus; on the second, he himself had provided the woman with an abortifacient for her consumption. The Inquisition did not pursue the case beyond his initial denunciation.[81]

Other cases reveal the Inquisition's lack of interest in allegations of abortions' procurement or enactment. A mid-eighteenth-century Inquisition trial from Zultepec involved Juana Incolaza Flores's denunciation of midwife Lucia Berrueta. Berrueta had previously declared to Incolaza that she had previously "lost" six of the seven babies to whom she had given birth. The seventh had disappeared from her womb when she was six months' pregnant. Berrueta described having awoken one night to discover the fetus's physical absence from her body, and deduced that it must have been because the fetus was a "Saurie [a spiritual being] and that at six months after conception in the maternal womb, while the mother is sleeping, Sauries leave the womb to seek graces, and once they find them, return to the womb to await the remaining months for the day they will be born into the world and attain, once born, the use of their divinatory gifts and the favors that await them."[82] Berrueta further related that the *Saurie* had been unable to return to the womb because, rather than remaining peaceful and quiet upon her discovery of the fetus's absence, she had become alarmed, shouting and screaming. As in Gregorio de Jesús María's case, whether incredulous about Berrueta's claim or unfazed by her loss of seven fetuses, the Inquisition court did not pursue the case.

The court also suspended its investigation of a late eighteenth-century Clarisa nun who claimed to have aborted a fetus with the assistance of the Virgin Mary. Sor Ana María La Cal's confessor denounced her to the Inquisition in 1788, stating that she had sometimes "executed lewd acts in front of others, speaking with the devil, as if she was sinning with him."[83] The convent's abbess swore that Sor Ana María had told another nun that she was pregnant and that the child inside her stomach would be called Juan, and that "he was destined to be another Baptist and another Messiah that would save the whole world."[84] Despite her impregnation with this miraculous progeny, however, Sor Ana María desired to abort her child. Her confessor told the court that he had heard Sor Ana María claim in public that "although I have been left pregnant, Holy Mary will save me."[85] He also attested that everyone in the convent knew that Sor Ana María had procured an abortion, and several other witnesses confirmed his testimony. Likewise, in other Inquisition cases in which the accused confessed to either providing or having procured abortions, the court of the Holy Office either dismissed the charges or did not focus on the issue of abortion in its judgments.[86]

Four criminal trials from the late colonial period involved abortion, but again, in these instances justices either ignored denunciations or did not sentence with severity those convicted. One undated denunciation of a military officer who had procured an herbal abortion for a woman he had impregnated was not pursued.[87] In a second case, tried by the Tribunal de Justicia de Indios, the curate of the town of Tultitlán, sentenced the indigenous woman María Manuela Ramos to *depósito* (supervised custody) after learning she had procured an abortion, but Ramos managed to flee before being confined.[88] A third trial, dating from 1784, concluded with a sentence of *depósito*, but in this instance the ruling was overturned. In this case the judges of New Spain's Real Sala de Crimen had originally convicted Matiana María, an unmarried Indian woman also from Tultitlán, to six years' reclusion in Mexico City's Santa María Magdalena *recogimiento*, a reformatory institution for women, for "having aborted in the countryside and having left the creature to be eaten by animals."[89] María claimed that she had not intentionally aborted but had suffered a miscarriage, alone. Leaving the remains of the fetus exposed, she had sought refuge in the parish church of San Lorenzo. From there, San Lorenzo's *teniente de justicia* had extracted María, requesting permission to interview her, and had then tried and convicted her. But San Lorenzo's curate vigorously objected to these actions, and eventually threatened excommunication to the *teniente* if he did not return María to his care. Concern over whether María had actually committed the crime was of secondary importance to curate Don Martin Josef Verdurgo. He was preoccupied, rather, with the threat the case posed to his jurisdictional privilege over María. Most of his correspondence dealt with questions of jurisdiction. In passing, he merely observed that "Matiana and the other witnesses have declared, in summary, that the only crime here was that of having had an accidental miscarriage and there is no fault in that, as well as not having procured that Holy Baptism be administered to the baby."[90] Eventually Verdugo succeeded in having María's *recogimiento* sentence overturned, retrieving her from secular authorities and placing her under his own care.

Finally, in a 1786 trial originating in San Antonio Xacala, judicial authorities sanctioned Juana Trinidad Márquez for having procured an abortion, but with a far lighter sentence than that ostensibly mandated by the law. According to the defendant's testimony, her second cousin, Antonio Márquez, had impregnated her under the promise of marriage and had then abandoned her. She had subsequently taken some herbs to abort the fetus. She was sentenced to perform public spiritual penance and six months' reclusion, while Márquez was exiled from his hometown for one year, required to perform public spiritual penance, and mandated to pay Juana one hundred pesos. In its investigation, however, the court was more preoccupied with the issue of the couple's contravention of incest sanctions and with Juana Trinidad Márquez's loss of her virginity than it was with her consumption of an abortifacient.[91]

Abortion in Practice: The Nineteenth Century

If the colonial documentation of abortion is remarkable in terms of its paucity, the nineteenth century, and more particularly its final two decades, is striking in terms of the skyrocketing cases of abortion brought before judicial authorities. Appendix 1 records cases involving abortion brought before various criminal tribunals in the nineteenth century; the vast majority of these involved Mexico City's Tribunal Superior de Justicia del Distrito Federal (TSJDF), which the 1857 constitution had created as the appellate court for the federal district. In comparison to the eleven cases of abortion uncovered in various archival collections for the seventeenth and eighteenth centuries, I have uncovered the existence of a total of eighty-five abortion cases in various collections for the nineteenth century. All but four of these occurred between 1880 and 1899, and all but five were brought before the TSJDF. Both the absolute numbers and the rate of growth in the late nineteenth century of those denounced for procuring or providing abortions when compared with earlier periods is impressive.

Two caveats that diminish the extent of this perception of dramatic increase in denunciations for the crime of abortion are in order, however. First, finding materials in the TSJDF collection at the time this research was conducted was difficult. The Archivo General de la Nación (AGN) has produced a computer-accessible finding aid that simply lists the title of the case and the year in which it occurred, but does not indicate where in the archival collection for each year the records may be found. Dozens of boxes of records exist for many of the years in the TSJDF fonds, and while a box-level index is now under production, it is not yet available.[92] It can—and did—take days to locate a single pertinent file. Thus, to date,

I have only located a small fraction of the total number of cases indicated in archival finding aids.[93] Second, since the existent case list for the TSJDF records provides only cursory descriptions, it is possible that some of the cases included in appendix 1 (some of which is based upon the existent annual case title inventory) should properly be classified as miscarriages rather than abortions.[94] Finally, because the last quarter of the nineteenth century, in particular, witnessed an increased rate of population growth (estimated at 1.5 percent per annum), with the country's overall population tripling from five to fifteen million between 1800 and 1910,[95] a similar rate of growth in the absolute numbers of abortions denounced in this time period would at least be expected.

Despite these caveats, the existent evidence permits several observations. First, it is clear that, particularly in comparison with the paucity of denunciations and prosecutions for the crime of abortion in the colonial era, the late nineteenth century witnessed a dramatic increase in the numbers of women, and some men, denounced for having procured or performed abortions. One explanation for the increase is that new state institutions might have themselves generated a growth in the crime, embodying Michel Foucault's observation that the objective of judicial apparatus is the creation of criminals.[96] Both the newly established reform-era appellate courts and the 1871 penal code, which created precise new regulations for the crimes of abortion and infanticide, may have played role in facilitating the growth—or at least the increased documentation—of the crimes of abortion and infanticide. The Tribunal Superior de México (the national appellate court), initially created by the first republican constitution of 1824 and reinvigorated in the 1855 Ley Juárez, and the federal district's supreme court, the TSJDF, founded in 1857, tried abortion and infanticide cases. Of the various criminal repositories examined for this project, the collections for these courts housed the greatest numbers of abortion and infanticide trials, and in both cases records for the crimes increased notably in the last three decades of the nineteenth century. As Sarah Chambers has observed in the Peruvian postcolonial context, it is difficult to determine the extent to which such increases might reflect better record preservation and increased vigilance by governing authorities rather than actual augmentations of crime rates.[97] Thus these courts' establishment, and their enhanced capacity for record retention, may partially explain the increased number of denunciations for the crimes.

This alone does not provide a satisfactory explanation, however. First, the judiciary that processed so few abortion trails in late colonial Mexico could not be characterized as one of comparative bureaucratic disorder. In 1710, the Bourbon regime founded a new court, the *acordada*, designed to operate independently of the existing *audiencias*. In 1756, the crown expanded the *acordada*'s jurisdiction from the countryside to cities as well. This tribunal, which had jurisdiction over all of New Spain, became particularly active in the late eighteenth century; from 1782 to 1789 it processed over two thousand cases annually, and was responsible for administering four-fifths of the cases tried in the viceroyalty. Nevertheless, the tribunal apparently prosecuted no cases of either infanticide or abortion,[98] as contrasted with the much larger numbers of cases brought before the TSJDF in the late nineteenth century. Second, even before the midcentury judicial reforms, a national appellate court did exist in Mexico City, but no trace of denunciations for abortion appears in the indexes available for the Supreme Court before 1899, even though other crimes are plentifully represented.[99]

Tellingly, such a stark rise in criminal cases prosecuted by various tribunals is much less apparent in other crimes, suggesting that the rise in numbers of abortion and infanticide cases reflects an actual rise in denunciations in the late nineteenth century. Little discrepancy exists, for example, between late colonial and nineteenth-century records of homicide. The AGN has records of forty-three cases of homicide that the *acordada* tried between 1777 and 1809; the *Ramo* Criminal (archival collection treating criminal cases) of the AGN turns up nearly 1,400 homicide cases for the period covering 1585–1844. The AGN's nineteenth-century *ramo* for the Suprema Corte de Justicia de la Nación contains 1,374 cases of homicide. So for this crime, the colonial and nineteenth-century data remain roughly constant in total numbers, whereas abortion and infanticide cases underwent dramatic increases in the late nineteenth century.

Modifications in the 1871 penal code's handling of abortion and infanticide may have influenced rates of denunciation and conviction for the crimes. The code reduced the punishment mandated for the crime and permitted the performance of abortions in order to save mothers' lives. In such cases, it is possible that both women's peers and community authorities would have been more comfortable investigating abortions than in earlier eras when the formal penalties (if not the judicial practices) mandated for the crime were greater. It also formalized and fostered the notion that the most valuable quality possessed by women of all stations was their reputation. The code provided harsher sentences to female defendants of ill repute suspected of committing either crime, as well as to women who had not made every effort to successfully hide their pregnancies in the period leading up to the birth (or death) of their infants. This legal development is particularly striking in comparison to perceptions of infanticide and abortion in other contexts. In England between 1624 and 1803, for example, the concealment of an illegitimate child's death was punishable by execution.[100] Just as contemporary medicojuridical tracts, particularly Francisco de Asis Flores y Troncoso's *El hímen en México*, celebrated the idea that virginity was a quality desirably preserved in women of all classes and races in the modernizing republic, the late nineteenth-century state encouraged Mexicans to promote the public reputation of sexual honesty for women of all stations. Judging by the increased numbers of abortion and infanticide denunciations that community members, women's employers, and state officials initiated, this message fell upon receptive ears.

One 1883 TSJDF abortion trial allows for some sense of the population's attitudes toward abortion and women suspected of its commission in the era of the Porfiriato. In this case, Adolfo Álvarez Gutiérrez, a Spanish soldier, denounced his former lover, Elvira Acosta, and her mother, Pomposa Acosta, for having intentionally aborted his offspring.[101] Álvarez testified that in a period of financial duress, he had left his pregnant lover in the house of her mother when he journeyed from Mexico City to Veracruz. Upon his return to the capital, he had encountered two distressed notes from Elvira. In these she declared that she mourned his absence, longed for his return, and announced that she had lost the fetus she had been carrying. Álvarez later declared that a female acquaintance had interrogated Elvira at the time of her alleged miscarriage about her physical state and Elvira declared that her mother had given her a "purge" that he suspected had provoked her miscarriage.[102]

Both notes that Elvira sent to Álvarez are included in her case's criminal dossier. In the first she begged Álvarez to return to her side, described the fetus's loss as accidental, provoked by a fall, and told of her emotional loss "for the daughter that might have provoked the return of your love for me."[103] In the second, which presumably followed receipt of a letter Álvarez had written accusing Elvira of intentionally aborting the fetus, she was more agitated and insistent. She declared that she "took no medicine" to provoke the miscarriage, and wrote that "if I told you I did so, it was only to see if this would push you to call me to your side since I cannot tolerate being separated from you." She commented that "nobody helped me except for my mother since [the pregnancy] was so little advanced I said it was not necessary for anyone to come," adding, "if my mother did it, I would take vengeance on my mother."[104] Her letter concluded with an indication of the strength of her era's perceived repulsion in the idea of abortion: "I swear, Adolfo, that I am not guilty and that God's curse should fall upon me if I lie."

Pomposa Acosta, Elvira's mother, vehemently denied the charge that her daughter had intentionally aborted, claiming that Álvarez was a swindler and a scoundrel who had invented "this terrible accusation, which is illogical in any case, given that it deals with the relations between a mother and daughter."[105] She countered that Álvarez had invented the charges as a way of seeking vengeance for the steps she had taken to terminate her financial support of the couple after Álvarez had begun physically assaulting her daughter, testimony that is consistent with her daughter's declarations. The closing documents in the file are, unfortunately, inconclusive, though the dossier does indicate that both Pomposa Acosta and her daughter would be found innocent of the charge of intentional abortion. A medical exam confirmed that no evidence remained of an intentional abortion and the court, which had earlier detained Pomposa Acosta, placed her in provisional liberty due to lack of evidence.

The increased numbers of denunciations for the crimes of abortion in the late nineteenth century also suggest—though there is more evidence about this idea in infanticide trials—that an increased sector of Mexico's population began to consider abortion a crime in a way that Mexicans had not done in earlier periods. While the medical texts discussed earlier indicate that knowledge about abortifacients circulated in the colonial era, Mexicans rarely denounced women in this period for seeking abortions. In the course of the following century, they learned to do so with increasing frequency. By the late nineteenth century, Mexicans like Elvira Acosta saw their offspring as valued beings who might serve to woo back estranged lovers. They may have also absorbed the nineteenth-century regime's concerns with populating the country with a productive and healthful citizenry. Finally, they may have understood, as Álvarez declared, that uncaring women of "bad sentiments" who committed or commissioned abortions were worthy of God's damnation.

This may explain why penal officers who encountered evidence of infant deaths initiated criminal inquiries more frequently than had been the case earlier. In one 1880 Mexico City case, for example, a police inspector initiated an investigation when on patrol he encountered a dead fetus in the home of a young single woman, Tomasa Escarcega.[106]

Escarcega testified that rather than having sought out an abortion, she had undergone an accidental miscarriage likely caused by the "shocks and afflictions" she had suffered, including the news that her brother had died unexpectedly. The investigating magistrate, supported with a physician's autopsy that the fetus had died in her womb several days before she had given birth to it, accepted her explanation.[107] Nineteenth-century midwifery texts show the acceptance of the explanation Escarcega provided for her miscarriage. The 1863 *Cartilla de partos* produced for Oaxaca's midwifery institute observed that "blows to the womb, excessive force, lifting heavy objects, anger, pleasure, and any moral impression the least bit violent" were the most frequent causes of miscarriage.[108]

This case illustrates that, despite the rise in denunciations for abortion that characterized the late nineteenth century, magistrates continued to exercise great caution in convicting for these crimes. In none of the nineteenth-century abortion cases located did judges convict women for having abortions. In a context of ongoing high rates of infant mortality, judges assessed that insufficient evidence indicated that fetal and infant deaths were necessarily intentional. They ruled that circumstantial evidence was too unreliable, and only accepted either eyewitness accounts or first-person confessions when they convicted. In 1842, for instance, in the city of Oaxaca, the first instance judge absolved Arcadia Martínez, accused of having willfully aborted, because of insufficient evidence. A judge in the superior court reviewing the case upheld the initial ruling due to insufficient evidence.[109]

A second case originating in the community of Yucayachi, Oaxaca, involved María Reyes, a nineteen-year-old, and María Anacleta, a mature married woman, who were accused of willful abortion and clandestine burial, respectively. Reyes was charged with having aborted at 7:00 A.M. on June 17, 1883, and Anacleta with having buried the corpse of the fetus one hour later. The judge of first instance absolved both women of involvement in the crime of abortion but found Anacleta, who confessed to the act, guilty of clandestine burial and sentenced her to three months' reclusion in the municipal jail. The appellate judge reviewing the case upheld the lower judge's ruling on both counts, noting that he had correctly sentenced Anacleta with a light punishment because her reputation for "good conduct" constituted an alleviating circumstance, as did the fact that she had confessed the crime and was also "so ignorant that she could not have known about the illicitness of the act that she committed."[110]

The Trajectory of Abortion's Criminalization

From the early colonial period through the nineteenth century, women in Mexico continued to use many of the same methods to provoke abortions. The earliest European chroniclers recorded that pre-Columbian midwives possessed botanical expertise about herbs, roots, and flowers, including *cihuapatli* and *altamisa*, that they used to provoke contractions in cases of stalled labor or to provoke miscarriages earlier in pregnancies. Knowledge of such medicines circulated without interference from medical or judicial authorities throughout much of the colonial period. Midwives and pharmacists provided their clients with medicines when they or their families requested them to provoke menstruation if it had been suspended, and colonial populations preferred to blur the line between the cessation of an early pregnancy and the innocent provocation of the menses delayed for other medical reasons. Although colonial law harshly condemned the act of abortion in theory, sentencing providers or procurers to the death penalty, in practice they rarely found pregnant women or medical providers guilty of the crime. Neither did members of the public—neighbors, family members, employers, or state authorities—frequently denounce women for it. When women aborted their fetuses, colonial sources suggest that their communities did not interpret the act as deserving of judicial inquiry as they did for other acts such as theft, assault, and homicide.

The second half of the nineteenth century brought changes to public views of abortion. First, Mexican physicians who lectured and wrote texts for professional midwifery and obstetrical training schools beginning in midcentury condemned women's contemporary practices of abortion. Second, Mexico's first national penal code, while liberalizing the penalties generally associated with the crime, created distinctions between those cases in which women had greater and lesser morally justifiable reasons to commit the crime. The 1871 code punished most harshly those women who before aborting their fetuses had lost their reputations of public decency, those who had failed to hide the fact that they were pregnant before they aborted, or those whose fetuses had been engendered within legitimate martial unions. Whether in reaction to these new imperatives on the policing of female morality or for some other reason, Mexican populations responded. In the first thirty years following the enactment of the 1871 code they denounced Mexican women for committing abortion to criminal tribunals in significantly higher numbers than they had for the entirety of the colonial period and the first seven decades of the nineteenth century. Despite this shift in public perceptions of abortion, the Mexican judiciary, even in the era of the Porfiriato, remained as cautious about convicting women and medical practitioners for the necessarily private crime of abortion as they had in earlier periods. As chapter 4 will reveal, many of the same patterns also characterized the colonial and nineteenth-century development of the practice of infanticide in Mexico.

4 Infanticide

. . . .

In July 1806, Mariana del Carmen Ventura, a *criolla* prostitute, stood accused of infanticide before Don José López de Anaya, the *teniente* charged with the administration of justice in the town of Zacualtiplan de la Sierra in the present-day state of Hidalgo. Having been denounced by a municipal official, Ventura revealed that since she had separated from her husband several years earlier, she had given birth to three children, all of whom had died immediately after birth. In the most recent instance she explained that, two months earlier, she had given birth to a boy

> in the middle of the night, when she was alone without a midwife
> or any other person except her legitimate son Pedro. The child was
> born alive, but showing signs that he was about to die, she took a
> mouthful of water and blew it into in his mouth, saying 'In the
> name of the Father and the Son and the Holy Spirit,' and then he
> died. The only one who saw this was her son, Pedro who, in the
> morning at about midday, made a hole at the foot of her bed
> where she ordered him buried and that is where his body remains
> to this day.[1]

The court ordered the infant's body unearthed for examination, imprisoned Ventura and assigned her a *curador*, a legal defender. Despite some of the damning evidence her case presented, including Ventura's decision to give birth alone and her subsequent private burial of her son's corpse, the court eventually acquitted her of all charges, concluding that all three of her children had died from natural causes.[2]

Ventura's case is representative of colonial and nineteenth-century infanticide trials in Mexico. Like most women accused of the crime, Ventura was poor and single, although at age thirty she was older than was the norm for defendants. As was typical, the infant she was accused of killing—her own—was illegitimate. Of sixty-three nineteenth-century infanticide trials containing biographical details of defendants, over 70 percent of the accused were the infants' mothers; these women ranged in age from fourteen to forty, but the median age of the accused was nineteen.[3] In Ventura's case, as in almost every other, the alleged crime occurred directly after the infant's birth. Elisa Speckman Guerra has observed that in other geographical contexts, the profile of women accused of infanticide and those of accused of abortion were normally quite different. While infanticide defendants tended to be young and unmarried, those accused of abortion were often older, married women who had established the network and resources imperative to the securing of such procedures.[4] In the cases examined here, however, the profile of women accused of both crimes was similar.

Despite some common characteristics of those accused of committing infanticide across time, the ways that both Mexican community members and judicial authorities perceived infanticide and its perpetrators changed dramatically between the late colonial period and the late nineteenth century. Residents of New Spain denounced notably few women for infanticide in the colonial era. In this period, too, magistrates acquitted nearly every defendant (see table 3).[5] Both denunciations and convictions rose as the nineteenth century progressed, peaking dramatically in the 1880s (see table 4). In the first half of the nineteenth century, criminal courts continued to acquit high proportions of those accused, but began convicting a higher proportion of the accused in the last decades of the century.

This chapter analyzes the evidence for the increase in both infanticide denunciations and convictions in the late nineteenth century, arguing that the rise reflects a change in popular conceptions of maternity and of female honor rather than merely a shift in the Porfirian state's increased vigilance about policing the criminal acts of Mexican society's lower orders. The documentation of infanticide cases suggests that as the nineteenth century progressed, Mexicans more frequently perceived infanticide, which most often involved a mother taking her infant's life immediately following childbirth, as a crime in a way they had not done in the colonial period. In that era, the small number of cases brought to the attention of judicial authorities suggests either populations' tolerance of its occurrence, their disinterest in the crime, or their inability to identify infanticide as a crime. By the late nineteenth century, however, members of the public had begun subscribing to altered conceptions of female honor, maternity, and children themselves that provoked them to denounce infanticide more frequently.

Just as physician Francisco de Asis Flores y Troncoso expressed his expectations about the important role Mexican virgins played in demarcating the country's national worth in his celebrated 1885 tract *El hímen en*

TABLE 3 Infanticide cases, Mexican Archives, 1699–1819

#	Reference	Date	Accused	Outcome
1	AHJO, Villa Alta, Criminal, legajo 6, exp. 8	1699	Juana Hernández	Convicted for infanticide; placed in *depósito* until married.
2	AHJO, Villa Alta, Criminal, legajo 10, exp. 8	1711	Juan Manuel de Yaé	Apparently convicted; died in prison.
3	AHET, legajo 28, exp. 16	1765	Pascuala Estefanía	Escaped before tried.
4	AGN, Criminal, vol. 96, exp. 16	1792	Juana Josefa Alsivar, Lorenzo Hernández	Suspected of infanticide; acquitted.
5	AGN, Ind. Vir., caja 1829, exp. 001	1800	Juan de los Santos	Suspected of infanticide; documentation is inconclusive.
6	AGN, Criminal, vol. 626, exp. 1	1802	María del Carmen Gusman	Suspected of infanticide; documentation is inconclusive.
7	AGN, Criminal, vol. 251, exp. 10	1806	María del Carmen Ventura	Suspected of infanticide; acquitted.
8	AGN, Criminal, vol. 98, exp. 9	1807	Prudencia Teresa Escobar	Suspected of infanticide; acquitted.
9	AGN, Criminal, vol. 52, exp. 12	1807	María de la Luz Lara	Suspected of infanticide; acquitted.
10	AHJO, Teposcolula, Criminal, legajo 49, exp. 32	1810	Angela Hernández	Not pursued.
11	AGN, Ind. Vir., caja 3503, exp. 001	1818		No-one charged.
12	AGN, Criminal, vol. 68, exp. 7	1819	María Dolores, María Felipa Urbana and María de los Santos	Convicted for infanticide; pardoned.

Sources: AGN, Criminal, Indiferente Virreinal; AHET; AHJO, Teposcolula, Criminal; AHJO, Villa Alta, Criminal.

Note: Not included were many trials for infanticide unrelated to circumstances of childbirth—those involving the deaths of older children, or homicides in which children were inadvertent victims.

TABLE 4 Denunciations and convictions for infanticide in Mexico by decade, 1820s–1890s

Decade	Total investigations	Complete cases	Acquittals (from complete cases only)	% of acquitted
1820s	1	1	1	100
1830s	2	2	2	100
1840s	7	5	4	80
1850s	8	5	4	80
1860s	28	16	10	62
1870s	16	1	0	0
1880s	62	28	13	47
1890s	27	4	2	50
TOTAL	149	62	36	Avg. 74%*

Sources: AGN, Criminal, TSJDF; AHJO, Ejutla, Penal; AHJO, Teposcolula, Penal; AHJO, Villa Alta, Criminal; AHMO; ACSCJ.

Notes: "Complete cases" refer to those files I have located copies of from the larger group of total investigations, which includes cases listed in the TSJDF box list inventory. *Discounting the zero percentage for the 1870s, since it represented only one case and was a statistical anomaly.

México, late nineteenth-century infanticide trials reveal the heightened expectations about the moral and sexual importance of all Mexican women's sexual virtue. At the same time as the state and medical practitioners were professionalizing and nationalizing the practice of obstetrics and gynecology, accused mothers, family members, employers, and municipal and judicial officials all contributed in the late nineteenth century to the development of ideas and definitions of both female honor and women's value. These they expressed most frequently in the language of *buenas costumbres* that differed markedly from notions of female honor in the colonial period in that they included heightened concerns over specifically plebeian women's compliance (or noncompliance) with such ideals.

Colonial Denunciation and Conviction Rates

The majority of the cases examined here that date from the colonial period originated in the Real Sala de Crimen, one of the three courts that operated under the aegis of New Spain's Real Audiencia. Located in the capital, the Real Sala de Crimen functioned as the court of first instance for crimes prosecuted in Mexico City and as both the overseeing body and appeals tribunal for local courts throughout the viceroyalty. In all the cases brought before the Real Sala discussed here, each of which transpired outside of the capital city, the court operated in this second capacity. As was the case with the abortion cases discussed in chapter 3, the vast majority of the nineteenth-century infanticide cases examined here were brought before the capital's appellate court, the Tribunal Superior de Justicia del Distrito Federal (TSJDF); smaller numbers of cases pertained to the country's central Suprema Corte de Justicia, to courts of first instance in the city of Oaxaca, or to courts in small municipalities in the southern state.

The small number of infanticide cases uncovered in the colonial period in the Real Sala de Crimen is surprising, particularly when viewed in contrast to the rising numbers of cases prosecuted in the nineteenth century. Why were there so few colonial trials? Why is there not even one case originating in Mexico City for the entire colonial period? Perhaps trials that occurred in the capital were destroyed in the fires, floods, riots, and wars that later ravaged archival collections there.[6] Perhaps the absence of trials is a reflection of poor record keeping by criminal courts, but why only records for these crimes should be particularly affected is not at all clear.[7] It is also possible that few records exist that originated in regional courts because these had little reason to communicate with the Real Sala on a regular basis in infanticide investigations because they were not complex cases. None of these explanations are particularly compelling, however, and initial research into the holdings of regional archives treating the crimes of abortion and infanticide has not uncovered large numbers of trials for either crime.[8]

The most obvious explanation for the paucity of trials might be that women in viceregal Mexico did not commit the crime, but various forms of evidence suggest that this was not the case. While reliable infanticide statistics for Latin America in the colonial period are nonexistent, our knowledge of colonial Latin Americans' widespread practices of child abandonment is much more complete and substantiates the fact that there were large numbers of children born in colonial Latin America to parents who were unwilling or unable to raise them. Mexico City's Casa de Niños Expósitos, for example, received an average of 118 infants per year in the period between 1786 and 1813.[9] We also know that, outside of the geographical context of colonial Latin America, contemporary infanticide statistics record criminal prosecution of infanticide at much higher rates per capita in places where judicial records are known to be complete.[10] We know also that the crime of infanticide is notable for its consistency across geographical contexts; prosecutions in England, France, Germany, Ireland, North America, and Poland all share many of the same features throughout the early modern period.[11] Is it likely that early modern Mexican women were less prone, for some reason, to murder their newborns than were their European contemporaries? I suggest that they were not. The small number of infanticide and abortion trials in late colonial Mexico is indicative not of the exceptionally low rate at which women committed infanticide in this setting but instead of the low frequency with which community members denounced them to authorities.

The law directed magistrates to treat infanticide with severity in the colonial period. The legal theory colonial magistrates consulted mandated that infanticide, like abortion, should be punishable by death. References to the Siete Partidas, a foundational thirteenth-century legal code, and to the colonial Recopilación de las Leyes de Indias (1680) persisted in legal judgments into the second half of the nineteenth century.[12] The Siete Partidas qualified infanticide, like abortion, as punishable with the death penalty, although it cautioned that infanticide was not considered a capital offense when it involved infants under the age of three days.[13] One eighteenth-century Spanish medicojuridical tract asserted that those who committed infanticide should, like all convicted of parricide (the murder of immediate blood relatives), be "sewn into a hide with a rooster, a dog, a snake and a monkey and tossed in the sea or a river."[14]

Colonial administrators denounced what they characterized as the common practice of infanticide in late colonial Mexico. In 1794, King Charles IV issued a real cédula (royal edict) addressing the plight of "exposed" (abandoned) children throughout his Spanish possessions. He sought to improve the lives of foundlings by providing them with several protections and declaring them all the legitimate "sons of the king." Charles also included in the decree a number of concrete measures to protect those apprehended while transporting infants to foundling homes "in the interest of avoiding the many infanticides that occur because of the fear that people who bring infants to foundling homes have of being discovered and persecuted, throw down and kill these children."[15] He instructed that a person who claimed to be transporting a child to a foundling home should not be detained or examined, lest fear provoke them to a rasher act. Instead, they should be accompanied to the home to ensure the infant's safe arrival.[16]

More locally, the founding ordinances of the (Orwellian-sounding) Department of Secret Births (Departamento de Partos Ocultos o Reservados), established in 1806 as part of Mexico City's Casa de Hospicio de Pobres declared that such an establishment was necessary to provide a place for Spanish women to give birth in private so they would not lose their honor. Otherwise, these women were liable to kill their offspring: "They are compelled to bury them secretly, to embrace the most cruel, bloody, and horrible acts against themselves and the innocent fruits of their wombs, unfortunate victims that they sacrifice to their own fear. They take powerful abortives and give birth in isolated places without help."[17] If such a characterization is to be believed, then again, it is odd that so few cases of infanticide or abortion surfaced to the attention of the Real Sala de Crimen or its local establishments throughout the viceroyalty.

Those few documents that do survive hint that women committed infanticide more often than the number of criminal cases might suggest. The bureaucrats who conducted one 1818 investigation into reports of infanticide originating in the Mexico City suburb of Popotla, where five infant corpses had been discovered during street cleaning, lamented mothers' ongoing practice of resorting to murder in cases of financial or social desperation.[18] As one of the women charged in a late colonial infanticide trial declared, "It is so common to hear when an infant cries that he should be strangled or murdered that there are hardly any parents around who haven't said such a thing."[19] Felipa Romero, a midwife accused of committing infanticide and brought before the municipal criminal court of the city of Oaxaca in the early postindependence era, echoed her thoughts. She commented that her investigators were searching in the wrong place when they charged midwives as those most often responsible for the crime, observing, "How often does it happen that mothers are responsible for the homicide of their own children?"[20] In the Oaxacan community of Ejutla in 1881, midwife Getrudis Ramírez denounced a parturient mother for suffocating her baby by clamping her legs together as he was being born. Another witness to the birth testified that the smothering had been accidental, provoked by the severity of the labor pains. At birth, the woman had cried out, "I cannot stand it! I'm dying!"[21] A defendant in an 1845 infanticide case from Teposcolula, Oaxaca, testified that mothers' desires to kill their own children was not only widespread in the aftermath of childbirth but also widely accepted. She said that one of her lovers had told her that if she became pregnant and "it was time to give birth, she should throw the baby out . . . and that no one would know about it and that some women took care of things this way and nothing happened to them."[22]

The discrepancy between these indications of more widespread practices of infanticide and the small numbers of surviving criminal cases suggests that women in New Spain did commit infanticide more frequently than the archival trail implies but that few of their peers denounced them for these crimes. Regardless of what legal codes and royal ordinances might have dictated, colonial Mexicans most often looked the other way when they learned that mothers aborted fetuses or abandoned or killed their newborns. Members of colonial society either did not consider infanticide grave enough to merit denunciation or did not suspect that women had actually committed such crimes, perhaps because women were adept at successfully concealing unwanted pregnancies and offspring. In several cases examined here, even witnesses who had intimate daily interactions with pregnant women testified that they were ignorant of these women's conditions, even very late in the gestational period. In Paula López's 1897 infanticide trial from Oaxaca City, for example, the young woman's uncle, José Hipólito López, declared that he had not realized his niece had been pregnant even though he lived with her up until her birth and despite a medical examination's confirmation that the infant she had carried and then either miscarried or killed had been born at term. Hipólito López's wife had also observed to another witness that she had been very surprised to learn that the young girl was pregnant, affirming "having believed only that she was fat."[23]

Judicial Leniency

Colonial magistrates were even more reluctant to convict women for infanticide than were members of the colonial public to denounce women for it. Of the twelve colonial infanticide cases studied here, only two resulted in convictions. Little information survives for either file. Virtually all we know about one case is that a man was imprisoned for the crime of infanticide in Villa Alta, Oaxaca, in 1711.[24] In the second case, also from Villa Alta, but dating from 1699, several of the neighbors of Juana Hernández, an indigenous widow from the town of San Juan Yalagui, described how she had hidden the birth of a child and had abandoned "what she gave birth to" so that it was devoured by dogs before it could be baptized.[25] In various settings in the colonial context, the horrific image of wild dogs devouring unbaptized "exposed" children functioned as a trope to support efforts for the construction of foundling homes.[26] However, as this case and several others illustrate, dogs were known to literally devour abandoned infants. As punishment, the *alcalde mayor* (magistrate and district administrator) for the town of Villa Alta de San Ildefonso determined that Hernández should be kept *en depósito* with the town jail's bailiff "until such time as the accused should marry . . . so that she avoid sins and live honestly and chastely."[27]

The outcome of four other colonial infanticide cases is not clearly indicated in the extant documentation.[28] But judges in local criminal courts or in the capital's Real Sala de Crimen either acquitted, dismissed, or pardoned the accused in each of the remaining five colonial infanticide cases, including the 1806 trial of Mariana del Carmen Ventura, with which this chapter opened. A few examples serve to illustrate. In one instance, a municipal official in the town of San José de Tula (Hidalgo) denounced a Spanish woman whom he had encountered in a roadway clutching a newborn's corpse with bloody hands. The mother, Teresa Escobar, declared her infant had been stillborn. Since no physicians were available in the town, the court called upon two phlebotomists and a midwife to examine the infant's corpse. They all attested that the baby had been born alive and had subsequently died. The midwife, María Josefa de Lara, said she had inspected the corpse and had seen a "blow close to the skull that had broken the bone" and another blow that had broken a rib. She judged that while likely premature, the infant had been born alive and then had been hit or dropped, and this had caused its demise, an interpretation also favored by Escobar's denouncer.[29]

Her eloquent *curador*, Francisco Ortiz Hidalgo, who had housed Escobar in the days before her miscarriage, introduced a different interpretation. He asserted that his discussion with two other phlebotomists has confirmed that Escobar's child must have been born prematurely and that both a very long walk and the jostling she received in a crowded church a few days before her labor had provoked her miscarriage.[30] The court sent copies of the case's testimonies to several doctors and requested their written opinions. These physicians concurred that there was just cause for believing Escobar's labor had begun prematurely and concluded that the infant could have been stillborn, supporting Otiz Hidalgo's interpretation. The court accepted this interpretation and released Escobar from prison.

In another 1807 trial from Temascaltepec, a mestiza servant, María de la Luz Lara, was accused of drowning her newborn. Two eyewitnesses described how they had discovered Lara alone on the banks of a river immediately after she had given birth. The saturated corpse of her newborn lay in a drenched basket beside her. Lara claimed that the infant had been born dead and said she had placed it in the basket, which had rolled into the river, and then she had fished it out. Her defense rested on the argument that if she had killed the newborn and wished to dispose of its body, she would not have dragged it out of the river. She also claimed that a fall from a ladder she had sustained a few days earlier had caused her miscarriage. Her employer testified that such a ladder did exist in her house, but said no one had seen Lara fall from it. Despite the possible cause for doubt her case raised, the court again accepted Lara's defense and released her. In this case, as in several others, the directive to declare the defendant innocent rested partly on a physician's assessment that she might have miscarried and partly on the ruling of a Mexico City official, here the *fiscal* (prosecutor) of the Real Sala de Crimen, who noted in this case that "it has not been possible to prove that María de la Luz Lara maliciously aborted and killed the fetus. Although there are some indications that she did, and upon these the case was founded, they are not decisive. Nor is there hope that the verification of the crime might happen in the future. For this reason, the prosecutor judges just the sentence of his inferior [the local administrator of justice], in which the said Lara is absolved."[31]

In a third case, originating in Tepeapulco (present-day Hidalgo) in 1819, the court ultimately pardoned three women accused of infanticide. An indigenous foreman of the Malpaiz estate, Juan Bartolomé, testified on August 4, 1819, that one year earlier, he and his wife María Dolores had taken three adolescent nieces into their home. They had not had "the slightest suspicion about their [nieces'] conduct until last Sunday night."[32] María Dolores declared that on that night, a baby's cry had wakened her. She soon discovered that one of her nieces, María Jacoba, had given birth "for which indignity she had given [Jacoba] a kick in the middle and a blow to the head." Dolores told her nieces to "silence this infant and mind what you do with it so that your uncle does not hear it."[33] Later testimony revealed that the father of the child was Dolores's son (María Jacoba's cousin), and that Dolores had wished to prevent the public dishonor that knowledge of the child's existence would bring to both her husband and son. Dolores asserted that she had given the order out of anger "in seeing that my niece had lacked respect for my house and . . . and would cause me to lose my honor."[34] Preoccupations with conformity to gendered codes of behavior and public morality concerned protagonists more greatly than reckoning with the criminal act of infanticide.

One of Dolores's nieces followed her aunt's grim directive. In her testimony, María Felipa Urbana, age fourteen, explained that Dolores had ordered Jacoba to "smother her child so that [Dolores's] husband would not hear it." When Jacoba hesitated, her aunt told Urbana to take the child and kill it, so she carried the infant to a nearby ravine where she "squeezed the air out of its little neck." With the assistance of another cousin, María de los Santos, she buried the corpse, marking the ground with some nopal leaves.[35] The court imprisoned all three women and investigated their case for two years, but in December 1821, in the first year of Mexico's independence from Spain, the *fiscal* judged the accused parties in the case to qualify for a general pardon that imperial Mexico had issued.[36]

In each of these instances, officials of New Spain's criminal court system treated those suspected of infanticide with leniency when any possible grounds for the dismissal of their cases existed.[37] Such leniency was at odds with the state's official position of condemnation of the crime. Mexican tribunals assessed those suspected of these crimes with greater clemency or indifference than either contemporary European courts or Latin American courts in later periods. In Paris, the records of the high court of appeal with jurisdiction over a population of eight to twelve million people revealed that from the sixteenth to the eighteenth centuries, approximately fifteen hundred women (and a handful of men) were executed for the crime of infanticide.[38] In the English setting, the Court of Great Sessions at Chester hanged twenty-seven of the 112 people accused for committing infanticide between 1650 and 1800.[39] Court and prison records from Nuremberg, Germany, document that eighty-seven women were executed for infanticide from 1513 to 1777.[40] Criminal courts in Buenos Aires, one of the few Latin American settings in which the history of infanticide has been documented, investigated twenty-five women for infanticide, convicting 80 percent of them, between 1871 and 1905.[41]

The leniency with which tribunals in New Spain treated those accused of infanticide and abortion is also apparent if conviction rates for these crimes are compared to general criminal conviction rates. In 1796, for instance, out of a total of 574 trials brought before the Sala de Crimen in Mexico City, only 1 percent resulted in pardons, and total of 31 percent in prisoners' release. In the period between 1800 and 1817, the *alcalde ordinario* of Mexico City's Cuartel Mayor No. 7 in the north of the capital, tried a total of 502 criminal cases, and of this group again pardoned only 1 percent, and released 35 percent of the accused.[42] In contrast, not one of the infanticide cases the Real Sala tried ended in a conviction. What could account for this discrepancy? Why were women getting away with murder in colonial Mexico? Did New Spain's popular and legal culture afford women greater autonomy in deciding whether or not to bare or raise children than we have previously assumed?

Several factors may account for both the public's reluctance to denounce and the court's hesitancy to convict women for these crimes. We might first consider that the high incidence of infant mortality that colonial Mexicans faced is an important contextual point that helps explain why both communities and court officials were disinclined to suspect women of committing infanticide. Across Latin America in the colonial period, infant mortality rates were astronomical. According to the 1683 Numeracíon General of Upper Peru, for example, life expectancy was only twenty-five years, and nearly half of the population died before age ten. In eighteenth-century Mexico, infant mortality was probably over 250 per 1,000 births.[43] Consideration of this factor surfaces in the trials examined here. In María del Carmen Ventura's infanticide trial, the *curador* acting for the accused characterized the charge against Ventura as unfounded and capricious. Women in his midst, he argued, frequently miscarried, "and was this always because they killed their babies?"[44] Mexican justices might also have been reluctant to find people guilty of either abortion or infanticide because legal theory (if not judicial practice) dictated that those convicted be awarded the death penalty.[45] Research on criminal sentencing in colonial Mexico reveals, however, that magistrates exercised considerable discretion in assigning sentences in the local context of New Spain, more often exercising clemency than legal codes dictated.[46] Therefore, a desire to avoid sentencing women with the death penalty—as was dictated by peninsular law—does not offer a full explanation of why the public would have been reluctant to denounce women.

Records of these colonial trials and those that followed in the nineteenth century also document that magistrates assiduously applied the law in assessing the guilt or innocence of the accused. Infanticide was a notoriously difficult crime to prove, because unlike other types of homicide that might occur in public or semiprivate conditions, these alleged crimes occurred in totally private settings and thus involved no eyewitnesses. Prosecution often relied upon the testimony of medical experts—midwives or physicians who examined both fetal corpses and mothers' bodies in an effort to provide circumstantial evidence about the likelihood that crimes had occurred. Medical examiners often attempted to assess whether a fetus and been born alive or dead by conducting the experiment of submerging a fetus's excised lungs in water. If bubbles appeared, this demonstrated the infant had drawn breath after birth and thus increased suspicion of infanticide.[47] Magistrates did not normally find such evidence sufficiently compelling to convict, however—especially in an era when the high natural rate of newborn mortality offered a reasonable explanation for even those deaths that might have seemed suspicious.

It is also possible that colonial magistrates did not hold defendants as accountable for their deeds as they did the accused in other homicide cases because they viewed the victims of these crimes—fetuses and newborn children—as less valuable than both the honor and the livelihood women would have had to sacrifice if their offspring had lived. This would at least have been the case for the infants and fetuses affected in the cases discussed here, who were uniformly illegitimate and poor and often of mixed race. The interpretation that these types of children were little valued in colonial society is borne out by some of the statistical information we have pertaining to the quality of life—and the frequency of death—they experienced in New Spain's orphanages and foundling homes. Child mortality in Latin American foundling homes could climb to as high as 80 percent in this era.[48] In the first eight years after its foundation in 1767, Mexico City's Casa de Niños Expósitos, for example, received 619 abandoned children, out of which 415 died in infancy.[49] Similar conditions prevailed in Havana's contemporary foundling home, where Ann Twinam observes, "for most babies, abandonment at the Casa proved a virtual death sentence."[50]

In other cases, awareness of accused parties' economic circumstances seems to have prompted justices to acquit suspects. In one 1792 trial from the town of Atitlaquia (present-day Hidalgo), both Juana Josefa Alsivar and Lorenzo Hernández were imprisoned for exposing a newborn whose body was discovered by neighbors and "whose face and head had been eaten by animals."[51] Alsivar, a poor nineteen-year-old Spanish woman, said Hernández had repeatedly forced himself upon her. She testified that the day before her appearance in court, she had been collecting water from the river when she had fallen facedown on the ground when frightened by a snake and had miscarried on the way back to her house. Since the infant was dead, she had wrapped her in some white cloths and hidden her on the path to her house. Three weeks later, with their trial still pending, Lorenzo Hernández's wife, María Ignacia, an Indian *cacique* (community leader), appeared before the court to plead that her husband "imprisoned in the royal jail for suspected illicit friendship" be released. She declared that she was pregnant, very sick, and "hardly able to walk." Although Hernández had confessed to having had a relationship with Alsivar, his wife claimed he was innocent and pleaded that he should be released "because I do not have anyone who can look after me in childbirth, nor anybody to provide me with food to eat."[52] Two weeks following Ignacia's plea, and having secured no further evidence from any party about either the illicit friendship or suspected infanticide, the court released both Alsivar and Hernández from prison, threatening both parties with future imprisonment if they maintained communication with one another.[53] In this case, then, the practical matter of addressing María Ignacia's economic circumstances, albeit themselves involving the future well-being of another newborn, outweighed the court's concern over his and Alsivar's suspected criminal actions.

Economic necessity also frequently surfaced as a central explanation for the commission of the crimes themselves.[54] Most of the accused came from impoverished families, and they were almost uniformly single— either unmarried or widowed. Their occupations were not always recorded in their trials, but several women investigated in the colonial era indicated that they worked as domestic servants, two were midwives, one was a nun, and another was a prostitute. In the postindependence era, most of the accused did not work outside of their homes, but two were midwives, one was a wet nurse, and one a servant. As their descriptions of the circumstances under which they gave birth or miscarried reveal, they were women with few temporal or material resources to spare. Angela Hernández, an Indian from San Agustin Tlautepeque, for instance, told the *alcalde* of Teposcolula in 1810 that she had miscarried alone, behind a house in the town of Achutla, since she had "no other refuge" and, since the child had been born dead, she had left it there and immediately returned to her own town.[55] María de la Luz Lara, the servant mentioned earlier, was working in the town of Temascaltepec in 1807 when she also gave birth by herself, reclined on the rocky banks of a river near her employer's house because, she claimed, her employer had refused her request to take shelter in her mother's house or in that of a neighbor.[56]

These were women who could not afford the luxury of recuperating from physical duress—whether in the form of childbirth, miscarriage, or abortion—and would have been similarly pressed, in some cases unsustainably so, had they needed to allot newborn child care into the schedules of their working lives.

A more explicit motivation the accused provided for their concealment of births—or in one instance, for the murder of a newborn—was the defense of honor. Hiding the birth of illegitimate children in order to preserve public reputations for chastity was a chief motivation for birth concealment, even among the lower-class women examined here. For lower-class women, the need to preserve a public reputation for chastity was also closely related to financial imperatives. In her 1807 trial, for instance, Prudencia Teresa Escobar, a woman of Spanish descent from the town of Tula, testified that, "carried away by her own weakness," she had been seduced by an Indian man, Antonio José, who had given her a promise of marriage. Once she had discovered she was pregnant, and "fearing the reaction of [those in] her house, feeling herself ready to give birth, she left the house where she worked with the intention of giving birth in the countryside."[57] Similarly, María de la Luz Lara also declared that she had made efforts to hide her pregnancy and birth from her employers.[58] For both of these women, Spanish employers were the audience before whom a successful staging of sexual virtue was crucial.

Financial pragmatism played a crucial role in the decisions Escobar, Lara, and many other reluctantly impregnated women in late colonial Mexico made about the conditions in which they would give birth. Evidence amassed from colonial criminal records, Inquisition trials, medical texts, and state decrees suggests that such women opted to end the lives of their offspring either prior to, or shortly after, their births rather more often than the scarce surviving documentation would suggest. Their peers may have declined to denounce women to state or church authorities for these crimes because of the frequency with which newborns died from natural causes in colonial Mexico. The fact that their peers were reluctant to denounce them, and that on those rare occasions when they were criminally investigated, they were convicted so infrequently, suggests that these mothers' assessments of the limits of acceptable maternal behavior was not far removed from those held by the wider body of New Spaniards, including the judiciary.

Beginning in the mid-eighteenth century, colonial authorities had begun championing a new, Enlightenment influenced discourse of the child, celebrating children's potential value as future subjects of the state, and this new discourse played a role in transforming Mexicans' attitudes toward acceptable maternal behavior.[59] Sonya Lipsett-Rivera has dated the link between elites' promotion of virtuous mothers and widespread social stability to the late eighteenth century, in the context of Bourbon administrators' reformist policies regarding child welfare and education. She found in her examination of divorce trials from 1750 to 1856 that in battles over child custody, women successfully argued that they had moral authority within the family.[60] Lipsett-Rivera links this to developments initiated in the last third of the eighteenth century to reassess women's social roles. Bourbon reformers began stressing female education to give women the proper training required to become responsible mothers. In the same period, the emergent republic also came to view mothers as having increased importance because they were understood as producers not only of children but of future citizens, and in this regard, at the close of the colonial era and first decades of the republican period, motherhood took on a "civic function."[61] Two decades after independence, the state reinforced this shift, legislating that education was obligatory for girls and boys ages seven to fifteen, although the actual shortage of elementary schools in practice made the law unenforceable.[62] By the era of the Porfiriato, the state more vigorously embraced the idea of the Mexican child in the formation of the nation through such programs as compulsory primary education and expanded public hygiene programs.[63]

At the close of the colonial era, administrators noted that the institutions and values they had constructed in colonial Mexico, which had traditionally valued Spanish and noble women's sexual chastity above those of all others meant that such women had the most ease of access to the social, fiscal and practical means of dealing with unwanted pregnancies other than through engaging in abortion or infanticide. The pubic discovery of a group of newborn corpses in the spring of 1818 caught the attention of Mexico's viceroy, its archbishop, and the president of the capital's police council, who launched an investigation into the reasons why young mothers committed such horrible crimes. They inquired into whether the Departamento de Partos Ocultos o Partos Reservados in Mexico City poorhouse was servicing impoverished pregnant women in need. The clinic had been founded explicitly for the explicit use of Spanish women. Its administrator reported that while they readily admitted women "whose circumstances qualified them," they did not have the resources to indiscriminately accommodate the "innumerable women of poorer classes" who appealed for their aid.[64] Such, apparently, became the women whom officials, employers, neighbors, and family members began denouncing with ever increasing frequency to legal authorities for the crime of infanticide as the nineteenth century progressed.

As the republican era dawned, then, Mexicans were changing those attributes they associated with idealized female virtue and were expanding their notions of the women they expected to embody this ideal. Earlier in the colonial period, as was discussed in chapter 1, sexual virtue was the primary indicator of women's value. In the earliest infanticide case treated here, the colonial state admonished that Juana Hernández, a widow, should remain *en depósito* until she should remarry in order that she learn to live "honestly and chastely."[65] But, by the outset of the nineteenth century, maternal virtue—for women of every rank and race—became increasingly predominant in legal discussions of women's value. The *curador* for Mariana del Carmen Ventura invoked this new discourse in his defense against charges that she could have killed her children. He argued that "the love that nature engenders in parents for the preservation of their children is so powerful that it surpasses their love of themselves, and even that of their own being. Neither her modesty nor her fear over the loss of her reputation could have conquered this force and persuaded her to commit the murder of any of the three infants to which she had given birth."[66]

Explicit articulations of the existence of women's powerful and inherent sense of motherhood appear with increasing frequency in nineteenth-century infanticide trials. In 1842, a court of first instance had sentenced María de Jesús Torres to six months' service in the kitchen of the local jail. Torres had been carrying her daughter in her arms when inebriated, and "because of her drunkenness, had given her daughter a blow against some rocks" that had proved fatal.[67] Her *curador* defended Torres's actions by asserting that the court should treat her inebriation in the same way courts perceived insanity—that is, as grounds for absolving defendants from responsibility for their actions—because, he argued, "who could imagine that a mother with the love that nature inspires in her toward her children could be capable of murdering in her arms that whom she had nursed with her breasts when she still had the use of her reason and movements?" Mexico City's superior court agreed, and released Torres from prison. By 1842, motherhood had become naturalized to the point that women who did not manifest maternity were aberrations.[68]

Curadores and justices (although not community members who appeared as witnesses or defendants themselves) advanced similar claims about motherhood in other nineteenth-century cases. The most spirited defense of women's natural manifestation of motherhood appears in Ignacia Teodora's infanticide trial, originating in the small community of Ejutla, Oaxaca, in 1855. The story was a sad one involving a man who did not have the means to care for a newborn son and journeyed from the neighboring community of San Martin los Cancecos carrying his child in his arms. He approached various women in stores and public byways in Ejutla, offering them the child. Several, including María Tiburcia, a thirty-eight-year-old witness, declared they were "too poor and without milk to maintain it," and thus refused him. But Tirubcia then described how "the imbecile Ignacia who was sitting there got up and asked for the baby and although she [Tiburcia] had told [the man] not to give it to her because she was crazy, he did not heed her but gave her the bundle."[69] Several days later, a *teniente de policia* discovered the drowned baby's corpse.

Various tensions, including divergent perceptions of insanity and normalcy, run through the transcripts of Teodora's trial. Her neighbors and family members testified repeatedly that everyone in Ejutla understood that Teodora was crazy. A nine-year-old boy, among others, passingly referred to her by her local moniker, "la loca Ignacia." Both her aunt and her father described her as "half crazy," and Ejutla's *alcalde*, who accepted the description, described her in the summary of the case he sent to his superiors in Oaxaca City as "out of her senses."[70] Judicial officials in Oaxaca City ordered medical professionals to examine Teodora to determine her mental state. There, two public professors of medicine and surgery challenged popular conceptions of the woman by certifying that she exhibited "no dementia of any kind."[71] Ejutlans continued providing testimony contradicting the assessment of the medical experts, describing her to the court as demented because "when asked why she was imprisoned, she answered that it was because she had battled with sacred animals." The two physicians stood by their earlier assessment, claiming that after five days' assessment of Teodora, they found "she showed not even the slightest symptom" of mania or insanity.[72] Witnesses and medical experts continued presenting conflicting assessments for many more days.

Teodora's *curador* pushed the court to accept the community's portrayal of her unsound mental equilibrium, arguing that the fact alone that she had drowned a child itself demonstrated she was insane. He declared that, motivated by the same instinct as prompts all women to nurture children, she had taken charge of the infant and pleaded, "there is not a woman alive who would deny a new born child her milk." Nor was there "a community on the face of the earth that would deny care to a child so destitute." The *curador* explained that when the baby's cries had become too unbearably long and loud for Teodora to endure, she had taken its life rather than give it over to the care of another woman or to a representative of the state. This act alone, he asserted, demonstrated her insanity. Although by his definition, all inhabitants of both the communities of Ejutla and San Martin los Cancecos who had refused to take responsibility for the infant when the father offered him to them should effectively be declared insane, the *curador's*'s argument convinced Ejutla's *alcalde* who absolved Teodora of all charges and released her into her father's care. By midcentury official discourse, if not always community action, decreed instinctive maternity was normal; its absence demonstrated insanity.[73]

Nineteenth-Century Denunciations and Convictions

Colonial patterns of denunciation and conviction for infanticide persisted in the first two decades after independence. Few women were denounced and courts routinely acquitted them. The 1840s and 1850s witnessed a small rise in both denunciation and conviction rates. Increasing frequency of denunciation and conviction became much more apparent in the 1860s, and peaked in the 1880s when courts processed over sixty infanticide in a single decade and convicted the accused 53 percent of the time, a rate significantly higher than in earlier periods.[74] Although the sources accumulated here document a decline in the prosecution of these crimes followed the peak in the 1880s, Speckman Guerra's research on these crimes shows that prosecutions continued at high levels in the 1890s.[75]

The frequency with which community members and state officials, most often police constables, denounced women for infanticide increased dramatically after midcentury, as did the reasons for such denunciations. In the 1830s, '40s, and '50s, community members did not initiate infanticide investigations at the moment of a child's death (or miscarriage), but only did so once the discovery of an infant or fetal cadaver rendered an official response to a suspected crime unavoidable.[76] For example, in February 1852, several residents of Caduaño, a small community on the southern tip of the Baja California peninsula, witnessed the gruesome passage through town of a dog carrying in its jaws the half-devoured remains of a newborn infant.[77] The corpse turned out to be the offspring of a woman named Petra Torres, who confessed to having given birth to a stillborn child one month earlier. Significantly, although various town residents testified they had known she was pregnant and then presumably observed that her pregnancy had ended without either the advent of a baby or the public acknowledgment of an infant's death, none had raised the matter with Torres, her family, or local authorities until the day, one month later, when the corpse's public arrival into town made ignoring the infant's death untenable.[78]

Later in the century, courts continued to pursue infanticide investigations when community members or state officials discovered newborn cadavers, but members of the public began denouncing women for their suspicious behavior at the moment the alleged crime occurred, even in the absence of such evidence. By the 1880s and 1890s, individual denunciations about women's criminal or immoral actions, rather than public discoveries of newborn corpses, served increasingly as the catalyst for infanticide investigations. This shifting pattern in denunciations indicates a change in either community members' perceptions of transgressive female behavior or in their understanding of their obligations to scrutinize such practices. In one Mexico City trial from 1880, for example, a police officer reported that he had initiated an investigation of one Lorenza Rodriguez for the crime of infanticide when he had overheard a woman doing her washing on a street corner remark that she pitied a "poor creature who was healthy at dusk and dead at dawn [anocheció bueno y amaneció muerto]."[79]

Prior to the 1870s, individual states within Mexico administered their own civil and criminal codes, and justices formed their legal opinions by referring to both colonial legal theory and nineteenth-century innovations. Mid-nineteenth-century reforms, as Linda Arnold observes, included mandatory appellate court reviews of major crimes after 1837 and 1841 legislation that required attorneys and judges to cite the legal foundations of their opinions.[80] The national constitution of 1857 further reformed the judicial system by guaranteeing protections for individuals accused of crimes and by abolishing court fees. In their judgments, nineteenth-century Mexican justices referred to Spanish and Italian criminal codes and legislation, French medical treatises, and diverse legal scholars, both domestic and European, but they also relied on older precedents.[81]

In theory, the punishment for infanticide without mitigating circumstances remained severe throughout the nineteenth century. Joaquín

Escriche's canonical *Diccionario razonado de legislación y jurispruden-cia*, first published in 1837 and then repeatedly throughout the century, declared infanticide should carry the death penalty. Ramón Francisco Valdés's *Diccionario de jurisprudencia criminal Mexicana*, published in 1850, concurred.[82] Mexico's first national penal code, created in 1871, mandated two important reforms in judicial understandings of infanti-cide as it did also with respect to abortion. It distinguished the killing of an infant up to three days after its birth from other acts of homicide, which were normally punishable by death. In such circumstances, it dra-matically reduced the severity of sentences for convicted parties from death to several years' imprisonment. It also mandated that accused par-ties' efforts to preserve their public honor should further mitigate the severity with which judges should treat them. Defendants could estab-lish and maintain their honor by maintaining good reputations, hiding their pregnancies and their children's births, and avoiding registering births in the civil registry. The killing of children from legitimate unions was to be treated more severely than the same actions in cases of illegitimate offspring, presumably because illegitimate children could bring dishonor to women`s reputations while legitimate offspring could not.[83] If such circumstances were not met, however, punishment in-creased accordingly, and defendants might be sentenced to up to eight years' imprisonment. Articles 224 and 225 of the penal code mandated further reduction in sentences for those who had not reached the age of majority.

Courts normally interpreted that one or more of these mitigating cir-cumstances existed and reduced a sentence to between a few months and four years. In one case dating from 1880, the TSJDF tried Tomasa Mon-tiel, a twenty-year-old servant whose newborn had survived her attempt to dispose of it through burial in "a mountain of manure."[84] The court ordered Montiel housed in the Hospital Juárez during the duration of her trial and required her infant to accompany her there in order that she might nurse it. A court of first instance had sentenced Montiel to four years' imprisonment, but the appellate court considered that she quali-fied for further mitigating circumstances because the child was illegiti-mate and because Montiel had enjoyed a good reputation and had hidden her pregnancy and birth; they reduced her sentence to one year and four months.[85] A municipal court in Oaxaca city mandated the max-imum imprisonment in only one nineteenth-century infanticide case, dating from 1885.

Scholars have not yet produced broad statistical analysis of criminal courts' prosecution or sentencing rates for pre-Porfirian republican Mexico.[86] We do, however, have such statistics for both the first decades of the nineteenth century and the Porfirian era. In both periods, available evidence suggests that criminal charges led to convictions in 60 to 65 percent of all criminal trials.[87] But in the infanticide cases amassed here, conviction rates were significantly lower, averaging 25 percent across the century. Apparently, then, courts found women accused of infanticide guilty less often than they found defendants in the entire pool of cases they tried. In the Porfirian era, while justices tended to treat female suspects accused of violent crimes with greater severity than they did male suspects, they did not extend this severity to their judgments against defendants in infanticide cases; they uniformly sentenced less harshly than nineteenth-century jurisprudence mandated.[88]

In nearly 75 percent of the nineteenth-century infanticide trials, justices acquitted defendants. In one case, for example, a local justice of Tlalintac, Oaxaca, initiated an infanticide investigation in 1853 when a bailiff discovered a dog carrying in its mouth the head of a baby. A midwife revealed that it must have belonged to the infant to whom María González had recently given birth. When she was questioned, Gonzáles declared that the baby had been stillborn at only four months and claimed that her mother had buried the corpse. But subsequent witnesses and a medical examination of the baby's head revealed to the court's satisfaction that the baby had been born at full term. Justice Juan José Serrano concluded in his judgment that even though the infant had been born at nine months, because there were no witnesses to a crime the evidence was insufficient to convict Gonzáles. He acquitted her of all charges.[89]

In another case dating from 1888, a police constable initiated an investigation after a city resident informed him of the location of the corpse of a one-month-old baby. Neighbors suspected that the accused, Guadalupe García, a single mother of three other children, had strangled the infant. Even though the presence of García's other illegitimate children might have preempted her from the claim of possessing *buenas costumbres*, both the judge of first instance and the appellate court absolved García of all crimes, citing a lack of evidence. In his final assessment the appellate justice observed that while some evidence did indicate García might have murdered her newborn, the possibility of her innocence existed. "In such cases," he continued, "it is better to leave unpunished a crime than to punish an innocent party, particularly in the present case, when we must acknowledge the moral habits [*buenas costumbres*] of the accused and the maternal love she possesses for her other children."[90]

Finally, there were several other instances when appellate courts, citing insufficient evidence, reversed convictions or lessened the sentences that courts of first instance had pronounced against infanticide defendants.[91] The most dramatic of these involved the case of María de los Santos de Pérez, convicted by the judge of first instance in her town of Zimatlán, Oaxaxa, in 1888 of infanticide and clandestine burial, for which he had originally condemned her to an exceedingly harsh sentence: twenty years of imprisonment in place of the death penalty. When the appellate court reviewed the sentence, however, the superior justice absolved Pérez of homicide charges based on lack of evidence and condemned her to only one year's imprisonment and a fine of one hundred pesos or, failing the latter, an additional three months' imprisonment. Pérez is pictured in her official prison photographic record, taken on the day of her release, posing with one of her other children (see fig. 5). Oaxaca City's municipal courts either did not have qualms or had no alternative to restoring women accused of such crimes to their positions as parent and caregiver to other small children.

Several factors offer partial explanations for the increased initiation of cases like Pérez's in the late nineteenth century. Possibly the change merely reflected the rise that would normally be associated with the overall population increase Mexico experienced over the course of nineteenth century or, alternatively, more thorough record-keeping practices that first courts and later archives practiced in the postindependence era. But neither Mexico's broad demographic trends nor changes in record keeping in the postindependence era offers a complete explanation.[92]

Changes in civil law and state administration may have played a role in fomenting the growth of infanticide cases. First, the initiative the Mexican state began pursing in 1859 with the creation of the civil registry's central record of births, deaths, and marriages may have served as an impetus to encourage more exhaustive documentation of childbirth and death.[93] Second, the enactment of Mexico's first national civil code in 1870 had significant repercussions on family structure and kin relations in Mexico. Among other measures affecting family law, the 1870 code terminated unwed mothers' right to file paternity suits, which they had previously used to leverage child support from fathers. The change increased the economic burden on single mothers and heightened the moral suspicion to which they were subject.[94] Nara Milanich concludes that the repercussions of the legal termination of paternity investigations enacted across Latin American republics in this era were potentially explosive because they "deprived illegitimate people of kin networks and drastically undermined the basis of their subsistence, especially as dependent children."[95] Ann Blum also concludes that the 1870 code's elimination of adoption as a means to bring illegitimate children into legitimate households would have also "weakened the claims of family members linked by informal relations, especially any claims that illegitimate children might make on their fathers."[96] Mexico's post-1870 legal context thus created an inauspicious environment for illegitimate children born into impoverished households.

Fewer legal means of ensuring economic and social stability for illegitimate children curtailed access to other methods of regulating pregnancy, as was discussed in chapter 3, and accelerated poverty may have induced women to commit infanticide more frequently in the late nineteenth century than they had in earlier periods. Scholars continue to debate the extent to which the economic modernization programs of the Porfiriato—railroad construction, land privatization, foreign investment, and extractive export development—negatively affected the living standards of Mexico's poorest classes. Moramay López-Alonso's research on the biological history of the Mexican populace in this era supports the predominant position that "the Mexican labouring classes . . . suffered a decline in their biological standards of living beginning approximately in 1870."[97] Francie R. Chassen-López qualifies this interpretation for the context of Oaxaca, demonstrating that the state's indigenous peasantry had considerable success in retaining traditional land tenure patterns despite the privatization of millions of hectares of land during the Porfiriato, although even she concedes that the gap between the rich and the poor grew wider in this era.[98] Laura Shelton has also argued that the economic changes that the development of mining, railroads, and urbanization wrought on late nineteenth-century Sonora disrupted traditional social networks that had previously facilitated systems of informal adoption and child circulation and made it harder to hide the births of illegitimate children, thus encouraging women to pursue other, more dramatic means of dealing with them.[99]

Decreased standards of living might offer a partial explanation for an increase of infanticide and abortion in the 1880s. As poor, unskilled, single women, those charged with these crimes formed part of a vulnerable economic sector. In the examined cases, nearly all defendants pled innocent of these crimes, asserting that their infants' deaths had been explained by unintentional miscarriages rather than intentional infanticide. Their trials, then, do not generally contain their own declarations of motives for the commission of the crimes. However, in contemporary exposure trials, women sometimes did admit that economic desperation motivated them to abandon their newborns. In 1870 in Oaxaca City, for instance, Agustina Sánchez, a twenty-two-year-old widow and midwife, gave birth to a child who she then entrusted to another woman to expose because "she did not have anything to pay for the expenses of caring and maintaining it." Other witnesses confirmed this, stating that Sánchez "is very poor, and they do not know of her having engaged in immoral behavior but rather until now few people knew she was pregnant, and it is known that she had given her son to an unknown person, that she has two children that her husband left her and can barely maintain them."[100] In another case from 1888, Joaquina Chávez's legal defender explained to the court that she had abandoned her three-week-old daughter because if she had not, "the baby would [have died] of hunger since she did not have anything . . . with which she could feed her."[101]

The Evolution of *Buenas Costumbres*

There are some grounds, then, for understanding women's greater economic desperation as contributing to an increase in infanticide in the late nineteenth century. But a more prevalent factor represented in the transcripts was defendants' articulated desire to hide evidence of their pregnancies and childbirths to preserve their reputations. After the introduction of the 1871 penal code, it is likely that defendants and their *curadores* invoked the language of moral habits and good reputation or *buenas costumbres* as an explicit strategy to secure mitigated sentences since the law decreed that defendants who did not have bad reputations (*no tenga mala fama*) should receive lesser sentences. Witnesses, defendants, *curadores*, and judges seemed comfortable invoking the phrase to describe women whose self-confessed or notorious behavior associated them with the very acts normally understood as contrary to *buenas costumbres*.

For instance, in the 1891 Oaxaca City infanticide investigation of Mauricia García, a sixteen-year-old single woman originally from Tlaxiaco, Oaxaca, the accused confessed that a premarital affair had left her pregnant. By the time that García had given birth (at full term) alone on the patio behind her dwelling, she had a new lover, Clemente Chávez. García declared she had successfully hidden both her pregnancy and the birth of her child from Chávez (who later testified that he had noticed her expanding waistline but had been satisfied with her explanation that she had an "inflammation"). García declared that the infant had been born alive, but said she had purposely left it outside, where it had died, in order to "avoid having a quarrel with her lover."[102] Thus, here a young woman declared she had engaged in premarital sex with two men, been impregnated by one, hidden her pregnancy from the second, and then abandoned her newborn infant, ensuring its death. Nevertheless, in his initial defense statement of his client, García's *curador* Ignacio Ramírez declared that she was a woman of *buenas costumbres* who deserved to be treated with the court's leniency.[103] The appellate judge who reviewed the initial sentence in García's case concurred; noting that she was a young woman "de buenas costumbres," he lightened her original sentence from two years and eight months' imprisonment to a fine of five hundred pesos or 280 days' imprisonment.[104] In an 1888 case, also from Oaxaca City, a twenty-five-year-old single mother, Guadalupe García, was accused of having strangled her one-month-old infant. Several witnesses appeared to declare that García was an "honorable woman of moral habits [buenas costumbres]," and "an honorable, hard worker."[105] In many late nineteenth-century trials, witnesses, defenders, and judges repeatedly made similar statements about women who had avowedly engaged in premarital sex, endured secret pregnancies, and either abandoned or killed their offspring.[106] If these acts constituted *"buenas costumbres,"* one might speculate, what did the behavior of morally suspect young women look like?

Pragmatic efforts to secure lighter sentences may account for some of the frequency with which accounts of *buenas costumbres* appear in late nineteenth-century trials, but this would imply that justices and defendants alike accepted the notion that the discourse of pious female conduct mattered more than its actual embodiment. This would also suppose that poor and most often illiterate Mexicans living in rural contexts or in small towns possessed a detailed understanding of the 1871 penal code, which seems unlikely, though it does seem to be the case that justices used the expression liberally to exercise lenience in their sentencing of convicted defendants.[107] Finally, it does not account for the term's presence in cases dating back to the early part of the century before the establishment of the 1871 code. Further examination of the meaning and evolution of nineteenth-century notions of female honor and reputation is merited.

In the first half of the nineteenth century, community members used the language of public honor in particular ways. In María Osorio's 1837 infanticide trial, her defendant, Felix López, requested that the investigating judge gather testimony from members of Osorio's community about all that was "public and notorious" about the accused. One witness, a male forty-year-old laborer, testified that it was well known that Osorio's parents "lived with piety" and had provided their daughter with "a good education and taught her the Christian religion and fear of God."[108] Another declared that he knew that Osorio's parents regularly "paid their taxes [contribuciones]," "fulfilled their civil responsibilities," lived "honorably as Christians," and had raised their daughter in the same way.[109] Three witness in an 1840 infanticide trial that was heard before Mexico's Supreme Court supplied a very similar account of another defendant's *buenas costumbres*. A laborer, notary, and merchant testified that they had known the accused for lengthy periods but had not known she was pregnant, and described her as being "of virtuous morals, upright, and belonging to an honorable, decent and god-fearing family."[110] Neither sexual practices nor declarations about appropriately maternal behavior figured into these 1837 and 1840 perceptions of *buenas costumbres*, which instead referred to membership in a good family, observance of Christianity, filial obedience, and civic responsibility. Such definitions resemble those that Shelton uncovered in criminal and civil suits she studied in the context of Sonora and Nuevo León in the period 1800–1850 where, rather than referring to honor through the inheritance of desirable bloodlines, *buenas costumbres* referred to conduct.[111]

By midcentury, public discussions of female honor for women of all classes became more linked to matters of sexual propriety, just as earlier scholars had argued was the case in the colonial era for women of the elite. Discussions of the *costumbres*, *buenas* or otherwise, are muted in the trials from the 1850s through 1870s, though they are present in some newspaper stories. In several articles from the 1850s, editors and journalists voiced public support for the creation of a maternity hospital in Mexico City that would continue to fulfill the mandate of the late colonial Departamento de Partos Ocultos o Reservados in providing a secret clinic for women to give birth in seclusion. One 1851 editorial commented that "considerations of domestic and social necessities, the instincts of modesty, shame, pride, and self-love all conspire against the most sublime and holy aspects of the hearts of women who, victims of seduction, inexperience, or powerful passions have had the disgrace to lose their purity."[112]

Such women, the text warned, were frequently led into prostitution and induced to abandon, abort, or murder the babies they carried. No matter the strictness of the punishment, the paper commented, it was nothing compared to the social condemnation such women experienced.

The discourse of sexual honor's connection to *buenas costumbres* appears frequently in trials from the last two decades of the nineteenth century, where it carried modified connotations. In one trial, an outraged man charged that his lover's mother-in-law had intentionally provoked his lover's miscarriage, but declared he did not hold the latter responsible for "she had always been a caring person of good sentiments."[113] In another 1888 trial from Oaxaca City, a neighbor denounced Guadalupe García to the police upon discovering a dead newborn whom García had allegedly throttled. In testifying to the court about García's character, one neighbor said she was "de buenas costumbres"; another declared that she had been "honorable and loving with her children because she had frequently seen the tender care that she professed for them."[114]

In testimony from the earlier part of the century, Mexican community members associated *buena conducta* with family, Christianity, and hard work, but by the late nineteenth century, witnesses invoked ideas about maternity, and feminine tenderness in their descriptions. By midcentury, Mexicans had accepted maternity as normative; in subsequent decades, its expression helped distinguish women of virtue from women of ill repute. More widespread acceptance of such values might thus also explain why higher proportions of Mexicans denounced mothers suspected of aborting fetuses or killing newborns to criminal courts during this period.[115]

Two other trials, one from midcentury and one from century's end, further illustrate changing associations with female sexual virtue and maternity. In the 1853 infanticide trial of María Gonzáles, one of the factors securing her absolution was the fact that at the time of the alleged crime she was already the mother of two other children. Her *curador* argued that this demonstrated that González's own parents had already accepted her other illegitimate children, and this fact negated the preservation of her honor as a motive for killing her baby. The justice trying the case agreed, observing that it was less likely González would have killed this third child since "she already had two before who are still living."[116] In contrast, in an 1888 case for the same crime, the presiding justice determined that the fact that defendant María de Petrocinio García was already the mother of three children at the time of her accusation proved that she was not "de

buena fama" (of good name). This no doubt contributed to Petrocinio's receipt of one of the most severe penalties in this group of trials: six years
and six months imprisonment in the women's prison in Oaxaca City.[117]
Whereas in the earlier case both community members and the ruling magistrate were apparently able to accept evidence of a woman's extramarital
sexual activities and still consider her a person of *buena fama*, by the close
of the century this was not possible—at least not in Petrocinio's case.

The Popularization of Maternal Honor

Petrocinio's case illustrates the idea that the stakes for plebeian women's
sexual propriety had increased along with expectations about their embodiment of perfect motherhood by the close of the nineteenth century.
In this period, women experienced increased pressure to protect these
claims, even if doing so was only possible through violent criminal action. If in the earlier colonial period society scrutinized elite women's sexual virtue and their reproduction of racially pure and civilly legitimate
offspring (as was detailed in chapter 1), by the late nineteenth century the
public reputation of sexual honor had become more imperative for women
of all social classes. Prestigious seventeenth- and eighteenth-century Mexican families sometimes found it necessary to launch "social virginity"
campaigns; in defending their claims to *buenas costumbres* in the late
nineteenth century, popular classes also participated in such campaigns.

Recent scholarship on criminal history often supports the view that the
modernizing state was the body chiefly responsible for disciplining, controlling, and scrutinizing national populations—particularly in the realm
of criminology. Robert Buffington, for example, describes the evolution
of a criminological discourse of increasingly controlling legal theories
that sought to control degeneracy and contain vice within the orderly institutions of the Porfirian state. In this period, writes Buffington, Porfirian elites, "whose optimistic dreams of progress were haunted by the
specter of national degeneration," expressed a "growing concern about
female criminality."[118] James Alex Garza has explored how, in an effort
to maintain moral superiority, Porfirian elites and administrators created
an imagined underworld of crime in Mexico City, erecting an ideological
barrier between the educated and popular classes and instructing the
middle class on appropriate behavior.[119]

The body of infanticide and abortion cases examined here suggests,
however, that the people themselves—scrutinizing one another's behav-

ior and making denunciations to the representatives of the state—played a more crucial role in this process than is often acknowledged.[120] In many of the cases, judges initiated criminal proceedings against those accused of infanticide and abortion at the prompting of members of the public— friends, neighbors, and even family members—who had observed or suspected these crimes' occurrence. A local magistrate initiated Felicitas Cruz's 1888 infanticide investigation, for instance, after Brigida Hernández—a woman who had assisted Cruz's birthing—requested help from a constable, claiming that Cruz had murdered her baby just after having given birth to it.[121] In some cases, such as María Natividad de los Santos's 1881 trial, it was a relative—in her case, her own father—who reported the alleged crime. In a minority of cases, a member of the medical profession (physicians or, in one case, a midwife) denounced a mother to the court.[122]

Frequently, local justices initiated their hearings when community members discovered the corpse of an infant and altered the authorities. But even in such instances, members of the public played prominent roles. María Ricarda Osorio's 1837 infanticide trial was initiated, for example, when a resident of her town discovered the body of a dead infant in the drainage channel of the mill. The local justice of the peace, José María Mendoza, brought three midwives with him to have them confirm the state of the body and give evidence about its identity. None of the women recognized the corpse, so Mendoza then ordered several local officials to solicit any news they might uncover in the town about the identity of the deceased infant or its mother. On the same day, the ministers and mayor returned to report to him that "the sought-after woman is the daughter of Matías Osorio and is called María Ricarda." They also noted that "this information is absolutely valid according to public knowledge [la voz pública]."[123]

The evidence from these trials suggests that such investigations would not have been initiated or could not have been pursued without the support of community members themselves. Furthermore, community members indicted these particular crimes as they did in no other types of criminal cases of the period. As Speckman Guerra observes, "We find in the infanticide cases a cooperation and mobilization of community members that is not present in any other type of crime. When they came to authorities' attention, an extensive network of informants had identified the guilty party and specified her whereabouts."[124] The tendency of community members to scrutinize the postpartum circumstances of new mothers (particularly single, unwed new mothers) and to denounce suspicions of misconduct to authorities in the nineteenth century stands in marked contrast to the evidence from the colonial era, when the smaller numbers of cases brought to the attention of criminal courts suggests community members involved themselves less often in such matters.

Both the legislation and evidence from legal transcripts suggest that over the course of the nineteenth century, the importance of sexual honor and public virtue for plebeian women—in these cases, poor, uneducated, and often likely indigenous women—became more imperative and more self-consciously articulated than they had at the close of the colonial period.[125] The cases also suggest that by the late nineteenth century, infanticide and abortion had become a matter of far greater concern to working-class Mexicans than it was to members of the judiciary itself.[126] In the late eighteenth century, colonial society policed female sexuality and reproduction because of that era's predominant fears surrounding race mixture and it quest for the reproduction of whiteness.[127] Plebeian notions of female sexual honor, in turn, principally turned on questions of race and the maintenance of one's assigned position in the racialized social hierarchy of New Spain. By the Pofirian era, however, elite and state preoccupations had transmuted. In an age primarily concerned with issues of economic modernization, women's sexual honor and reproductive practices were scrutinized in these terms. As such, scrutiny was brought to bear more dramatically to women of all social classes.

This finding is consistent with other scholars' conclusions about non-elite Oaxacan society's increased efforts to embody Porfirian notions of honor. Kathryn Sloan's research on nineteenth-century *rapto* (abduction) cases from Oaxaca demonstrates how young women from the city's popular classes insisted on their possession of honor in their communications with each other and their testimonies to the city's civil courts.[128] Mark Overmeyer-Velazquez describes how in the late nineteenth century Oaxaca City's commercial and political elite engaged in a protracted campaign to modernize their city, a place where a lack of female sexual honor "was deemed a threat to basic domestic stability that would in turn corrupt society and stymie progress."[129] One important element of this campaign involved the policing of sexual respectability, particularly in public health campaigns to survey and scrutinize sex workers. In Mexico more broadly, William French has shown how those who embodied Porfirian notions of female sexual honor—the maternalistic "guardian angels" of Mexico's domestic sphere—had a crucial role to play in the mental topography of Pofirian economic prosperity, for they produced, raised, and inculcated temperance, industry, and obedience in a generation of workers and citizens necessary for the modernizing nation.[130]

Of course, the perceived link between female sexual honor and broader social stability, and the imperative role mothers played in producing and raising citizens of Mexico, predated the Porfiriato. In midcentury, as Robert Buffington observes, Mexican intellectuals including José María Luis Mora and Mariano Ortero increasingly viewed the family as playing a crucial role in maintaining order, law, and morality. As one commentator discerned in the pages of Ignacio Cumplido's 1852 *La ilustración Mexicana*, when "proletarian classes failed to live in families . . . children will have no parents, women will have no husbands, and the corruption of customs will cause misery, barbarism, and vice."[131] The crucial change during the Porfiriato was the extent to which elites and administrators tied this notion of women's obligations to (re)produce Mexico's citizenry to their visions of economic modernization, which moved elite preoccupations with sexual practices and reproduction down Mexican society's social hierarchy.

In her analysis of nineteenth-century criminal jurisprudence, Arnold has argued that Mexican judges were extremely cautious in their assessments of cases of all violent crimes: "Those charged with administering justice . . . recognized the need to adher[e] rigorously to rules of evidence lest an accused become a victim of revenge rather than be held accountable to society and its laws."[132] She notes that justices assiduously applied the rules of evidence and judicial reasoning in such cases, which they valued over the "moral outrage" that accompanied public awareness of a heinous crime, and asserts that "it is time to recognize Mexican law as innovative and recognize Mexican protection of the rights of the accused and condemned as part and parcel of an innovative tradition in Mexican law."[133] Arnold's point is well taken, but it alone does not explain everything about the reasons why justices in these kinds of trials in particular were so hesitant to convict women accused of infanticide and abortion with whom they treated with less severity than they did criminal defendants in general and female defendants in particular.

Second, these trials are characterized more by the absence of moral outrage than a preoccupation with their heinousness. Perhaps this attitude is best expressed in the photograph and circumstances of the photograph of María de los Santos de Pérez taken on the day of her re-

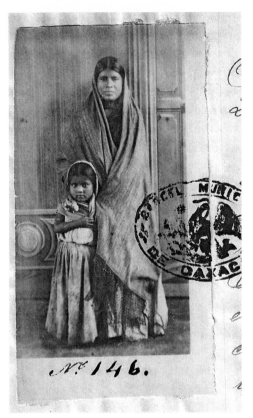

FIGURE 5 María de los Santos de Pérez (1889). Carceles, Registro de extractos de presas, libro 12, fol. 24, 1889, Oaxaca. Credit: Archivo Histórico Municipal de la Ciudad de Oaxaca.

lease from prison (see fig. 5). Pérez stands next to a small child, presumably her daughter. The child has slid her arm under her mother's shawl, and glances a little nervously at the camera. The framing of the photo and the backdrop are identical to idealized family portraiture of the era, and if we did not know its context, we might assume it an iconic mother-and-child portrait. Neither the subjects, the photographer, nor the administrators who affixed the image alongside the summary of Pérez's sentence saw any contradiction between creating this normative depiction of Pérez and her daughter and associating it with a suspect convicted of infanticide.[134]

How might we interpret the discrepancy between community members' increasing concern with the crimes of infanticide and abortion and justices' continued reluctance to condemn women for the crimes? Perhaps the crimes of infanticide and abortion did not form a central part of Porfirian elites' preoccupations with Mexico's criminal underworld. Their energies were devoted to policing a Mexican criminal underclass associated with the public crimes of robbery, vagrancy, and drunkenness, rather than the private acts discussed here.[135] Of greater concern to the nineteenth-century justices who presided over these investigations, besides upholding the letter of the Mexican penal code of 1871, was the maintenance and defense of the public face of female honor and its centrality to the foundation of familial stability, which was deemed essential to the forming of a prosperous and modern Mexico.

Part III **Populating the *Patria***

. . . .

5 Monstrous Births

From the late eighteenth century to the late nineteenth, Mexicans expanded their scrutiny over the sexual and reproductive practices of women in their communities. As this chapter and chapter 6 will examine, this was also an era of substantive change in the largely unstudied arena of popular and scientific understandings of both routine and aberrant births and birth procedures.[1] Consider, to begin with, two newspaper announcements publicizing the birth of monstrous babies, one from the beginning and one from the end of the period examined here. The first, printed on February 8, 1785, in the *Gazeta de México*, one of New Spain's first news periodicals, celebrated the birth in the city of Guanajuato of a pair of twins joined at the head: "They received the holy waters of baptism and were christened Joseph Nepomuceno Guadalupe and Joseph Ignacio Guadalupe. . . . Many people, admiring these rare effects of nature, have visited them, and there has been no record in these twins of any deformity or defect in their separate and agile bodies . . . every day more news circulates about their existence and longevity, causing ever more admiration for them given that the first one was born foot first, and in delivering him, the midwife discovered the knot that joined the two heads."[2]

The second, published in the Mexico City daily *El Siglo Diez y Nueve*, reprinted an article that originally appeared in the northern paper *Revista Internacional*. It described how—on February 9, 1893, in the small town of Bavispe, Sonora—a woman had given birth to a "singularly horrible being." The article recounted that this creature had been born with "a head like a bladder, straight hair resembling that of a pig, two horns, about three inches long, the eyes of a rooster, a perpendicular mouth, which was in a straight line with the nose, and a kind of ostentatious plume halfway over the head; the feet and hands each bore six digits of equal size; and it had one of these along with its heels, on the top of the instep of each foot." The article concluded that the unhappy woman who had carried inside her this "assembly of members of all class of animals" had died from horror at seeing it and that the spectacle was so atrocious the community even feared for the life of the midwife who had delivered it.[3]

The differences between the two articles' characterizations of these births and of the reactions of community members to the newborns illustrate many of the changes typifying evolving perceptions of monstrous births in Mexico that this chapter will examine. First and most notably, the stories convey very different associations with monstrosity. The late eighteenth-century *Gazeta de México* article and the citizens of Guanajuato whom it described rejoiced in the singular phenomenon its notice detailed. This was an attitude common to many of the fifty notifications of unusual births published in the *Gazeta* between 1784 and 1803. Both contemporary sources and modern scholars have reported that monsters and monstrous births in colonial Latin America evoked loathing or freak show curiosity. But the *Gazeta* notices often depict New Spaniards rejoicing in the advent of unusual births. The *Gazeta* announcements, which originated in both large cities and rural communities, drew attention to women's production of multiple offspring, including twenty cases of triplets and six of quadruplets, and to their birthing of progeny the paper often classified as "monstrous"—infants born with sub- or supernumerary limbs, unusual facial features and, in one celebrated case, a child born with her heart on the exterior of her body. The *Gazeta* notifications conveyed attitudes of wonder, affection, and pride. The paper's authors, readers, and the urban and rural communities depicted in its pages celebrated such births as evidence of New Spain's prodigious fertility, a perspective that reflected both the particularized manner in which the Enlightenment developed in Mexico and the late colonial development of "creole patriotism" traceable in historical and scientific productions of the period.[4]

At both the start of the colonial era and the apex of late nineteenth-century liberal modernity, conceptions of monstrous births reflected broader preoccupations with the production and reproduction of Mexico as a nation, the country's standing on the international stage, and its handling of its own internal populations. Anxiety over childbirth and deviations from its normal, healthy occurrence were issues of heightened preoccupation in the last decades of colonial rule when Europeans and creoles alike scrutinized the Americas, monitoring and analyzing the new peoples, identities, and nations these territories were in the midst of producing.[5] Increasing numbers of newspaper articles and reports in scientific journals treating the occurrence of aberrant childbirth over the course of the nineteenth century indicate that Mexicans' preoccupations with monstrous productions continued to intensify and transform in tone over time, culminating in the 1895 establishment of the teratology (birth malformation) salon in the Museo Nacional de México.

Along with the intensifying scrutiny and spectacle of monstrosity over the course of the nineteenth century, and particularly by its end, Mexicans developed new attitudes toward monstrous productions. First, although not a uniform reaction, the later notices convey a popular attitude of revulsion and horror toward birth monsters rather than the wonder and pride of earlier notices. Second, whereas the late colonial *Gazeta* notices restricted speculation as to the origins of unusual infants to "the rare effects of nature," by the late nineteenth century, scientists and physicians turned their focus directly onto (and into) the bodies of the mothers who had produced such phenomena. They increasingly monitored the biological conditions of aberrant embryos' development in the female uterus. This shift, as chapter 6 will discuss, paralleled contemporary obstetrical developments in all aspects of childbirth. Like their contemporaries in the fields of eugenics and criminology, late nineteenth-century obstetricians studied the conditions of embryotic development to search for clues about whether birth abnormalities were inherited or acquired. Eager to defend Mexico's status in the field of international opinion, the field's most central spokesperson, obstetrician Juan María Rodríguez, advocated for the notion of monstrosity as acquired. This view allowed for the possible biological regeneration of monstrous productions but also contributed to the construction of the inherent pathology of Mexican women's reproductive anatomy.

Mexican Monstrosity in the Era of the Enlightenment

Late eighteenth-century monstrous birth announcements exemplified various aspects of both the baroque religious culture and the enlightened initiatives typifying the publication in which they were published. Manuel Antonio Valdés's *Gazeta de México*, the third of New Spain's eighteenth-century periodicals to take this name, was an emblematic product of the Mexican Enlightenment. Valdés first requested permission to publish the paper from New Spain's viceroy Don Matías de Gálvez in 1783, arguing that the periodical would serve the dual goal of fostering civic loyalty and ameliorating the lives of regular citizens through its publication of edifying and useful materials. The paper would include such material as notices of elections, major construction projects, public works, reports on harvests and the prices of commodities, and legal matters of public interest, as well as "rare happenings."[6] The viceroy conceded his license, no doubt aware that Guatemala City, Havana, and Lima, as well as many European cities, were already producing similar papers.

Publication commenced on January 14, 1784, with annual subscription set at twenty-two reales. In an era when an unskilled worker might earn two reales daily, the *Gazeta* was thus aimed at a wealthy, literate audience, though scholars have yet to determine the extent of its readership. Initially the *Gazeta* was published twice each month, but beginning in January 1806 it appeared as often as twice weekly. Most readers received their editions through regular subscriptions, but the paper also had a vending stand in the Portal de Mercaderes along the west side of Mexico City's *zócalo* (central plaza), where it could be purchased until 9:00 P.M. on the evening of publication.[7] The *Gazeta*'s readership was drawn from members of the viceroyalty's civil and ecclesiastical bureaucracy and the larger body of the literate elite in the capital and other urban centers. The paper's sales, rather than its advertising revenue, constituted its principal fiscal support, so for financial motivations, the *Gazeta* was likely to be particularly responsive to the reading tastes, expectations, and attitudes of its readership.[8]

Valdés himself was the principal author and editor of the *Gazeta*. His writings were interspersed with reprints of civil and ecclesiastical decrees and communiqués as well as treatises written by local physicians and scientists, including José Ignacio Bartolache and, most notably, the secular priest and eminent scientific writer José Antonio de Alzate y Ramírez, who worked as the paper's science editor. Valdés also sought contributors from local bureaucrats and members of the public. In his original proposal to Gálvez, Valdés had requested that the viceroy direct civic officials in outlying regions of the kingdom to deliver "notices" for publication each week or fortnight to either the office of the viceroy or to the printer himself.[9] Valdés facilitated this procedure by preparing a set of guidelines, an *instrucción*, outlining his requirements for publishable notices. On a number of occasions he also appealed directly to his readers, requesting that they keep the *Gazeta* notified of happenings in their regions. A prologue Valdés published in his periodical in August 1784 "pleaded to all people who might participate with notices appropriate to a *Gazeta* that they not neglect to report them under any circumstances, since doing so results in the honor of the fatherland, and the good of the public."[10] In a second notice, published in January 1786, he instructed readers that he hoped to receive reports on various events including fires, floods, the erection of buildings, the invention of new machines, the deaths of people of advanced age or public prominence, and—notably—monstrous births.[11] Not all local administrators were enthusiastic about complying with Valdés's requests for news. Mexican viceroys had to reissue their directive and recirculate Valdés's *instrucción* at least three times in the first decade of the paper's existence.[12]

Despite such resistance, both bureaucrats and members of the public were willing to write to the paper with notifications about monstrous births that had occurred in their districts, which Valdés presumably edited before publishing. Only occasionally did he provide an indication of the original authors of the notices he published—for instance, commenting, on February 11, 1784, that "D. Josef de Cubas Bao, citizen of Cuernavaca, who is responsible for the news from Chilpancingo" had transcribed a paragraph from a letter he had received from Acapulco recounting the birth of quadruplets.[13] On another occasion, Valdés noted that "the administrator of the mail" from the town of Irapuato had reported that an Indian woman of fifty-eight or fifty-nine years, the wife of an eighty-year-old man, had given birth to triplets.[14] Midway through a third notice, Valdés recorded that a "somewhat educated and very reliable barber" had provided a description of a monstrous girl who had been born without nostrils, arms, or legs.[15]

The most explicit indication of the origin of unusual birth reporting was a letter the *Gazeta* published in February 1789 written by Don José Manuel de Zárate, a senior public clerk for the city council of Querétaro, at the behest of a *regidor* (city councilman), Pedro Antonio de Septién.[16] The letter explained that Septién, charged by Querétaro's municipal council to collect "interesting news" for the greater illumination and use of the *Gazeta*, had learned that a "monstrous child" existed in the vicinity of the city and appointed Zárate to report on the details of the case. With varying degrees of success, then, Valdés encouraged far-flung correspondents in the viceroyalty to observe and record *hechos gazetables* (newsworthy items) for his paper.

Valdés captivated his readers, but also enlightened them, for his *Gazeta* operated as a vehicle to promote the Bourbon administration's larger goals of modernization, edification, and reform. From the start the journal was an important publisher of civil and ecclesiastic proclamations, decrees, and reports. The paper's extensive inclusion of official state material in its pages has contributed to the mistaken idea that the paper originated as a state organ. In fact, the paper, did not become the official journal of the government until January 1810, when it was rechristened the *Gazeta del Gobierno de México*, and it carried on under this name until September 1821.[17]

Beyond its publication of official state notices, the *Gazeta* also answered other mandates. Drawing from the European tradition of *hojas volantes* (news flyers) and the more recent and scientifically illuminating *periódicos científicos*, the paper also published news and notices designed to both facilitate and enlighten the lives of New Spaniards. In its first years of publication, the *Gazeta* was oriented particularly toward addressing scientific and medical issues of public interest—particularly those treating food shortages and the series of epidemics sweeping the viceroyalty in the late 1780s.[18] In its capacity as reporter of local news, science, and politics, Valdés's *Gazeta*, like its antecedents and other contemporary journals, also manifested a sense of creole patriotism. Mexican writers, including Alzate, a stalwart defender of the abilities of creole scientists to generate innovation, rather than to merely absorb European innovation, used the *Gazeta* as a venue in which to promote the accomplishments of Mexican writers and to publicize their familiarity with the most current science.[19] In the Mexican context, such patriotism was intrinsically associated—notably, in the era of Bourbon modernization—with local manifestations of Catholic devotion.

In the European context, enlightened modernization is often coupled with secularization, but in various ways, eighteenth- and early nineteenth-century political and scientific modernization in Mexico retained its religious roots. For example, José María Morelos's 1813 revolutionary constitutional proposal decreed first that Mexico should be "free and independent from Spain" and second that, in this new republic, "the Catholic religion should be the only one, without tolerance for any other." Morelos's final resolution mandated that Miguel Hidalgo's Grito de Dolores (Cry of Dolores) be solemnly observed every September 16, while his nineteenth decree enshrined December 12 as a day reserved for the celebration of the Virgin of Guadalupe.[20]

Baroque religious expression and empirical science coexisted unproblematically in late eighteenth-century Mexico. So although the paper brimmed with news of science, medicine, and revolutionary wars, as David Brading notes, to read the *Gazeta* is also "to enter a world in which the Mexican elite appeared immersed in a cycle of theatrical devotion in which new churches and convents were consecrated, images paraded through the streets, and devotion to our Lady of Guadalupe grew ever more fervid."[21] Alongside treatises on the botanical world of New Spain, notices publicizing religious festivals and public devotions filled the *Gazeta*'s pages. Neither Valdés nor his readers saw any contradiction in publishing a treatise in January 1784 on the advent of a caudate comet, which the paper determined was merely an astronomical event to be understood as "neither a miraculous thing" nor one that "should be attributed with ill fate" adjacent to the news of an epidemic of pleurisy sweeping Mexico City, which the city council elected to address by resolving to solicit assistance from the Very Holy María de los Remedios through a nine-day prayer cycle.[22]

A sensibility that was both baroque and patriotic also characterized the presentation of childbirth in the *Gazeta*. The continuity of counter-reformation religious concerns within a scientific framework explains one feature of the birth notices the paper published with striking consistency. Such notifications varied in terms of the details they included (or ignored) about the class and caste of newborns' parents, and they only rarely described the medical personnel and procedures utilized in these atypical births, but they consistently treated the question of newborn baptisms. When newborns received baptisms, even if they died shortly thereafter, the notices reported the births in a positive light.[23] One 1793 notice, which detailed the brief life of a bicorporal monster, celebrated the happy fortune (*felicidad*) that at least one of the heads to emerge from the womb had been baptized while still showing signs of life.[24] The notice's attention to recording whether baptism had occurred reflected the cultural preoccupation, in early modern Mexico, with the prevention of eternal damnation through the enactment of the sacraments.[25] More specifically, it likely reflected the viceroyalty's embrace of a mandate, originating from within the Catholic Church and championed by Spain's reformist monarch Charles III, requiring that caesarean operations be performed on all mothers who died during childbirth in order to ensure the baptism of all fetuses trapped within their wombs.[26]

Colonial Monsters

Sources documenting how colonial Mexicans perceived monsters beyond the *Gazeta* notifications are rare, but the scattered references to monsters in late colonial texts vary significantly from the *Gazeta*'s celebratory portrayal of their advent in New Spain. Other contemporary sources associate monstrosity with diabolism, freakish spectacle, and repugnance.

Images and descriptions of the devil that surfaced in Inquisition trials from seventeenth- and eighteenth-century Mexico document popular associations of diabolism with animal-human hybrids and monstrosity.[27] For instance, a 1789 engraving, published on the occasion of the beatification of Sebastián de Aparicio, a sixteenth-century conquistador who became a muleteer and subsequently a Franciscan friar, depicts winged devils whose bodies enmesh human and animal elements tormenting Aparicio.[28]

Historian Martha Few discovered a similar instance of monstrosity associated with diabolism in Antonio Fuentes y Guzmán's 1690 history of Guatemala, *Recordación Flórida*. In this work, Fuentes y Guzmán included the story of an indigenous woman who had exhibited her refusal to convert to Catholicism by defiantly roasting and eating her infant; she then died while giving birth to a monstrous snake. The Guatemalan chronicler, writes Few, used the story as a warning about the repercussions of rejecting Catholicism.[29] In an 1803 legal case, Few located another Guatemalan "monster," this time a hermaphrodite whom she believes threatened contemporaries through its connotations of social transgression. Few writes, "What was dangerous about monstrous female bodies and body parts was the possibility that this would lead to transgressive female sexual behavior . . . that challenged gendered social roles of colonial society, and the heterosexual relations that structured it legally, religiously, and socially."[30]

Few's interpretation and much current scholarship addresses how the discourse of monstrosity has acted as an agent of social control in various early modern contexts. As Laura Lunger Knoppers and Joan B. Landes observe, "Monstrous bodies carry the weight of political, social, and sexual aberration or transgression: the borders of the known and the acceptable are marked by the construction of the monstrous Other."[31] Thus the specter of monstrosity functioned as a means of policing deviancy, often in terms of religious practice or idealizations of gender. In her examination of monstrosity in post-Reformation England, for instance, Julie Crawford traces how monsters and their mothers, frequently associated in popery with the horrific physical manifestations of divine punishment, acted as "objects for Protestant education, reflection, and repentance."[32] In the early modern era, as in the medieval period, such negative readings of monsters dominated interpretations of monstrous births; as Jennifer Spinks concludes, they were overwhelmingly understood as "divine punishments for sins, or ominous warnings."[33] Similarly, in their definitive treatment of the evolution of popular and learned understandings of monsters and other "natural wonders," Lorraine Daston and Katharine Park assert that both popular and learned audiences associated monsters most pervasively from the medieval period to the end of the seventeenth century with divine punishment, thus provoking a response of horror in those who viewed them.[34]

As well as operating in terms of religious control, in the first waves of Europe's colonization of the New World, monsters served as a mechanism of imperial domination. In the first period of contact, cartographers imagined the terra incognita outside the known boundaries of Europe as peopled by monsters.[35] According to Peter Burke, monsters offered Europeans a means "to define their identities and to confront cultural differences at a time when knowledge of these differences was becoming more widespread thanks to the spread of printing in general and printed maps and newspapers in particular."[36] Such ideas provided moral and intellectual justification of European colonization and helped assure Europeans' ability to gain or maintain power over colonial subjects, territories, and populations. The discourse of monstrosity also helped promote European self-conceptions. In her study of the early eighteenth-century conjoined twins Judith and Helena, discussed further below, Maja-Lisa von Sneidern has suggested that the public voraciously consumed the spectacle of the twins such that they operated as "wonders overwhelmed with signs at a time when the metropolis was overwhelmed with wonders from around the world."[37] She argues that priests, lawyers, and physicians, in particular, used the circulation of knowledge of such monstrosities to provide them with "authoritative law while Mother England experienced both epistemic instability and a proliferation of novel and weird imports."[38]

As well as serving as a means of policing difference, Von Sneidern's portrayal of a public that hungrily consumed the spectacle of the twins suggests another meaning for monsters. Daston and Park argue that within particular contexts—as early as the thirteenth century, and flourishing in the sixteenth—monsters were capable of provoking pleasure rather than inducing horror in viewers.[39] Monstrous spectacles, including conjoined twins, giants, dwarfs, and people with missing or supernumerary limbs, brought viewers pleasure when they understood such creatures in purely natural terms rather than as manifestations of divine wrath. As such, medieval and early modern spectators viewed monsters as objects of wonder—in other words, as beings that demarcated the "outermost limits of the natural" whose existence might demonstrate "the playfulness of nature" or be interpreted as "signs of nature's fertility."[40]

Patricia Drwall Adank contends that the monsters whose images were reproduced in the pages of the *Gazeta de México* should be understood in crasser terms. She argues that Valdés's inclusion of these notices echoed the sensationalistic tradition of the *hojas volantes*, writing that such lurid inclusions were designed to entice a wider readership to the *Gazeta*.[41] But, Adank observes, rather than eliciting a reaction of pleasure in the wonder of nature, one notice about the birth of a one-eyed creature "lacked intellectual or scientific observation or speculation and clearly had been selected to titillate an interest in curiosities and deformities which Valdés perceived among his subscribers."[42]

Whether operating as wonder over nature's complexity or the lurid titillation of freakishness, an element of the pleasure of the spectacle of monstrosity—and its potentially revenue-generating appeal—certainly existed in colonial Mexico. Documentation from 1799 has survived that describes how an Indian tributary in the town of San Francisco Chamacuero persuaded the Mexican viceroy to grant him a license to charge admission of one real to any man who wished to view his son, a boy "aged nine years who has four feet and two virile members whose imperfection excites curiosity." The viceroy cautioned that Antonio José could only exhibit his son after a physician had ensured that the "peculiarity or rarity found in the boy is worthy of the public's paying to see him," while vehemently restricting admission to male viewers only.[43] Here the public's potential pleasure in viewing the boy's "curiosity" was removed from any association with divine punishment and was also distinctive from mere titillation. The desire for certified rarity here is akin to Park and Daston's descriptions of awe in the natural world's unpredictability.

During the Enlightenment, a new view of monsters emerged among the European intelligentsia. Park and Daston write that Europeans developed a novel conception of the order of the natural world, understanding it as absolutely uniform and subject to no exceptions. In this era, then, monsters were increasingly perceived as natural errors—or deformities—and so inspired repugnance in their viewers.[44] Thus, in the writings of one of the most important writers of the period, French naturalist Georges-Louis Leclerc, Comte de Buffon, monstrous productions were those debased or impaired in nature. In his massive treatise *Natural History, General and Particular* (1759–89), for example, Buffon likened the production of the mule to that of monstrosity, describing it as "a vitiated production, as a monster composed of two natures, and for that reason has been thought to be incapable of reproduction."[45]

We might assume that responses of repugnance would have character-ized monstrous productions in the pages of the *Gazeta de México*. After all, the periodical was a product of the Bourbon Enlightenment, and a publication in which creole intellectuals strove to demonstrate their familiarity with the latest European medical and scientific literature. However, the *Gazeta*'s portrayal of monstrous births, although embracing aspects of scientific rationalism, depicted their advent in pleasurable terms. This occurred not because Mexican writers who lived on the geo-graphic periphery of the Enlightenment were reluctant to embrace Euro-pean rationalism, but rather because they rejected the inferior status that this intellectual movement assigned to the locale in which they operated. Recent scholarship has problematized an earlier teleological framework that portrayed scientific empiricism obfuscating older, supernatural ex-planations for monstrous creations. In England, France, and Germany, as elsewhere, understandings of monsters as divine portents continued to exist in the midst of the Scientific Revolution.[46] Most current scholars of Europe write today that three central responses to monstrosity—horror, pleasure, and repugnance—have coexisted across time, just as the term "monster" itself retained its Latin meanings of "marvel, prodigy, wonder" and its reference to the horrific into the eighteenth century in many European languages.[47] Instead, the *Gazeta* announcements treated monstrous births as natural wonders and objects of pleasure because this view was consistent with the dominant creole vision of the natural environment of the New World, a land of health, prodigy, and fertility not only equal to but surpassing that of the Old World.

The *Gazeta* Announcements

Monstrous birth notices in the late eighteenth-century *Gazeta de México* adopted a tone that was both rationalistic and celebratory in their descrip-tions of unusual births. The paper employed the term "monster" to de-scribe offspring in only half of the notices describing unusual rather than multiple births and consistently included meticulous descriptions of the irregularities observed in the infants' formation, explicitly or implicitly drawn from descriptions provided by local administrators or medical per-sonnel. Thus, for example, on January 25 1785, the paper reported that in the town of Pachuca, a girl was delivered "of a body perfectly formed and organized, except the head, because she had only the right eye in its cor-rect place and in the place where the left should be, a mark on the skin, flat, like a scar, without the ball of the eye, nor an indentation nor cavity appearing . . . the nose in the form of a pear, without any nostrils in it, nor any sign of them. . . . In place of the mouth there was another little mark like a scar, flat on the skin, with no lips, and lastly there were six digits on all hands and feet."[48]

On other occasions, Valdés included details about the births recorded by physicians who examined the infants—recording, for example, that on March 10, 1784, in Cuernavaca, "the wife of D. Joseph Pobrete gave birth to a monstrous but dead infant. A somewhat educated and very reliable barber gave the following description: There were no nostrils, but rather two holes in their place. The hands came out of the elbows, and the feet from the knees. The eyes were small and perfectly round, and the brain (as suggested the external mass) was duplicated, because on top of the normal shape of the head, a prominence was projected of the volume of a second one, that joined the front and the back sides of the infant."[49]

Along with their clinical tone, the *Gazeta* notices convey an understanding of monstrosity as a natural rather than supernatural phenomenon. The viceroyalty's medical establishment supported dissection of deceased infants' bodies, and physicians sometimes performed these and published their findings—understood as useful for the public's instruction—in the *Gazeta*, though occasionally, as in the case of the child born with her heart outside the body, infants' parents refused to grant permission for the procedure. The *Gazeta* also conveys a naturalistic attitude to unusual births by including notices of the birth of "monstrous" livestock in its pages, whose announcements paralleled, in tone and diction, its treatment of monstrous human births. For instance, a notice on July 12, 1785, declared that at the Fernández estate in the curate of Guanajuato "two rams were born, completely united by the area behind the chest from the first vertebrae or first bone of the spine to the crown of the head."[50]

The perception of the similarities between monstrous human and animal births is articulated most explicitly in a contemporary manuscript source. Among the works housed in the rare book collection of the Biblioteca Francisco de Burgoa, located within a former Dominican monastery in Oaxaca City, is an edition of the eminent naturalist Francisco Hernández's tract *Rerum Medicarum Novae Hispaniae Thesaurus. Plantarum Animalium*, published in Rome in 1651. A single (two-sided) handwritten page and drawing (see fig. 6), evidently taken from a longer manuscript, has been inserted into Hernández's work, following a page in which he

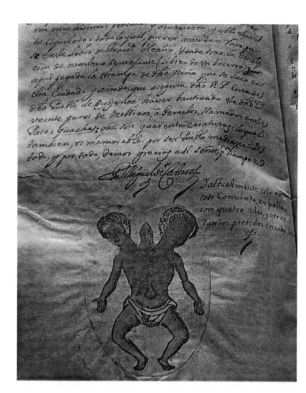

FIGURE 6 Monstrous birth: girl with two heads, Oaxaca, 1741. Credit: Biblioteca Francisco de Burgoa de la Universidad Autónoma Benito Juárez de Oaxaca.

discussed a calf born with two heads. The text announces that on June 14, 1741, in the town of Santa Catharine Quijenee in the bishopric of Oaxaca, "Doña Pasquala Chaves, legitimate wife of Don Manuel de Aguilar, *indios caciques* and residents of the said town, gave birth (having started to labor at eight the night before) to a dead girl that had two heads that were perfect in every way, and between them was something like a little arm."[51]

The manuscript's author wrote that he had elected to insert it into the pages of Hernández's text next to the latter's description of a "similar monster although a calf." Beside the image of the monstrous baby, a further notation reads, "At present, there is in this monastery a chicken with four wings and as many feet, two on each side."

As well as associating the two-headed infant, naturalistically, with the birth of a two-headed cow and a four-winged chicken, this manuscript's author used language and conveyed details consistent with the tone of notices in the *Gazeta de México*. Far from conveying an attitude of repugnance toward such productions, these sources attest to the estimation and even affection that colonial Mexicans felt for their community's monstrous babies, suggesting further reasons why their contemporaries enjoyed reading about them. One striking feature of the Burgoa manuscript is the author's use of the term "perfect" to describe the two-headed newborn; he declared that the baby's body was "perfect in all its elements (except for the heads)." Once its internal organs were examined, these were declared "cabales" (without defect). For eighteenth-century writers, the term "perfect" carried multiple meanings: high moral virtue, beauty, the quality of being well formed, agility, superiority, and also "complete or fulfilled in its line."[52] Whatever the meaning, however, the connotations of the term were positive.[53]

So too did the *Gazeta* notices emphasize the various "perfect" elements of the monstrous infants whose births they chronicled. Most often, the paper's descriptions of "monstrosity" consisted in its identification of those instances in which infants' bodies deviated physically from the norm. However, the *Gazeta* adopted an admiring attitude toward these infants insofar as while meticulously detailing the exceptionality of their bodies, its notices also highlighted each infant's many "perfections." In the announcement about the conjoined twins joined at the skull described at the opening of this chapter, for instance, the *Gazeta* observed that "there has been no record in these twins of any deformity or defect in their separate and agile bodies."[54] In another case from 1789, the paper reported that an Indian woman had given birth to a child "who had three very perfect tongues, with the distinction that the superior one protruded above the mouth and occupied the place of the superior lip (that it formed) and then was attached to the nose like the point of a needle prick, and the other two [tongues] were very perfect."[55] Another *Gazeta* notice recorded how one Mónica Josefa Nataren had given birth after an intensive labor of four days to a "bicorporal monster, composed of two females united by the chest from the clavicles to the navel, both completely perfect, except for the left hand of one, in the internal side of the thumb in the first phalanx was joined to two phalanxes of another finger."[56]

The twins, as depicted in the *Gazeta*'s accompanying image, are illustrated in figure 7. As with the Joseph Guadalupe twins, the fact that these two girls were conjoined did not negate their "complete perfection." Another announcement described a girl born with prominences extending from both temples and from the crown of her head "resembling the crown of a turkey or rooster," but whose other body parts were "very perfect and regular."[57] Several other accounts of similar "perfections" characterize the infants' descriptions.[58]

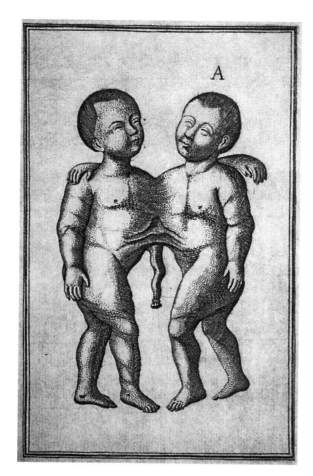

FIGURE 7 Monstrous birth: bicorporal infants, 1793. "Vicorpóreo compuesto por dos hembritas unidas por los pechos desde las clavículas hasta el ombligo." AGI, MP-ESTAMPAS, 20 (2). Credit: España. Ministerio de Educación, Cultura y Deporte. Archivo General de Indias.

Pride is, not unexpectedly, displayed in communities' reactions to news of robust women who successfully birthed and nourished triplets or quadruplets. One 1803 notice reported that María Mónica Moreno of Zimapan had given birth to triplets, each measuring one *vara* and one *pulgada*: "They were born healthy and well formed. The birth was successful, and the mother is so robust, that at present, she is nursing not only all three babies, but also a son who she had continued to nurse during her pregnancy."[59] Another recounted how one María Rosa Domínguez, an Indian woman from Córdova, had given birth to three boys without the assistance of a midwife. Two days after this feat, two public notaries followed by two surgeons visited the mother.[60] A 1786 announcement described triplets born in Chalco whose parents were so proud of their offspring that they "presented the children, still living and robust, to the most excellent viceroy."[61] The intendant of Yucatán wrote the viceroy and archbishop of New Spain, Francisco Javier de Lizana y Beaumont, in February 1810 to report the "extraordinary news" that an Indian woman had given birth to three robust babies.[62] Two announcements from the last years of the *Gazeta's* publication described the phenomenal fecundity of women in New Spain, celebrating how one woman, a Silesian immigrant, had given birth to an astounding forty-four children, while another, an indigenous woman from San Ángel, had given birth to a single boy and girl, and then to a set of quadruplets followed by a set of triplets. In the latter case, the *Gazeta* noted the parents were humble cultivators who lived from what they grew in the *chinampas* (floating gardens), circumstances that demonstrated that "luxury and property are not the principal source of fecundity."[63]

Communities also used the birth announcements as vehicles for the inclusion of other optimistic observations about the fortitude and longevity of its citizens. Far from showing themselves to be the enfeebled inhabitants of an unhealthy clime, as contemporary Europeans might describe them, a correspondent from Puebla reported to the *Gazeta* in October 1784 that a woman had given birth the previous month and that the "Licenciado D. Christoval Montiel, a subject of 86 years of age" was the child's godfather, and among those present at the baptism was his "fifth" grandmother [*quinta abuela*] of more than 101 years of age, a woman who continued to "enjoy health and strength."[64]

This pride and affection in the fecundity of New Spain was even extended to the arrival of monstrous offspring. After the birth of Rafaela Cortés's conjoined twins in Guanajuato in 1785, as noted above, "many people went to visit them, admiring in them the unusual effects of nature." The longer the twins lived, the paper continued, the more admiration they generated. A second announcement published two months later informed readers that although the public had already been told the "agreeable" news of the twins' birth, the *Gazeta* was obliged to announce their unfortunate demise.[65] A notice from Sombrerete published in November 1785 opened by exclaiming, "In this Kingdom María Ruisa (alias la Larga) gave birth with joy (*con felicidad*) on the 24th of the past month to a child whose monstrous face provoked a meeting of the medical professionals."[66] Members of the community of Tuxpan, Veracruz, also expressed awe and wonder at the birth of a monstrous child stillborn in that town in 1792. On this occasion, although one Juan de Dios Savala denounced a midwife for the witchcraft she had used to curse his pregnant wife, he also commented that the stillborn child was "marked so strangely that she had caused great admiration in all who had seen her."[67]

The *Gazeta* notices also convey a sense of pride in the spiritual and medical expertise with which newborns were received. The *Gazeta* reported, for instance, how one municipal official, the senior *alcalde ordinario* (town council member) of Córdova, deduced that an indigenous woman would be incapable of nursing each of the triplets she had birthed in October 1794 and had promptly dispatched a wet nurse to assist her, paying for the cost himself.[68] In the case of conjoined twins born in Oaxaca in 1793, the *Gazeta* reported that the mother would not have been able to expel the bodies "if the doctor [*facultativo*] who assisted, and had predicted twins, seeing that the patient was fainting because of the repetition and duration of the labor . . . had not decided, as a last recourse, to break the skull that had fully advanced . . . and although at that time he did not succeed in extracting it, he succeeded a few hours later, with the increase of uterine contractions brought on by tonics."[69]

Pride and affection for monstrous offspring is also explicit in the case of one set of conjoined twins born in Querétaro in 1789 whose detailed birth announcement, composed by a Querétaro city council clerk, Don José Manuel de Zárate, was published along with an image (see fig. 8) that depicted a baby whose body was normal from the waist up but from whose groin protruded a second set of buttocks, genitalia, legs, and feet.[70] Two doctors who accompanied Zárate wrote the following description of the infant: "The said child is monstrous, and his monstrosity consists in having four legs and feet, with twenty-three toes, four buttocks, two penises [*miembros viriles*], [and] two testicles (one associated with each virile member)." They then described the exact formation of the "monstrosity," which involved the number and position of the extra legs and buttocks that they termed "preternatural." They cataloged the various peculiarities of the legs, feet, and genitalia, reporting with great interest that the child, who at the time of writing remained "robust and healthy," urinated from both penises simultaneously with no apparent discomfort.

The report and drawing so enticed *regidor* Septién, who had encouraged Zárate to report on the birth, that he sent the image on to the viceroy of New Spain, Manuel Antonio Flores, later that month, indicating he hoped it might be sent on to King Charles IV. Septién declared that he was including it as a demonstration of his veneration ("en obstantación de mi veneración"). He described the infant as a model of the "admirable

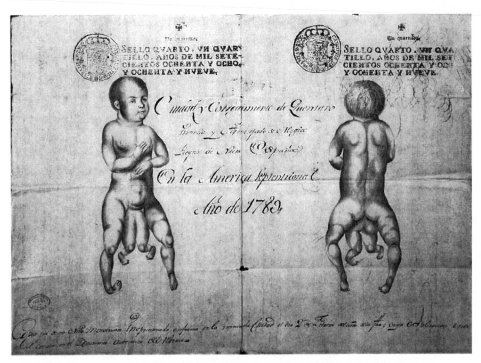

FIGURE 8 Monstrous birth: infant with four buttocks and legs, 1789. "Diseño de una criatura deforme que nació en la jurisdicción de Querétaro." AGI, MP-MEXICO, 420 BIS. Credit: España. Ministerio de Educación, Cultura y Deporte. Archivo General de Indias.

features of nature, because of its unusualness, and because it is an exotic production [producción peregrina] of this remote hemisphere, I have deemed worthy of sending to his majesty through your hand. . . ."[71] The language Septién used here is significant because the term *peregrina* refers to "the exotic" but is also the adjectival form of a religious pilgrimage—a *peregrinación*. Such pilgrimages to holy sites embedded in particular local contexts constituted one of the most important early manifestations of New World local identity and "creole patriotism."

Viceroy Flores, in turn, transmitted news of the child to Charles in June 1789, writing that he had sent to his majesty the drawing and details of the circumstances of the "monstrous boy that nature has produced in the district of this jurisdiction."[72] We do not know what the king made of this declaration, but we have more information about the reaction of his predecessor, Charles III, who in 1780 received similar notification about a monstrous child—from his possessions in the Philippines—whose shoulders and chest were blanketed in fur-like hair and who had patches of hair growing from various parts of his body. In this earlier case, the Spanish king ordered the child's transportation to Spain that he might be "cared for and given an education and a useful destination."[73] In his choice of language, the king explicitly adopted the emergent view of children and childhood. The Bourbons instituted an array of reforms designed to increase the state's material and intellectual control over its youngest subjects. As one contemporary royal decree expressed, the state needed to assume control over supervising children's education so that "they might learn some trade or useful occupation."[74] This utilitarian-inflected response may express nothing more than the utilitarian perspective of child-rearing emergent in this period, but the *Gazeta* announcements conveyed a distinctive attitude to the production of these unusual babies. The publications convey the curiosity with which readers and community members viewed monstrous productions, but also the attitudes of reverence rather than repugnance with which such children were greeted.

Creole Patriotism

The intellectual climate of the European Enlightenment fostered the articulation of what scholars have termed creole patriotism, the quest for an American identity that in Mexico was developed out of pride in the region's indigenous past and its natural wealth.[75] The Enlightenment saw the proliferation of deprecatory views about the climate and territory of the Americas. Both the European theory that the New World was a "degenerate" territory and creole rejections of the notion of their territory's inferiority dated back to at least the mid-seventeenth century.[76] But numerous influential writers of the Enlightenment, including the Count de Buffon, Abbot Guillaume-Thomas Raynal, the Dutch cleric Cornelius de Pauw, and the Scots historian William Robertson redeployed the notion of American degeneration in the eighteenth century.

Creole friars and scholars just as vigorously rejected it. These writers, anxious to defend their social positions in the face of European disparity, frequently turned to the very elements upon which Europeans founded their notions of American inferiority as the source of their unique identity. European authors viewed the Mexican climate and natural life as the root of New World inferiority, but for Mexican writers, including José Antonio de Alzate y Ramírez, Francisco Javier Clavijero, and Juan José de Eguiara y Eguren, they became the foundations of a novel and desirable identity. Exotic indigenous civilizations were, for De Pauw, "a race of men who have all the faults of a child, as a degenerate species of humanity, cowardly, impotent, without physical force or vigor, and without elevation of spirit."[77] For creole patriots, who championed the first excavations of New World archaeological cities and monuments in the last quarter of the eighteenth century, however, indigenous civilization became a cultivated model of sophistication. Creoles articulated this identity in the science, history, and art they produced, but they also expressed it in their perceptions of unusual childbirths as described in the *Gazeta de México*'s birth notices. These announcements document that patriotic defense characterized New Spaniards' responses to unusual childbirths in their midst, the very occasions that Enlightenment Europeans identified as manifestations of the degeneration of the New World.[78]

Eighteenth-century European writers, and in particular the French naturalist Buffon, argued that the inferior climate of the New World caused infertility and the degenerative reproduction of its inhabitants. In his *Natural History*, Buffon developed contemporary environmentalist beliefs shared by such writers as De Pauw and Robertson about the influences of climate on the fertility and health of territories' animal populations. Buffon believed that climactic determinism had formed an America characterized by both savagery and impotence, writing that the region's inferior humidity had sentenced its life forms to degeneration, because "animated nature is less active, less varied and even less vigorous" in the New World.[79] The animal species of America, he asserted, were smaller, weaker, and less plentiful than in Europe, and European livestock "degenerated" when exposed to the debilitating climate of the New World. De Pauw also berated the putrid vegetation that infected the inhabitants of the New World, producing effeminacy, impotence, and torpidity in its males and sterility in its females.[80]

For Buffon, central evidence for the fact of American degeneration lay in the absence of white skin pigmentation in its inhabitants. "Nature," he wrote, "in her full perfection, has made men white, and Nature reduced to the last stage of adulteration, renders them white again."[81] Nonwhite populations, he deduced, must have originated as white but "degenerated" away from whiteness through their lack of exposure to invigorating cold climates, and he proposed that if such people were transported to superior environments (suggesting Denmark as a possible setting), their whiteness would reemerge after several centuries. The absence of whiteness in America was thus proof of its imperfection.[82]

Manuel Antonio Valdés and other writers published in the *Gazeta* were obviously familiar with the writings of Buffon and his European cohort. A February 1784 edition detailing the discovery of some "elephant bones" found in Tepeyac referred to the classification system Buffon employed in *Las épocas de la naturaleza*.[83] More explicitly, the December 30, 1793, edition included a lengthy notice originating from Oaxaca about a woman who had given birth to the two-bodied monster illustrated in figure 7. After including a detailed physical description of the twins, it then discussed Buffon's description of Judith and Helena, a pair of conjoined twins born in Hungary in 1701 whose fame had spread across Europe and, obviously, to the New World as well.[84] The citation began, "Despite the fact that the Conde de Buffon in his *Natural History*, on page 326 of vol. 5, treats another birth of two girls united at the waist verified in Hungary in 1701, and says that they lived until the age of 21, it was a momentous occasion [gran dicha] that one of ours lasted until she was baptized, since, as they were united at the chest and with only one heart, it would have been difficult for either of them to live, although there are doctors who believe the opposite."[85] In explicitly comparing the Oaxaca-born conjoined twins to Europe's longer surviving Judith and Helena, the *Gazeta* conveyed both pride and compassion, referring to New Spain's two-headed baby as "las nuestras" (ours) and explaining that it was no wonder that Mexico's conjoined twins had perished faster, since in sharing one heart they had faced a greater biological challenge than Judith and Helena's shared use of the buttocks and urinary passage.[86]

Creole Mexicans, most famously the Jesuit scholar Francisco Javier Clavijero, rejected European notions of inherent American inferiority that they confronted. Clavijero refuted Buffon, De Pauw, Robertson, and others in his *Historia antigua de México* (1780–81), a celebratory account of Mexico's history up to the era of Spanish conquest in which he ridiculed the inaccuracies of Buffon and other Europeans who claimed to have understood American realities "better than we who have been for so many years in America."[87] Clavijero defended the diversity and abundance of Mexico's natural world, put Mexico's indigenous population at the center of Mexican identity and material achievements, and generated glowing reports on the health, fecundity, and moral virtues of New Spain's population. He noted that many of his compatriots lived until eighty, ninety, or one hundred years, which could "only be attributable to their sobriety with regard to food and to the health of the climate."[88] Mexican scholars also addressed the inaccuracies of European science in the *Gazeta*, where, for example, Alzate published a scathing critique of Linnaean taxonomy, which had just been introduced in Mexico, charging its use of Latin botanical labels as fatuous and unhelpful and championing instead the virtues of Nahua systems of naming, as well as the writings of Francisco Hernández and Francisco Jiménez, earlier botanists who had worked extensively in Mexico.[89]

The *Gazeta* was initially created to foster loyalty to the Spanish crown and advocate the adoption of Enlightenment perspectives in Spanish America. The crown aspired through the foundation of such initiatives to modernize its New World territories and to augment the political and fiscal usefulness of its citizenry. Inadvertently, one of the most tangible results of these modernization programs was the creation of a public community of Mexican citizens. Producers, consumers, and protagonists of such works as the *Gazeta de México* learned to identify with each other through the common experiences reported in its pages, whether these were notices on the current price of lard, recent advances in medicine, or maneuvers in the Napoleonic Wars plaguing relatives and business interests on the Continent.

Nineteenth-Century Monsters

While the *Gazeta de México* announcements conveyed late colonial attitudes of pride and awe toward monstrous births in the last decades of the colonial era, shifting perceptions of monsters are apparent in sources documenting Mexican monsters over the course of the nineteenth century. Notices of monstrous births—and occasionally monstrous adults—continued to appear in newspaper articles in various publications in the republican era, primarily the Mexico City daily *El Siglo Diez y Nueve* in the period from 1842 to 1895.[90] Second, more specialized scientific journals, such as *El Museo Mexicano, ó, Miscelánea Pintoresca de Amenidades Curiosas é Instructivas*, a weekly review that aimed to diffuse advances in culture and education to Mexican citizens of all strata, began carrying extensive reports on monstrous births in the 1840s. Monstrous births received their most attentive treatment in the medical discussions of the emerging field of teratology, the study of birth abnormalities, which became a central topic in medical journals, most notably the *Gaceta Médica de México,* the official organ of the Academia Nacional de Medicina, beginning in the late 1860s. Finally, interest in birth anomalies culminated in 1895 with the inauguration in the capital city's Museo Nacional de

México of a *salon de teratología*, where the museum advertised that visitors could observe seventy-five examples of anomalous birth specimens, both human and animal, "some preserved in alcohol, others dried, and others represented by photograph."[91] Subsequent to the salon's inauguration, doctor Román Ramírez published the accompanying *Catálogo de las anomalías coleccionadas en el museo nacional.*[92]

Some elements of late colonial representations of monsters in Mexico endured in these later treatments, including the understanding, at least until midcentury, that divine intervention might be responsible for their production. In a learned treatment of a two-headed baby published in 1844 in *El Museo Mexicano*, one of the journal's editors identified the paper's scientific ambitions for publicizing and analyzing the monstrous production. The physician who penned the article, Juan Nepomuceno Bolaños, used it to explore the evidence for and against the medical theory of epigenesis, the understanding that organisms passed through a sequence of distinctive phases in their development from eggs. But Bolaños also declared that he understood the root cause of such developments as divine in origin. "Nature," he wrote, "is nearly always profound and undefinable in its works as in the thinking of the creator, who executes . . . not molecules or principals or systems, but individuals of the human species realizing at once, before our eyes, that which is written on the immortal page: *You will be two in one flesh* (Genesis chap. 2, verse 24)."[93]

Diabolic understandings of monstrosity also persisted through the latter part of the nineteenth century, when some Mexicans continued to understand "monstrous births" in supernatural and explicitly demonic terms. One 1887 Mexico City birth notice published in *El Siglo Diez y Nueve* classed a fetus born with one eye located below its nose as the advent of "El Antecristo."[94] An announcement from Cosalá, Sinaloa, in the same paper described how a "curious phenomenon" had occurred in that town when a woman had given birth to twins "and one of them suffered a fit of rage and threw up a great deal of blood and then . . . horror! The fetus still showed signs of life." Some local inhabitants who learned of these events "had become very alarmed, believing that the fetus was an augury of the end of the world."[95]

Despite the persistence of supernatural interpretations of monstrous phenomena in the late nineteenth century, newspapers and medical journals predominantly presented these in terms that celebrated the scientific understanding of human development. Such announcements also promoted the desire to preserve and display monstrous productions as spectacles for public and learned consumption. One 1854 notice reprinted from Colima's *El Orden* described a fetus born with a lump of flesh in the shape of a nose in place of its head. While the town curate had sought to send the corpse to the local museum, the creature's indigenous parents energetically opposed its exposure there, and he was forced to bury it.[96] More frequently, parents consented to the preservation of such corpses, and by 1868 their display had become a matter of national patrimony.

Obstetrician Juan María Rodríguez published an article that year in the *Gaceta Médica de México* detailing the birth of "monstrous human quadruplets" in Durango two years earlier. The attending physician who supplied the account to the *Gaceta Médica* explained that he had delivered a five-month-old fetus and a "placental mass, upon which were developing a number of other fetuses (five well visible), and . . . rudiments of another multitude!" The physician also reported that two Americans who had learned of the birth "had made great efforts to purchase the fetus to take it with them to the United States, but calculating that my fatherland was also worthy of possessing such a curious monstrosity, I resolved to keep it, and these gentlemen had to content themselves with only taking with them some dozens of photographs that they planned to send to their wives."[97] Rodríguez observed approvingly to his readers that the physician and his superiors in Durango had shown "love for the fatherland and for the School of Medicine" in transmitting the specimen to the Museum of Pathological Anatomy housed in the capital's Escuela de Medicina de México.[98] Such collections received their most prominent home in the Museo Nacional's 1895 *salon de teratología*.

Physicians and curators may have increasingly sought to preserve and display monstrous productions, but newspaper articles from this period reveal the increasingly negative connotations these creatures evoked among members of the Mexican public. An 1872 report published in the *Gaceta Médica* described how exaggerated stories had circulated in the public about the "horrific shapes and exaggerated size" of a pair of conjoined twins born in Oaxaca.[99] One 1885 notice reprinted in the Mexico City paper *El Monitor Republicano* but originating in the state of Morelos described a woman who had given birth to a "horrendous" fetus who was regular in formation from the neck down with the exception of all its fingernails and toenails, which resembled those of a canine. Its head, as well as being oversized, was missing one ear and one eye; its nose was imperceptible; and it was crowned by a boney protuberance adorned with two horns. The notice closed by remarking that "fortunately, the creature could not live and was buried so its mother did not have to see her deformed child."[100]

In another article, the same paper reprinted a letter that had first appeared in *La Revista Mercantil de Chihuahua* that told of how a woman had given birth to a "horrible fetus that had the body and four paws of a dog; the head of a cat; a pointy snout, with many teeth and very sharp canines; ears a little rounded like those of humans; with long, coarse whiskers on the snout, like those of a cat; a very large and rough tongue like that of a cow; with very large, round, and yellow eyes; and with a little fur on tops of the feet and hands; the face is that of a badger." The article reported that the frightened people who had witnessed the birth had buried the creature but that, four days later, the state governor had ordered it disinterred for a judicial inspection.[101]

An 1893 broadside by famed engraver José Guadalupe Posada similarly evokes the repulsion that Mexicans had, by the close of the nineteenth century, learned to associate with monstrous productions (see fig. 9). The engraving depicted a baby pictured with an extra set of eye sockets, hairy legs, and a tail. The headline, however, described the child as the "child born without a skull." The accompanying article described how the baby's birth had caused a "horrible sensation in all classes of society" that had learned of its existence, and described how the creature's mother, "full of the most punishable shame," turned the fetus over to the local authorities to transfer to the Museo Nacional, where the public could view "all the curiosities they may wish to learn about."[102] The horror and repugnance of popular news coverage in the second half of the nineteenth century differed dramatically from the pride and affection running through monstrous birth notices appearing in the *Gazeta de México* and dating from the last decades of the colonial period.

Other features of nineteenth-century news stories about monstrous births rendered them distinctive from those of a century earlier. In the late colonial period, the *Gazeta* notices generally limited speculation as to the causes of monstrosity to their origins in the awesome powers of nature. But as the nineteenth century developed, popular and scientific sources alike sought more detailed explanations for the causes of monstrosity. Both scientific works and popular imagination increasingly speculated about the women whose bodies had produced such creatures. Like their continental peers, Mexican physicians' understanding of the roots of monstrosity shifted from external (divine or climactic) to internal (biological, psychological or moralistic) causes as they sought to understand

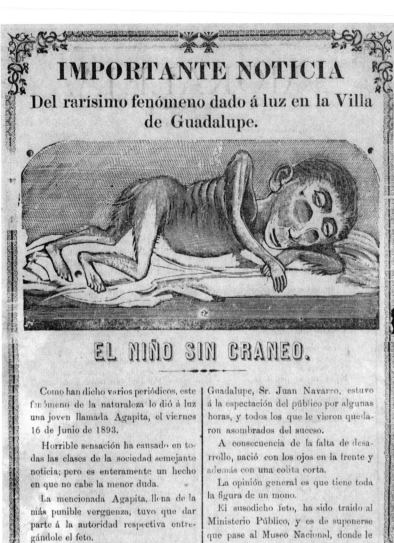

IMPORTANTE NOTICIA

Del rarísimo fenómeno dado á luz en la Villa de Guadalupe.

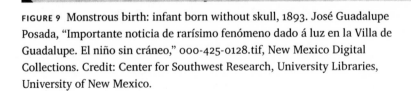

EL NIÑO SIN CRÁNEO.

Como han dicho varios periódicos, este fenómeno de la naturaleza lo dió á luz una joven llamada Agapita, el viernes 16 de Junio de 1893.

Horrible sensación ha causado en todas las clases de la sociedad semejante noticia; pero es enteramente un hecho en que no cabe la menor duda.

La mencionada Agapita, llena de la más punible vergüenza, tuvo que dar parte á la autoridad respectiva entregándole el feto.

Debido á la muy buena disposición del Alcaide Municipal de la Villa de Guadalupe, Sr. Juan Navarro, estuvo á la espectación del público por algunas horas, y todos los que le vieron quedaron asombrados del suceso.

A consecuencia de la falta de desarrollo, nació con los ojos en la frente y además con una colita corta.

La opinión general es que tiene toda la figura de un mono.

El susodicho feto, ha sido traido al Ministerio Público, y es de suponerse que pase al Museo Nacional, donde le verán todos los curiosos que deseen conocerle.

FIGURE 9 Monstrous birth: infant born without skull, 1893. José Guadalupe Posada, "Importante noticia de rarísimo fenómeno dado á luz en la Villa de Guadalupe. El niño sin cráneo," 000-425-0128.tif, New Mexico Digital Collections. Credit: Center for Southwest Research, University Libraries, University of New Mexico.

whether aberrations in women's reproductive anatomy or particular conditions that embryos experienced in their development in the uterus might account for the production of anomalous fetuses.[103]

Paralleling the expansion of the social scrutiny of women's sexual practices discussed in chapter 4, nineteenth-century announcements occasionally commented on the sexual reputations of the women who bore monstrous offspring. One 1853 article published in *El Universal* reprinted a story originally published in a paper from the Saône-et-Loire district of French Burgundy about a poor woman, "exemplary in her customs," who had given birth to a monstrous three-headed baby. The woman had been widowed for ten years preceding the birth, but had developed a mysterious tumor in her belly at about the time of her husband's death. Anticipating its readers' speculation that only illicit sexual activity might explain the widow's apparent pregnancy so long after her husband's death, the article discussed an eighteenth-century treatise, *Lucina sine concubitu*, which established that "posthumous babies could be born many years after the death of the father, for purely accidental reasons."[104] Another article, reporting on the birth of an animal-like fetus in Chihuahua, opened with the observation that the woman who had produced the creature was "of irreprehensible conduct."[105] The notices presumably included the commentaries to dispel any speculation that extramarital (or extraspecies) sexual unions had engendered these women's monstrous prodigy.

In the pages of professional journals and in presentations before their peers, Mexican doctors debated the meanings of monstrosity with one another. By midcentury, their preoccupation with refuting the European association between New World monstrosity and degeneration had receded and new preoccupations surfaced. One article published in *El Museo Mexicano* in 1844 is particularly instructive because it refers explicitly to one of the late eighteenth-century *Gazeta* notices treated above. The original 1793 announcement had publicized the birth of the conjoined twins, united from the chest to the navel, that are pictured in figure 8. After their extraction, physician Juan Figueroa had performed an autopsy on the twins and had preserved their bodies. Fifty-one years later, a professor of medicine in Oaxaca, Juan Nepomuceno Bolaños, had acquired their mummified remains, and had notified the mid-nineteenth-century publication. His article reveals the different concerns that monstrosity held for physicians by the time of its publication.

Following trends in the developing medical field of teratology, the 1844 article sought primarily to categorize monstrosity according to the classification system developed by Gilbert Breschet and others, and accordingly labeled in terms of *agenesios* (imperfect development), *hipergenesios* (monstrosities with excessive parts), and *diplogenesios* (organic deviation, owing to the union of two germs).[106] Bolaños's article concluded by offering a commentary on the meaning of these phenomena, "so interesting for nature and fecund in ideas for philosophy and medicine but so sad and desultory for the human species!" While Judith and Helena had endured the "odious and tyrannical" weight of several years of existence, Mexico's monstrosities had perished immediately. Bolaños consoled readers that "fortunately such freaks of the natural world were seen so rarely that they can be read as warnings from the Omnipotence [God], so that we can thereby understand his immense gifts."[107] The eighteenth-century article had conveyed a tone of pride in Mexico's ability to produce wondrous twins who faced greater biological challenges than did their European counterparts. This later text instead conceived of them as deviant productions whose aberrational examples served to reinforce the beauty and regularity of normalcy.

In a lengthy separate article published in the same journal that discussed the birth of a two-headed baby in 1844, Bolaños again prioritized the importance of classifying the monstrous twins along with detailing his observations of their internal anatomy in comparison to similar cases originating in Europe.[108] He cited the writings of Étienne Geoffroy Saint-Hilaire, the French physician who founded the formal study of birth malformations in the 1820s, whose son Isidore pursued this research and coined the term teratology in the 1830s.[109] Bolaños grappled with various contemporary debates in his report. Much of his analysis focused on determining whether a two-headed but single-bodied creature would have operated biologically as one or two distinctive entities had it survived. But he also probed the implications of such a being in terms of contemporary civil and criminal jurisprudence. Would such a creature inherit wealth as one or two distinctive heirs? If the hand of one side of the creature committed a crime, would the other side also be held responsible? Finally, he questioned the extent to which the particular phases of an embryo's development in the womb might serve as the primary force in determining the existence of abnormalities. In other writing, Bolaños asserted that monstrosities served to contrast with normalcy and thus to reinforce the beauty of regularity. Here, however, he allowed himself to contemplate the disturbing possibility that epigenesis rendered possible: that monsters, rather that representing beings essentially distinctive from the rest of creation, instead denoted only the most extreme gradations of tendencies that all organisms might share. Bolaños noted that in his research Saint-Hilaire had proceeded by comparing "the most ordinary type of an organism or an animal and followed it through all its aberrations and possible deviations . . . studying their relations, analogies, and differences."[110]

The determination of whether monstrosity was best understood as an exception to normalcy or as a shade of normalcy became a central focus of the science of teratology in the mid- and later nineteenth century in Mexico, while discussions about the implications of monstrosity continued to interlink with the nation's articulations of its national identity. Like his predecessors in the pages of the late eighteenth-century Mexican *Gazetas,* Bolaños revealed that he understood the study of monstrous productions as a reflection of his country's broader national development. Pausing to consider the march of scientific progress in all fields of study, Bolaños saluted Mexico for its emergence in his own day into an era of momentous scientific achievement. He observed that other countries at other points in history had been "the sources of important knowledge and the lands that had fertilized this thinking are reduced today—to nothing." In the present, however, new nations like his own "have left behind their infancy, which had obscured them in metaphysical darkness." Scientific study produced in these new nations had brought them into a new "era of glory and virtue for the human race."[111]

Monsters and Obstetrical Medicine

Juan María Rodríguez, the most influential obstetrician of late nineteenth-century Mexico, researched and published extensively on the study of monstrosity. Rodríguez earned his medical degree in 1855 and, for over twenty years, served as a physician in the Departamento de Partos Ocultos o Reservados (Department of Secret Births) in the Mexico City poorhouse and later in the Casa de Maternidad, where he assisted women in childbirth and directed the training program for obstetrical students. He became a professor of obstetrics at the Escuela de Medicina and was elected president of the National Academy of Medicine in 1880. In 1870 Rodríguez published the first edition of the *Guía clínica del arte de los partos,* an obstetrics manual that saw many editions and became the standard reference work for several generations of Mexican midwives and doctors.

Rodríguez's work in clinical obstetrics led to his investigations in the science of teratology, for monstrous births often presented obstacles to safe deliveries.[112] In his inaugural discussion of the field of teratology published in the *Gaceta Médica de México* in 1869, Rodríguez described his attendance at the birth of a pair of conjoined twins whose bulk had required extraction with pincers and the application of powerful traction on all four limbs in order to avoid the performance of either a craniotomy, cephalotripsy, or embriotomy.[113] He followed this piece with two dozen subsequent articles in the same journal and others over the next twenty years. In the course of this body of research, Rodríguez articulated definitive positions on the nature and causes of monstrosity, the relationship of such aberrant productions to the total sphere of organic creation, and the implications of monsters for the development of obstetrics—and, in turn, for the ongoing development of his country's overall population.

Rodríguez drew extensively in his writings on Saint-Hilaire's research on teratology. Like Saint-Hilaire, he focused primarily on the question of classification in all of his examinations of monstrous productions. In this he endorsed the French physician's notion that monstrous productions could only be understood through the precise isolation of each anomaly they presented.[114] In the first article he published in the *Gaceta Médica*, for example, Rodríguez painstakingly used Sainte-Hilaire's categories to classify a "monstruo humano diplogenésico, monocéfalo, autositario, onfalósito, no viable," (a two-bodied creature that gave an outward appearance of possessing one head, but whose internal formation revealed the union of two entwined entities).[115]

Central to Saint-Hilaire's theory of monstrosity was his doctrine of the "unity of organic composition," which, as Miranda Gill explains, posited that "animals demonstrated the same relationship between their different parts, thereby emphasizing the 'analogies' between different species."[116] At its most extreme, the position implied that all living creatures embodied varieties of the same original archetypal species. Similar to naturalists Jean-Baptiste Robinet and Jean-Baptiste Lamarck, Étienne Geoffroy Saint-Hilaire advocated a theory of organic development that emphasized the continuities of development between various life forms. He understood monsters as "transitional forms binding together the chains of beings and helping the 'correct' combinations to emerge over time."[117]

Rodríguez, like Saint-Hilaire before him, advocated that embryonic development held the key to best understanding the development of monstrous abnormalities. He believed that rather than having inherited perversions of a germ or seed present at creation, monstrous deviations must have developed from healthy seeds that experienced accidental damage before birth. French teratologists attributed monstrosity to a theory of "arrested development," which indicated that all human specimens, in their own embryonic development, had passed through a stage of monstrosity en route to normalcy.[118] Saint-Hilaire defined monstrosity as "a very serious form of anomaly which makes the accomplishment of one or many functions impossible, or which produces amongst affected individuals an aberrant physical structure [conformation vicieuse] very different from that which its species ordinarily presents." But he also wrote, "Monsters are merely normal beings; or rather there are no Monsters, and nature is one."[119] In supporting this view, Rodríguez and other Mexican teratologists adhered to the notion that environmental conditions—factors affecting embryos within the uterus during their development—rather than hereditary factors lay at the source of monstrosity. In this way, their thinking paralleled those of their Mexican contemporaries who championed Lamarckian rather than Mendelian interpretations of genetic development in the field of eugenics, for these gave greater allowance to the role of environment rather than inheritance alone played in human development.[120] Both the theory of epigenesis and the determinative role of environment in generating birth anomalies predominated medical and scientific understandings of monstrosity in Mexico by the close of the nineteenth century.

Monstrosity Naturalized

In his writings about monstrous productions, Rodríguez sought to refute the popular disparagement into which monstrous productions had fallen in Mexico. At the close of the eighteenth century, creole patriots refuted the pejorative degeneration Europeans associated with Mexico's climactic and racial environment and celebrated unusual births productions in their midst as demonstrations of fertility and natural prodigy. Over the course of the nineteenth century, however, monsters developed new connotations. The general public received them with horror and repugnance as they had not done in the late colonial period. Drawing from the science of French teratology, Juan María Rodríguez argued that rather that understanding monsters as horrifying anomalies, such creatures "demonstrate the principle of unity within the diversity of phenomena, and establish the harmony that exists between entities that develop together that differ in form, constitution, or in terms of the force that animates them."[121] Rodríguez, then, advocated a theory of monstrosity that did not relegate birth anomalies to classification as aberrational exceptions but defended the notion that they formed a part of the spectrum of normalcy; by better understanding the forces that had produced aberration, it was possible to improve obstetrical medicine and the health of the country's overall population.

His position is reflected in the unsigned monthly medical reports the Casa de Maternidad produced detailing monstrous births that had occurred in the institution. The report for July 1877 remarked that, along with a premature birth, the birth of twins, and a woman who required dilation of the cervix for the surgical removal of her placenta, "in this month, one woman gave birth to a monstrosity" whose extraction—first with forceps, and then manually—had produced a perinatal infection that had killed her shortly thereafter.[122] The monstrosity, which merited no further discussion or description in the records, was for the recorder—possibly Rodríguez himself—unremarkable. Rodríguez understood such births as reflecting a shade of normalcy rather than as radical aberrations.

At a time when Darwinian-inflected debates about descent, adaptation, and race dominated Mexico's scientific community, such questions featured centrally in the Museo Nacional's *salon de teratología*, which opened in 1895. Román Ramírez, the physician who produced the catalog accompanying the salon, observed in it that monstrosity should be understood as an extreme manifestation of "hereditary tendencies" present in all humanity.[123] Like contemporary eugenicists in Mexico and beyond, the salon and the museum that housed it adopted as a central premise the examination of whether the country's production of monstrosities demonstrated that the nation belonged to the racially normal stock of Europe or whether such monstrosities represented a pathological variety of the species.[124]

In Ramírez's day, unlike in the late colonial period, both public and scientific communities took an increased interest in mothers' roles in producing monsters. Such developments paralleled both the increased sexual scrutiny to which Mexicans subjected a wider body of their country's female population and the development of a pathological view of Mexican women's reproductive anatomy, a subject treated further in chapter 6. Juan María Rodríguez, like Ramón Ramírez after him, determined that the biological site responsible for fostering monstrosity was the uterus.

While on the one hand he worked to redeem monsters from the negative associations they had developed in his period, Rodríguez's conclusion that monstrosity was best explained by studying either abnormal deviations of the uterus or extraordinary experiences it underwent during pregnancy conflated the association between aberrant motherhood (whether moral or biological) and the production of abnormality.[125] Ramírez, for his part, asserted that biological malformations appeared in the course of an individual's embryonic development but that the greater the anomaly, the more immediately it appeared after the fertilization of the egg.[126] The views of both physicians, and their notion that anomalous births were best understood as aberrations of Mexican women's reproductive anatomy, were emblematic of changes in broader patterns of the apprehension and treatment of both regular and irregular childbirth that Mexican women experienced over the course of the nineteenth century.

6 Obstetrics, Gynecology, and Birth

· ·

Of all the dimensions of childbirth and contraception, the history of routine births is the most difficult to apprehend. Before the mid-nineteenth century, routine births transpired outside the domain of existent documentation. Midwives, who delivered most infants born in Mexico, did not keep written records of their work, and before the mid-nineteenth century, medically or criminally exceptional births were virtually the only ones that generated written acknowledgment. Physicians in Mexico were not active in obstetrical medicine until the close of the eighteenth century. Comprehensive censuses, which would at least indicate changes to birthrates and statistics about infant and maternal mortality, do not exist for years prior to 1895. In contrast to Anglo America, the Spanish American context does not supply a tradition of personal records in which women recorded details about birth and birth control in journals, memoirs, and letters;[1] they either could not or would not produce records about such intimate matters.

In the colonial period, a public discourse about routine childbirth that the majority of Mexican women experienced was virtually nonexistent. The Archivo General de Indias in Seville, one of the richest archival repositories of colonial history, houses few records that deal with childbirth in Spanish America. The bureaucrats, magistrates, and notaries who generated the ocean of documentation that constitutes the archive did so during the conceptions, pregnancies, and childbirths of their wives, lovers, daughters, and sisters across the viceroyalties of Spanish America and yet virtually no record of these fundamental events required acknowledgment in the administrative documentation they produced. The state rarely imposed regulations on childbirth. Besides the initiation of the licensing of midwifery after 1750, one of the few state regulations involving childbirth in the Bourbon era was a proclamation Viceroy Branciforte issued in 1797 urging midwives and surgeons in New Spain to use the balsam of the copaiba tree instead of the other materials—tallow, cinders, salt, or grease—that they habitually applied to newborns' umbilici. Cuban health practitioners had discovered that copaiba balsam alleviated the *mal de siete días* (seven days' illness), which caused convulsive fits and death in newborns, and also that it proved effective on all manner of skin disorders.[2]

The absence of documentation about routine childbirth in the colonial record carries significance beyond the challenge it poses for the reconstruction of this history. It is also indicative of colonial Mexicans' attitudes toward childbirth. In the colonial period, birth was at once a private matter and an event so ubiquitous that it fell below the purview of state, medical, or public notice. Childbirth was thus everywhere and nowhere. Most deliveries occurred in private settings where midwives and family members attended laboring women. Some women also gave birth alone. The mechanics of birth were unacknowledged aside from unrecorded conversations that occurred among those in attendance. While the questions and concerns that we occasionally glimpse in criminal and Inquisition trials indicate that expectant mothers in eighteenth-century Mexico sometimes felt trepidation and anxiety in the weeks approaching childbirth and thus brought such concerns to their midwives, the overwhelming impression the colonial record conveys is that mothers and other community members viewed the act of giving birth as a pedestrian event.

From the perspective of most Mexican mothers, the uneventfulness of giving birth endured through the nineteenth century. For example, Tomasa Montiel, a servant in Mexico City tried for infanticide in 1880, testified that she had given birth in a matter of moments in the middle of the night, silently and totally alone, in the kitchen of her employer's house after slipping out of the room she shared with her employer. Members of the household in which she lived and state officials who tried her case both accepted Montiel's experience as normal.[3] Yet while many women continued to understand birth as an affair undeserving of particular notification, over the course of the nineteenth century the public discourse about birth within the realms of the state, the popular press, and the medical establishment changed significantly. In such arenas, childbirth transformed from its former status as an unremarkable and private matter at the end of the colonial period to an event of intense public concern by the close of the nineteenth century. Such is evident, as this chapter discusses, in the new prominence of nationalist obstetrical medicine in republican Mexico, the establishment of maternity hospitals in the last third of the nineteenth century, and the prominent discussions of childbirth that appeared in popular news and scientific publications from the mid-nineteenth century onward.

Some patterns common to the various dimensions of childbirth and contraception examined in earlier chapters also characterize the history of birth in the period from the mid-eighteenth to the late nineteenth century. First, the heightened awareness nineteenth-century Mexicans paid to the sexual and reproductive practices of a wider portion of the country's female population discussed in chapters 3 and 4 coincided with and was partially responsible for the greater scrutiny Mexicans directed at childbirth over the course of this period. Second, as treated in chapters 1 and 2, various medical practices dating from pre-Columbian and early colonial contexts endured though the nineteenth century, although both early modern European midwifery techniques and national medical procedures modified these in the setting of newly established maternity hospitals in the last third of the nineteenth century.

Mexico's experience presents some counternarratives to the prevalent story of the modernization of childbirth in other contexts whereby physicians wrested control over childbirth from traditional midwives. While it would be distortive to present midwife-physician relations in Mexico as exclusively harmonious, neither were their interactions always characterized by unilateral domination. By the close of the nineteenth century, professional physicians delivered increasing numbers of babies using new birth procedures in institutional settings and urban centers—but not always to the betterment of women's health. High rates of fatal puerperal infection accompanied physicians' increased use of surgical interventions during childbirth. But neither professional obstetricians nor the modernizing medical practices they used did away with midwives, who continued to deliver most children born in Mexico to the turn of the twentieth century.

Midwifery and Childbirth in the Colonial Period

Virtually the only sources that record the occurrence of prosaic births in New Spain were those printed in state circulars—royal *cédulas* or viceregal *bandos*—that announced the advent of royal and noble births. Administrators frequently considered their occurrence significant enough that they ensured the distribution of such news to the most local administrative level. *Bandos* announcing royal births were read aloud in individual communities across New Spain throughout the colonial period. Needless to say, such notices were totally devoid of all mechanical details about the births they heralded beyond the joyous acknowledgment that they had occurred. King Charles III notified his subjects on September 28, 1772, for example, that "divine mercy had deigned to grant a happy and blessed birth to the Princess, my cherished daughter-in-law, who gave birth at twelve minutes past five in the afternoon of the nineteenth of the current month to a child (who has been named Carlos Clemente)."[4] Similarly, on August 9, 1794, the *Gazeta de México* announced that "at 6:15 in the morning, the most excellent Señora Virreina Marquesa de Branciforte gave birth to a darling girl";[5] this was followed with lengthy details about all the guests in attendance at the baptism. Beyond encouraging the celebration of the continuity of royal lineage, community listeners might have had other cause to celebrate these births, for they were occasionally associated with acts of regal benevolence. Thus the *teniente general* of the small community of Yanquitlan, Oaxaca, announced on July 30, 1708, to "every resident and inhabitant of all estates and conditions" that all prisoners of the jails of New Spain were pardoned and set at liberty and acknowledgment of God's grace in assuring the happy childbirth of the queen, María Luiza Gabriela.[6]

In the colonial period, births of royal heirs and of the upper nobility were events worthy of public notice because they involved the generation of members of the powerful families who ruled colonial society. New Spaniards considered few other births in this light, however. The retreat of discussions of childbirth from New Spain's public record marked a change from pre-Columbian Mexico's communal recognition of childbirth at less lofty levels of Mexican society. In that period, midwives had occupied an important practical and symbolic position because of their work in ensuring the reproduction of children of all classes. Commoners and nobility alike had revered childbirth and its participants. Early postcontact sources also provide detailed coverage of birth practices and of the respect the Nahua—whose religious pantheon included Tlazolteotl, goddess of birth and filth—held for birth, birthing women, and birth assistants. According to Bernardino de Sahagún's sixteenth-century informants, midwives were skilled in various procedures to be used in difficult births. For instance, in cases in which childbirth could not occur because the fetus had died within the mother's womb, midwives might perform an embryotomy (an operation involving the dissection and removal from the uterus of an embryo). In such instances, once having obtained permission from the laboring woman's family, a midwife, "who was skilled and able in her work, when she saw that the baby had died inside its mother, because it was clear that it was not moving, and that the patient was in great pain, then put her hand in the patient's place of generation, and with a knife of stone, cut the body [of the fetus] and took it out in pieces."[7]

Women whose families prohibited embryotomies and who died in childbirth for this or other reasons were subsequently known as goddesses, *mocihuaquetzque* (valiant women), and were honored for having died as warriors.[8] Nahua communities were so convinced of the supernatural powers of *mocihuaquetzque* that the robbing of their tombs was a frequent problem.[9] But whether they died in childbirth or survived it, the Nahua recognized and respected the fundamental and difficult societal contributions made by all women who gave birth, describing the successful act of birth in that belligerent society's most respectful tones as a "manly victory."[10]

Sahagún and others recorded extensive details about the medical practices pre-Columbian and early postconquest midwives employed. We know they encouraged laboring women to adopt vertical birth positions—crouching, squatting, or sometimes kneeling while suspended from an overhanging beam.[11] As labor became more intense, they instructed *tenedoras*, or occasionally male *tenedores*, to support women in upright positions and physically restrain them while they labored. Midwives intervened to facilitate stalled labor by massaging and turning the fetus and by the manual dilation of the vulva. They also fumigated the vulva at birth with a vapor created from boiling the herb rue.[12]

During the colonial period women increasingly adopted the use of birthing stools favored by early modern European midwives. By the turn of the nineteenth century, physicians often encouraged women to assume the supine position while laboring and giving birth, but their patients resisted this change. In his 1910 history of obstetrics, obstetrician Nicolas León reproduced the observations of a late nineteenth-century obstetrician who practiced in the city of Puebla. With regard to the positions Mexican women assumed during the act of childbirth, doctor Antonio Villanueva commented, "In our society, one custom endures that is the cause of serious obstacles, whose existence belies civilization and progress." The offending act was *Poblana* midwives' custom—"origin and consequence of the gravest evils and the most absurd preoccupations"—of placing women in labor upon the "birthing chair." Worse still, on other occasions they positioned women on thin mats, and in positions of great discomfort and suffering, they gave birth on their knees. "Only in very few cases," Villanueva concluded, "do we see women assuming for this supreme act the only acceptable position, the only rational position: the horizontal position." Later he observed that in such cases when the women did assume the supine position, the midwife was "almost always subordinated to the direction of a surgeon."[13]

In the pre-Columbian era and throughout the colonial period, midwives prescribed various substances to accelerate contractions if labor was stalled, including the labor accelerator *cihuapatli*. Midwives' ubiquitous usage of such medicines present one explanation for Mexican women's enduring patronage of these health care providers when faced with European alternatives. A 1788 Jesuit medical tract printed in Mexico counseled that women could facilitate birth by "drinking the urine of their husbands when they were on the point of giving birth."[14] Another remedy that European medical sources endorsed, as recorded in the *Boticario general* of both Spain and New Spain in the late colonial period, was a solution of horse manure diluted in wine that laboring women were encouraged to drink, perhaps because it was a substance so disgusting that it provoked vomiting and in turn accelerated labor contractions.[15]

Drawing from a practice long used in both European and pre-Columbian midwifery, colonial midwives might also provoke contractions when labor was stalled by puncturing the amniotic sac with either their fingernails or hooked instruments. In 1775, physician Ignacio Segura issued a tract in which he chastised those who used this method, cautioning that the operation should only be undertaken in the most desperate circumstances.[16] In his *Cartilla nueva util y necesaria*, published in Mexico in 1806, however, Antonio Medina indicated that the Protomedicato (medical board) endorsed midwives' performance of the procedure.[17]

One important duty that midwives performed in pre-Columbian central Mexico was the blessing of parturient women and their offspring.[18] After cutting off newborns' umbilical cords, midwives explained the roles and expectations that awaited male and female Nahuas: "If it was male, she gave the umbilical cord to soldiers so they would take it to the place where they battled . . . so the boy would have a love of war. If it was female, they buried it near the hearth and . . . in this way, she would love to be home and make things that were necessary for eating."[19] Baby girls, like boys, were bathed and welcomed to their communities, but were also warned of the works and fatigue that awaited them in the labor of their lives.

A second early colonial source describing pre-Columbian birth procedures among the Nahuas, the 1541–42 *Codex Mendoza* (see fig. 10),

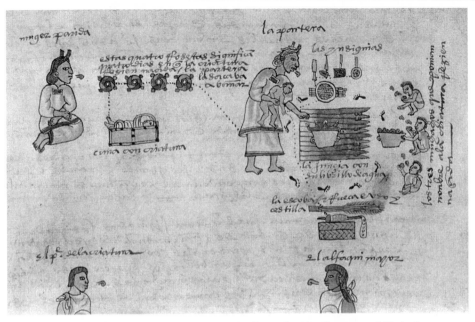

FIGURE 10 Midwife in naming ceremony in the *Codex Mendoza*, 1534. MS. Arch Selden. A. 1, fol. 57r. Credit: The Bodleian Libraries, The University of Oxford.

described how four days after the infant's birth the midwife bathed the infant and performed its naming ceremony: "If it was a boy, they carried him with his symbol in his hand; and the symbol was the tool used by the infant's father, whether of the military or professions like metalworker, woodcarver, or whatever other profession . . . if the infant was a girl, the symbol they gave her for bathing was a distaff with its spindle and its basket, and a broom, which were the things she would use when she grew up."[20]

Indigenous, Spanish, and mixed-race midwives continued to preside over most births throughout the nineteenth century. León conflates the past and the present when addressing Mexico's indigenous population's birth practices in the first one hundred pages of *La obstetricia en México*, where he treats "the pre-Columbian, colonial, and present obstetrical customs of the various Indian tribes of our territory."[21] Even in complicated births, such as were recorded in the birth notices of the late eighteenth-century *Gazeta de México*, upper-class women still often opted to be attended by midwives rather than physicians.

In his satirical portrait of life in New Spain during the last decades of colonial rule, Mexico's first novelist, Joaquin José Fernández de Lizardi, detailed the earliest hours of the life of his eponymous protagonist in the novel *El Periquillo Sarniento*, translated into English as *The Mangy Parrot*. Born in Mexico City in the early 1770s to parents of middling but modest means, Sarniento relates,

> After I was born, following the baths and other necessities of the hour, my aunts and grandmothers and other old-fashioned ladies wanted to bind my hands and wrap me up as tight as a bottle-rocket. . . .
>
> They then drew from a basket a length of ribbon that they called an *amulet sash*, adorned with *deer's eye seeds*, *azabache hand charms*, *crocodile teeth*, and other such trinkets, so as to dress me up with these relics of superstitious paganism on the same day that had been set aside for my godparents to profess, on my behalf, my faith in the holy religion of Christ.[22]

The tokens and charms the women used derive from both Old World and New World traditions.[23]

The engraving depicting this scene in the 1830 edition of *El Perquillo Sarniento*, attributed to illustrator Luis Montes de Oca, shows a parturient woman reclining in the corner of room, tended by a second woman who offers her a bowl of broth (see fig. 11).[24] A third woman holds a tightly swaddled baby, and a fourth, presumably a midwife, holds a strip of cloth, perhaps a belt or possibly a mask. A well-dressed man waves off the women, and the caption reads, "Lord help me! How my father had had to fight against the old ladies' prejudices!"[25] The rare snapshot Fernández de Lizardi provides of a postnatal scene in late colonial Mexico illustrates both the man's frustration at the superstitious customs of the "benditas viejas"—older women whose beliefs and practices were drawn from earlier traditions originating in both Spain and ancient America and the extraordinary persistence of such customs that middle- and upper-class urban creoles continued to employ through the eve of Mexican independence.

Physicians and their understanding of obstetrics and gynecology played a marginal role in most women's experiences of childbirth in colonial Mexico. As was discussed in chapter 2, by the end of the colonial era a small number of elite women in urban Mexico presumably preferred the services of male physicians to those of female midwives. *El Diario de México* published an article in 1806 in response to a foreign reader's query about where he might locate a competent surgeon to assist his wife in

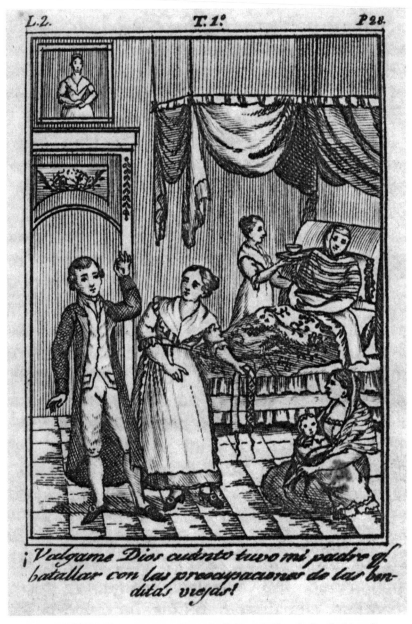

FIGURE 11 Birth chamber, ca. 1830. From José Joaquín Fernández de Lizardi, *El Periquillo Sarniento*. Credit: Nettie Lee Benson Latin American Collection, University of Texas Libraries, the University of Texas at Austin.

childbirth. The paper advised that he should visit hospitals in the capital city where he would be directed to surgeons practiced in delivering babies in natural and complicated births.[26] But, as Nicolás León observed, the adoption of European obstetrical medicine occurred in this period "only among inhabitants of cities and significant towns, for everywhere else, even today, colonial customs mixed with survival of Indian customs survive."[27]

Physicians may have connoted status and education, but pregnant women in late colonial Mexico—even those of high status—most often trusted midwives rather than doctors with assisting them at childbirth. In a letter published in 1805 in *El Diario de México*, one recently widowed father bewailed his late wife's insistence that a midwife should attend her during childbirth. His wife had refused to have a male surgeon attend her birthing "because our general custom is to entrust ourselves to barbarous women, without more schooling than that of having themselves given birth, for the assistance of our wives at this most critical moment, which is invested with their lives, our happiness and that of our children."[28] A letter "a husband" sent to the paper the following year complained of the disastrous custom that "innumerable women" in the kingdom retained of visiting midwives on a monthly basis during pregnancy to have their wombs manipulated in order to ensure the correct placement of the fetuses they carried; such operations, he contested, resulted frequently in miscarriages, difficult labors, and disease or deformity in the offspring after birth.[29]

These two men despaired of midwives' medical practices at childbirth, but other community members criticized them for the religious acts they enacted in colonial bedrooms. The *castiza partera* Isabel Hernández, for instance, testified to the Inquisition in 1652 that on one occasion she had assisted at the lengthy labor of a slave woman. To provoke her labor, midwife Hernández had given her the "huevo de la Ascención," explaining that she had previously learned that a hen's egg preserved from the day of Christ's ascension (celebrated on the fortieth day after Easter) until the same day the following year had medicinal qualities. After drinking part of such an egg dissolved in wine, the slave woman had succeeded in giving birth to her child.[30] In a set of cases dating from 1627, several witnesses denounced a group of mulata midwives to the Inquisition for superstition. Witnesses described the midwives' practice of inducing the women to quickly produce the afterbith by removing religious relics the birthing mothers had kept close to them during labor.[31]

One early eighteenth-century mestiza midwife, María Calvillo, apparently placed "old shoes and a horn" under the beds of women she attended in an effort to facilitate their deliveries.[32] As in this case, many of the midwives brought before the Holy Office were accused of having cast spells or used supernatural powers to provide physical or spiritual help or harm to members of their communities.[33] Although physician Ignacio Segura encouraged midwives to "pray and ask God for a happy outcome in deliveries," he chastised those who used "prohibited and suspicious prayers in their work."[34] In the colonial era, the church sanctioned dozens of prayers and devotions to various saints to ensure happy outcomes at childbirth, but the Inquisition investigated other ritual practices deemed heterodox, including the custom of feeding women wafers inscribed with prayers to the Immaculate Virgin at the moment of birth.[35]

Besides tending to women in labor and to their newborns after birth, midwives in late eighteenth-century and nineteenth-century Mexico also performed baptisms on newborns, as they had done in the pre-Columbian era. Newborns who died before they could be baptized risked their souls' perdition, so midwives performed these rites as emergency measures. When Oaxaqueña midwife Felipa Romero saw that the newborn she had delivered after a protracted labor in 1837 was struggling to breathe, she promptly baptized him.[36] Both Inquisition and criminal trials reveal, however, that members of the public occasionally complained to authorities about errors in the manner in which such baptisms were performed. In 1713, midwife María Calvillo was denounced for using hot water mixed with salt to baptize newborns, and in 1774, one woman who had recently given birth brought midwife María Guadalupe Sánchez to the attention of the Holy Office for having arranged for her newborn to be baptized two times.[37]

In the second half of the eighteenth century, the Bourbon state explicitly supported midwives' performance of the rite of baptism in urgent situations. In 1749, Charles III (then King of Sicily but later King of Spain as well) issued a *pragmática* requiring that fetuses be extracted live from the wombs of mothers who died in childbirth in order to ensure newborns' celestial salvation through the rite of baptism. In this text, Charles decreed his support for a medicoecclesiastical tract first published seven years earlier by Sicilian canon and inquisitor Francisco Cangiamila.[38] Cangiamila's text declared that in instances where women died during pregnancy or childbirth, fetuses must be extracted from their mothers' bodies through the "caesarean operation." When no doctor was available, priests themselves must be ready to perform the task. (Cangiamila advised them to equip themselves with sharp knives so they would always be prepared to act.) Charles republished his *pragmática* in 1761, accompanying it with a Latin version of Cangiamila's text and decreeing that those who were not prepared to perform the operation could be charged with infanticide and prosecuted under penalty of death.

Ecclesiastics and statesmen embraced the task of publicizing the decree in New Spain; Cangiamila's text was reproduced in two different translations in Mexico in the 1770s. Franciscan friar Joseph Manuel Rodríguez translated the tract and published it in Mexico in 1772 under the title *La caridad del sacerdote para con los niños encerrados en el vientre de sus madres difuntas y documentos de la utilidad y necesidad de su práctica.*[39] Both Viceroy don Antonio María de Bucareli and Archbishop Alonso Núñez de Haro y Peralta endorsed Rodríguez's text. The archbishop advised all curates and vicars to buy Rodríguez's "little book" which would equip them "in a convenient and simple way" how to perform caesareans.

Ignacio Segura issued a second translation of the work in 1775, under the title *Avisos saludables a las parteras para el cumplimento de su obligación* (Healthful counsel for midwives in the fulfillment of their obligations). This edition, as its title implies, was directed much more explicitly at midwives. Segura's text is one of the few extant sources that discusses the birthing procedures Mexican midwives used—or at least were instructed to use—in the late colonial period, though because it was a written text it would have been accessible only to a small proportion of midwives operating in the viceroyalty. Rather than counseling priests on how to perform caesarean sections, Segura's tract focused on midwives' obligation to extract fetuses from deceased women and baptize them themselves: "If the baby is born but there is a danger it will die before being taken to church, the midwife must baptize it."[40] Midwives were to be vigilant in cases when babies were born prematurely or without crying, those who had difficulty breathing, those who appeared weak, or those whose mothers' labor had been overly strenuous. They should also be prepared to intervene if they feared that the infant's parents might kill it, "as occurs with some illegitimate babies."[41]

The first reports of the performance of caesarians on live women were published in the pages of the *Gazeta de México*. The May 29, 1779, edition of the paper contained a report from the Santa Clara Mission in California, where two missionaries had performed the operation on an indigenous woman eight months pregnant and afflicted by a violent fever. "Neither their ignorance of anatomy, their lack of medical texts, nor the fact that they had never witnessed the operation deterred them from their goal," the *Gazeta* commented. Immediately upon the laboring woman's death, the friars performed the operation, "whose success exceeded the expectations of the fathers, who were delighted they were able to baptize the extracted child . . . who only survived for seven hours after the operation."[42] Over sixteen years later, the *Gazeta* reported that one Brígida Ruíz from the town of Chiautla de la Sal had died when a caesarean operation was performed on her. A five-month-old infant was extracted live from her womb, but died shortly thereafter.[43] Two years later, in September 1798, missionaries in Sonora again performed the operation on an Indian convert to Christianity. The Mission of San Antonio de Oquitoa in Sonora reported that

> María Antonia Zapatito, wife of Cristóbal Bravo, an Indian from this mission, died here on this date. She was five or six months' pregnant and Father Ramón López, desiring to bless the fetus with holy Baptism . . . instructed the midwife and retired sergeant Francisco López de Xeres, that according to Cangiamila's instructions, they would be the agents of the operation. . . . The sergeant, prepared with a vessel of water, proceeded to open her right side with a shaving knife. The midwife inserted her hands into the womb, and in the short time of two minutes, removed the pouch containing the baby [criatura], who was baptized, surviving afterward for eight minutes.[44]

These eighteenth-century reports of caesareans' performance were highly exceptional, however. Despite the various types of surgical interventions at childbirth that the Mexican medical establishment embraced in the last third of the nineteenth century, caesarean sections were rarely performed in that period or in the decades before it. Francisco de Asis Flores y Troncoso commented that the first occurrence of a caesarean operation in which a mother managed to survive did not occur until 1850, and this only under highly exceptional circumstances: a physician at the Hospital of San Pablo in Mexico City had managed to extract a fetus from the gaping wound that a kicking cow had inflicted upon a woman's navel. He cleaned and closed the wound, and bled the patient. Six hours later, she had expelled the placenta vaginally. Subsequently the woman survived a severe infection of her abdominal walls.[45] This unusual case is one of the few references to the operation in nineteenth-century sources.

Caesareans are not discussed in the records of either the Casa de Maternidad or the Escuela Nacional de Medicina. Unlike such procedures as embryotomies, the caesarean operation was the topic of no nineteenth-century medical publication in Mexico.[46] The operation is rarely discussed in the premier medical journal founded in 1864, the *Gaceta Médica de México*, although there are passing mentions of the operation's execution in hospitals in 1866 and 1867, the latter instance in a postmortem operation.[47] References to caesareans in nineteenth-century news periodicals occurred in two 1853 notices in *El Siglo Diez y Nueve*, when the Bishop of Puebla issued a pastoral declaring that the priesthood should continue to perform caesareans on mothers who died in labor, reprinting long passages from Cangiamila's 1742 text.[48] The small number of caesarean births occurring in nineteenth-century Mexico was not unusual; the operation was not performed widely in the United States or Europe, either, until the mid-twentieth century.

Nineteenth-Century Continuities

Caesarean births were rare and unsuccessful novelties in late colonial and nineteenth-century Mexico, but many of the medical practices relating to childbirth in this period are striking in terms of their retention of pre-Columbian medical knowledge and practice. Various medical and obstetrical texts published in the colonial era and in nineteenth-century Mexico included directions for preparing medicines for laboring or for women in the postpartum period that included ingredients used in the pre-Columbian era. Sixteenth-century writers, including Martín de la Cruz, Francisco Hernández, and Gregorio López, for instance, all described the various analgesic and obstetrical conditions for which Indians in the pre-Columbian and colonial period had used *toronjil* (giant Mexican hyssop).[49] In his important eighteenth-century medical treatise *Florilegio medicinal*, Juan de Esteyneffer detailed various treatments that could be administered to newborns. When a baby suffered from a sore on his head, Esteyneffer recommended the application of a plaster made from the child's mother's milk and the finely ground powder of copal, a tree resin whose medicinal use originated in the pre-Columbian period.[50] Several late colonial *boticario* and medical manuals contain remedies for treating parturient women that maintained midwifery practices from earlier periods. One handwritten medicinal guide from 1750 counseled that "discomfort at birth" could be treated by making a "tortilla of eggs, rotten cheese, rose oil, and a powder made from tequesquite [a mineral salt used since pre-Hispanic times]. This is put on the stomach, and [the patient] should drink guava syrup."[51]

Such continuities endured through the nineteenth century as well. Even as medical authorities such as Flores dismissed the barbarity of indigenous-influenced midwifery practices, evidence survives of the extent to which such practices continued, and even of their incorporation in state-regulated medical texts. One 1863 obstetrical text created for Oaxaca's official medical licensing course, the *Cartilla de partos escrita esclusivamente para que sirva de testo en el curso que debe darse a las parteras en el Instituto del Estado* (Reader on childbirth written exclusively for use as a text in the course that midwives must take in the state institute), provided an extensive list of medicines and remedies midwives might administer to women during and after labor. For fits of intensive trembling, midwives might provide a mixture composed of four ounces of "flor de tilio," twelve drops of "licor andonino de Hoffman," (a mixture of alcohol and ether) and one half-ounce saffron syrup. Flor de tilio (*Tilia americana*) refers to the flowers from a tree indigenous to Mexico used as a sedative in the pre-Columbian period.[52] An inventory of the medicine Mexico City's Casa de Maternidad stocked in 1876 also contains the names of several medicines midwives administered in the precolonial and colonial eras, including *manzanilla* (chamomile), *tilia*, *beleño* (a toxic nightshade), *flores de sauco* (elderberry flowers), and *tintura de pimienta* (tincture of pepper).[53]

In 1867, physician Aniceto Ortega commented on the efficacy of pre-Columbian obstetrical practices he had witnessed in his field practice in the countryside of the north central district of San Luis Potosí. He noted that "the certain effects of a few teaspoons of mezcal [distilled agave alcohol] are commonly known, although few medical practitioners operating in this country have had occasion to witness there near infallible effects." He went on to explain that he had frequently witnessed mezcal's administration in the countryside of San Luis Potosí and had also observed the rarity of puerperal infections in that population: "In five years that I have practiced obstetrics in the countryside of this province, while having to use forceps and perform fetal inversions, often several days after the leaking of the amniotic liquid and the death of the fetus, and in the midst of such unfavorable and difficult conditions that I have sometimes feared the rupturing of the uterus, I have never seen the introduction of metroperitonitis [the inflammation of the peritoneum around the uterus], nor any other serious puerperal infection."[54] Along with praising mezcal's efficacy, Ortega suggested that the pre-Columbian delicacy *cuitlacoche*, a fungus grown on corn, likely possessed the same chemical properties— and the ability to induce uterine contractions—as *cuernecillo de centeno*, the drug derived from a fungus grown on rye.[55] Finally, it is noteworthy that Juan María Rodríguez, for all the contemporary despair his contemporaries expressed over midwives' dangerous administration of *cihuapatli*, observed in his canonical *Guía clínica del arte de los partos* (1878) that an extract of the plant could be usefully administered after the expulsion of both the fetus and the placenta to prevent hemorrhaging.[56]

Surgical Interventions

While elements of pre-Columbian medicines persisted in nineteenth-century institutional obstetrics, one broad obstetrical change this period witnessed was an increase in surgical interventions during birth. In the colonial era, physicians who published obstetrical tracts in Mexico advocated the cautious use of medical interventions. Juan de Esteyneffer, writing in 1713, observed that a normal period of labor might extent up to twenty-four hours; only if labor extended beyond this time did women require medical intervention.[57] Antonio Medina noted that in most cases, no assistance was needed to encourage the fetus's exit from the womb beyond the "forces of nature."[58] José Ventura Pastor advised allowing nature to take its course during normal births, but noted that an exhausted woman with a rapid pulse who was having difficulty breathing might be bled from the heel.[59] In most cases, however, Ventura prescribed nothing stronger than broth for laboring women. For pain relief, he counseled that a cloth soaked in warm, unsalted lard might be placed on the womb.[60] He also described how he sometimes administered purgatives for women whose labor was stalled. European physicians also began endorsing the use of a naturally occurring chemical compound, ergotamine, (in Spanish also called *cunernecillo de centeno*) to precipitate women's labor when it was stalled, although midwives had already been using it for this purpose and for its antibleeding properties for some time.[61] Pedro Vidart and others recommended applying pressure on the mother's perineum during contractions to diminish the risk of tearing when the fetal head crowned.[62] Physicians advised that fetuses inauspiciously positioned for easy birth might be turned via manual manipulations.[63] With the possible exception of the bleeding, all the procedures colonial medical texts described would have been practices already familiar to most midwives.

By the 1780s, and increasingly over the course of the subsequent century, the types of procedures obstetricians could and did perform became more distinctive. Physicians began to increasingly advocate the use of surgical instruments to perform more vigorous interventions than they had in earlier periods. Writing in 1789, Ventura advised that if the cervix of a woman in labor failed to fully dilate on its own, it was sometimes necessary to make two or three incisions in it to facilitate birth. More dramatic interventions required the use of instruments, including the *tenazas corbas* (curved pincers), *tenazas en cuchara* (spoon-shaped pincers), and various types of forceps in cases where the fetus became lodged in the pelvic cavity of the mother.

With unsterile conditions or improper application, the use of such instruments could be disastrous. When used correctly, they could and did save both women's lives and those of their children. Scarce evidence survives about their employment in colonial Mexico, but Ventura's tract, which was influential in Mexico, provides considerable detail on such experiences in Madrid. In his *Preceptos generales* he included detailed clinical notes about individual births he attended, including his frequent application of his preferred instrument, the spooned pincers, to extract both live infants and dead fetuses trapped in his patients' uteruses. On one such occasion in 1763, Ventura had attended an exhausted woman whose labor was arrested because her fetus's very large head could not pass through her narrow pelvic cavity. The woman, who had lost a baby in a previous birth in identical circumstances, had already labored for twenty hours. The fetus's head was so far advanced in her pelvis that Ventura was unable to insert his hand and turn it in order to perform a foot-first extraction. Taking the precaution of baptizing the fetus by means of a syringe, Ventura introduced the "smooth spoons" (pictured in fig. 12) into his patient's vagina, positioning them on the fetus's head. He successfully extracted a large girl who, at the time of his text's publication, twenty-six years later, was still living, and whom he declared had experienced no graver repercussions from her difficult birth than two small scars that had quickly healed.[64] Over the course of the next two decades, physicians on the Continent and abroad received more frequent training of instruments like those Ventura advocated. By 1805, Mexican doctor

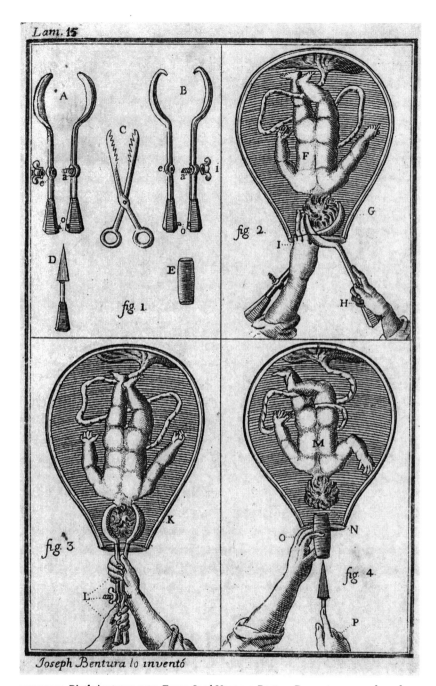

FIGURE 12 Birth instruments. From José Ventura Pastor, *Preceptos generales sobre las operaciones del parto* vol. 1 (1789), plate 15. Credit: Wellcome Library, London.

José Miguel Muñoz, for example, had established a reputation of success with forceps deliveries.[65]

As surgical interventions became more common, the state moved to restrict the kinds of procedures midwives could legally perform. In 1794 the viceregal state issued a circular declaring that doctors, *boticarios*, and midwives were required to assist patients who needed their aid, but that in life-threatening cases such medical personnel were also obliged to provide the details of the cases to local magistrates.[66] The Protomedicato received occasional complaints requesting that it enforce the prohibition, which midwives and their clients likely ignored in most instances.[67] After the turn of the century, medical professionals—including the director of the Real Escuela de Cirugía, Antonio Serrano—continued to lobby for stricter professional regulation.

Professional training and regulation of all branches of medicine intensified at both the state and federal levels in the nineteenth century, particularly after the 1833 founding of the Esctablecimiento de Ciencias Médicas and the 1841 creation of the Consejo Superior de Salubridad, the federal public health regulatory board.[68] In the postindependence era, each state in the republic followed its own regulations in terms of medical training and licensing. Various cities established formal midwifery training programs in the first half of the nineteenth century including Mexico City (1833), Mérida (1835), Guadalajara (1837), Puebla (1841), and Morelia (1848); others followed later in the century.[69] While the number of formal midwifery programs and the rate at which women enrolled in them certainly grew over the century, licensed practitioners continued to represent a minority of those who practiced midwifery. Between 1841 and 1888, only 140 women enrolled in the program at the Establecimiento de Ciencias Médicas, and in 1866, municipal records indicated that a total of only twenty-four licensed midwifes were practicing in Mexico City.[70] Some foreign midwives claiming they had license to do so, also practiced in at least the country's urban capitals by midcentury. For example, one Mexico City daily published an advertisement in 1849 of one "Señora C. Simon, a midwife from Paris's faculty of medicine, accredited in Mexico, who offered her services to anyone doing the honor of confiding in her."[71]

Over the course of the nineteenth century, legislation routinely prohibited all midwives (licensed or not) from performing any procedures prescribed for arduous childbirths, though the fact of the oft-repeated legislation indicates that midwives persisted in performing prohibited operations. In 1845 the Consejo Superior de Salubridad decreed that "no one was permitted to perform the duties of a midwife who has not acquired the principals and studies that the art requires."[72] The following year, the same body declared that *parteras* should restrict themselves only to the tasks of receiving the baby, cutting the umbilical cord, giving first aid in case of asphyxiation, and informing parties when the services of a doctor were required.[73] Legislation dating from 1852 mandated that midwives call a *professor medico-cirujano* (doctor of medical surgery) to assist them in cases of complicated deliveries.[74] In 1857, the Consejo Superior de Salubridad prohibited midwives from "applying any remedy of any kind, and from practicing any operations."[75] In 1892 the Ministerio de Gobernación, operating under president Porfirio Díaz, explicitly decreed that midwives could not use instruments in their deliveries, nor could they administer anesthesia or intrauterine injections.[76] Midwives responded to the regulation with public indignation. A short article in the anti-Porfirian newspaper *El Hijo del Ahuizote* reported on May 15, 1892, that "the midwives have protested against the regulation that the Consejo Superior de Salubridad has imposed on them, which they see as tyrannical. These Tuxtepecos are tyrannizing humanity even during the birth, before the birth, and after the birth (hasta en el parto, antes del parto, y después del parto)."[77]

The particular choice of language is telling, for *El Hijo*'s writer was making an ironic reference here to a line from the Catholic catechism as articulated first by Pope Paul V's 1555 decree that Jesus Christ "was born from the virginal womb of the Holy Virgin Mary, who was herself a Virgin before the birth, during the birth, and after the birth."[78] The connotations of both virginity and childbirth to which the phrase alluded had shifted dramatically from its colonial meaning of the Catholic doctrine of Mary's perpetual virginity and the particular significance this held for women operating in the social and racial context of colonial Mexico to its concrete evocation in the 1892 usage of a woman in the literal act of giving birth. In the second setting, it referred specifically to women's physical production of children, and its importance in the generation of a modern nation, a state that Díaz's critics understood his policies to imperil.

Opponents of the Díaz regime apparently supported midwives' abilities to participate in medical interventions at birth, but other nineteenth-century Mexicans sporadically initiated legal suits over their ability to perform these. In 1837, for example, a medical doctor initiated a criminal investigation of infanticide against Oaxaqueña midwife Felipa Romero.

The physician declared that he had been called to the home of María Josefa Nuñez, a single woman, twenty years of age, who had just given birth. He said he found her with her "vagina torn and her uterus completely maimed." Nuñez herself testified that during the birth she had felt excruciating pain in her "parte pudenda [vagina]" but could not ascertain what class of instrument Romero had used upon her. A second physician who examined Nuñez declared that she had an inch-long incision on the lower part of her vulva "apparently made with an instrument." As for her baby, Nuñez asserted that it had been born alive, but that the midwife had baptized it for fear it was on the brink of death. Fifteen minutes later it stopped breathing.[79]

Ignacio Castañeda, a municipal judge, ordered Romero apprehended and demanded her explanation. Romero asserted that she had used no instruments on Nuñez and that the infant's death had been caused by the severity of Nuñez's intensive two-day labor and because of a blow Nuñez had suffered a few days before going into labor. She further declared that shortly after it was born, she had observed that "the baby started to make movements as if it was suffocating, for which reason [she] had sucked out its nostrils and taken other steps to stabilize it, and she noticed that a yellow substance was dripping from its nostrils."[80] Despite her efforts, Romero testified that the newborn died soon thereafter. After interviewing several other witnesses, including a male *tenedor*, the court ordered Romero imprisoned in the *casa de recogida* (house of female correction) while it completed its investigation.

A few days after her confinement, a third party, likely her *curador* drew up a powerful defense of her practices and submitted it to Castañeda. Although apparently illiterate (Romero did not know how to even sign her own name on the defense), the letter exemplifies Romero's extensive obstetrical knowledge. "How could it be otherwise," she asked, "than that a woman should suffer an extraordinary extension [to these parts] when not only the head of a naturally corpulent fetus, but also its lengthier span from shoulder to shoulder had forcibly passed through her vulva? Could this happen without detriment to her parte pudenda?" Later she argued that if the interpretation the best doctors of anatomy asserted was true—that the fetus naturally attempted to force itself out of its "maternal prison" during each contraction—it was also possible that mothers, because of exhaustion, fear, shame or malice, might attempt to stifle this expulsion. In such cases, as Romero believed had happened here, the fetus might dilate its chest and initiate the movement of its lungs but its mother might, with repellent motion, suffocate it before it was expelled.[81] Castañeda was sufficiently concerned to request that three different physicians provide their own evaluations of the parturient mother. Two determined that no instrument had been used, while the third concluded that a one-inch long incision on the lower part of the woman's vulva had been "apparently made with a cutting instrument—either [a piece of] glass or a knife."[82] Romero's judge, however, sided with the majority opinion. Acquitting Romero of all charges, he set her free.

In a second case, originating in 1879 in the rural community of Ejutla, Oaxaca, the father of Merced Carmona, a woman who had recently given birth, accused *partera* Getrudis Ramírez of making three incisions on his daughter.[83] In Ramirez's trial, Isabel Altamirano, another midwife who had examined Carmona, confirmed that the latter had three wounds in her genital area, all of them made with a cutting instrument.[84] In her defense, Ramírez testified that the baby, Carmona's first, had ripped the mother's inelastic perineum upon expulsion from her vagina. In a second examination nine days later, midwife Altamirano indicated that Carmona was faring so badly that she feared she might die.[85] A short time after this, however, Ramírez informed the court that obstetrics professor Doña Luz Riojano had examined and cured the recently delivered mother and begged the court to interview Riojano about her opinion of Carmona's wounds.[86] The court did not succeed in locating Riojano, and the resolution to Ramírez's case is not contained in her dossier. However, other evidence exists that the court released Ramirez and permitted her to continue working as a midwife, for two years later she again appeared before the court of Ejutla, this time to denounce one of her clients for committing infanticide.[87]

Both of these cases suggest that although members of the public and physicians were vigilant against the possibility of midwives undertaking medical procedures beyond those within their legal jurisdiction, judicial officials were liable to give the benefit of the doubt to midwives themselves, acquitting them of such charges when they judged them unfounded. These and other cases also indicate that although both the federal and state governments increasingly restricted those procedures that midwives could lawfully perform, and increasingly scrutinized their professional certification, neither endeavor was particularly effective. An 1894 news story reporting on the death of an infant at the hands of an "inexperienced midwife" lamented the absence of a law that "clearly specified which professionals required a legal title."[88] In fact, Mexico had had such a law with respect to midwifery for nearly a century and a half; the population simply did not adhere to it.

The Era of Obstetrical Institutionalization

Physicians' augmentation of surgical intervention over the course of the nineteenth century marked a significant shift in attitudes and practices toward childbirth in this period. While physicians had disdained the medicine of childbirth in the colonial era, in the second half of the nineteenth century obstetrical medicine became a central concern for the profession. In this era reproduction and childbirth—previously understood as private matters, unobserved and undocumented in public contexts—became a significant and respected area of medical expertise that was linked to state interests in the articulation of Mexico's national identity. Obstetrical issues featured prominently in the *Gaceta Médica de México*. The Casa de Maternidad (the capital city's first maternity hospital, founded in 1866 and equipped with an obstetrical clinic after 1870) and the *cátedra* (professorship) in gynecology the Escuela de Medicina de México created in 1887 provided venues in which physicians could study and train others in obstetrics. By the late nineteenth century, obstetrics and gynecology had become, in Laura Cházaro's estimation, central to "the problems of a nation in the process of becoming."[89] Verena Radkau similarly observes that in this era, Mexican physicians sought to construct a form of "medical nationalism" and contends that obstetrics became the most prominent branch of medicine that fomented this notion of national distinctiveness.[90] It was no coincidence that it was an obstetrician, A. J. Carbajal, whom the Porfirian state selected to represent Mexico in the first International Medical Congress held in Moscow in 1897.[91]

At the height of the Porfiriato, the mechanics of childbirth emerged as a matter of intensive public discussion and scrutiny in Mexico. In an intriguing contrast to the context of nineteenth-century Anglo America, where—two generations of scholars have argued—the nineteenth century marked the relegation of childbirth to the private realm away from its earlier, more public, position in pre-revolutionary America, childbirth became a central preoccupation of state and public concern in nineteenth-century Mexico.[92] The publicity of childbirth is most apparently marked in the increased role discussions about birth and obstetrical medicine played in daily publications. Mexican dailies covered news about the Casa de Maternidad from the 1850s to the 1890s, but also published frequent and detailed discussions about developments and services in ob-stetrical medicine, and frequently published advertisements directed at a readership of pregnant women.[93]

Included among them were such notices as an 1855 advertisement from one Dr. Hipólito Villaret announcing to Mexico City women "Healing—Quick and Dramatic or the art of healing punctually and without pain by this new method for illnesses of the womb, irregular menstruation . . . bloody or yellow flux . . . gonorrhea . . . narrowing of the uterus . . . and impotence."[94] An 1891 notification publicized the development of a new portable obstetrical table.[95] One lengthy 1870 article by Juan María Ro-dríguez referred to other contemporary periodical coverage of the capi-tal city's newly opened Casa de Maternidad. Rodríguez refuted articles in the *La Orquesta* and the *El Monitor Republicano* that suggested that medical staff at the Casa humiliated and shamed its patients by subject-ing them to "scientific study" that the "modesty of women prohibits not only in practice but even in thought."[96] The paper allotted Rodríguez over four columns of space to defend the Casa's motivations and operation, in which he explained that the growing numbers of women who sought the institution's medical services did so not to be subjected to nefarious sci-entific probing but instead to take advantage of the medical expertise offered to them there. These services, he wrote, were available to the "most virtuous women from the loftiest families to those most destitute and fallen."[97]

Beyond the growth of obstetrics in the public imagination depicted in such newspaper coverage, records from the Casa de Maternidad give some indication that Mexican women of various classes began adopting differ-ent attitudes toward childbirth in the last third of the century. We see this in their willingness to frequent the establishment. Although births at the Casa represented a fraction of the total number of births in the capital city, the fact that the institution was often filled to capacity in the 1870s through 1890s indicates that growing numbers of women considered a public hospital, as opposed to a private home, a suitable location for child-birth. The Casa's maternity ward was constructed to house thirty women. While in 1869, three years after its foundation, only thirteen women en-tered the Casa each month, ten years after its foundation that number had climbed to thirty per month. One decade later, an average of thirty-three women entered the facilities on a monthly basis.[98]

In the last quarter of the nineteenth century, a growing number of women in Mexico's urban centers thus chose to give birth in public, institutional settings, attended by state-regulated health practitioners. The increased publicity of childbirth and pregnancy is also apparent in the more frequent and explicit appearance of discussions of obstetrical medical practices in contemporary periodical literature and newspapers. But it was particularly within the venue of medical publications—theses, research reports, and procedural manuals—that the augmentation of gynecology and obstetrics to matters of national public concern is most apparent. In the last third of the nineteenth century, a new field of medical research that focused on understanding the reproductive biology that was nationally unique to Mexican women emerged. Documenting the gynecological distinctiveness of Mexican women became a central concern for many prominent late nineteenth-century practitioners.

Chapter 1 discussed how this preoccupation featured in Francisco de Asis Flores y Troncoso's 1885 tract *El hímen en México*, but his was only one of many such studies. In 1881 Florencio Flores, a contemporary of Francisco Flores and another student of the celebrated obstetrician Juan María Rodríguez, produced *Ligeros apuntes de pelvimetría comparada* (Brief points on the pelvimeter compared) as his medical thesis for the general examination in medicine, surgery, and obstetrics in 1881.[99] In this work Florencio Flores asserted that by comparing Mexican women's pelvises to those of European women described in medical textbooks, he would uncover "the reasons why childbirth is often difficult, if not dangerous, in Mexico."[100] He argued that such difficulties were due to the "resistance of the pelvic canal because of its crammed arrangement" in the bodies of his countrywomen. He concluded that the "Mexican pelvis presents a particular formation [from that of Europe], caused by the general reduction of all its dimensions, and especially that of its reduced height, and in the exaggerated slope of the pubic symphysis."[101] He also observed that the reason for Mexican women's differently formed pelvises was "the mixture of races," although he admitted it was difficult to determine how this had occurred.[102]

Both Francisco Flores and Florencio Flores derived their notions of Mexican women's distinctive reproductive anatomy from their mentor, Juan María Rodríguez, professor of obstetrics and maternity at the Casa de Maternidad and director of the Escuela Nacional de Medicina's museum of anatomy. Beginning in 1864, Rodríguez began publishing articles describing what he called "the fatal secret" of his nation's women: their pathologically narrowed (*acorazada*) pelvises.[103] Whereas European texts indicated women's pelvises normally measured ten to eleven centimeters, Mexican women's pelvises, Rodríguez declared, measured substantially smaller: from six to eight centimeters. Under such circumstances, the physician explained, it was essential for the medical profession and the Mexican public to embrace more interventionist birth procedures that alone could assure that women could safely give birth.[104] Rodríguez's disciples, furthering their mentor's claims, concluded that narrow pelvises were a distinctively national attribute of their developing mestizo nation.[105] Francisco Flores detailed elsewhere that along with their smaller pelvises and distinctively shaped hymens, Mexican women also had distinctively angled pelvises, vulvas that pointed in different directions from those of women from other nations, and shorter perinea.[106] All of these distinctive features of Mexican women's reproductive anatomy required the development of a specifically Mexican obstetrical practice, or in Flores's terms, a "tocológica mexicana."[107] Manuel Ramos, a Porfirian practitioner, published a paper in a national medical review in 1880 that described the existence of "a Mexican obstetrical school, that is to say that obstetrics is the branch of medicine that has created independence for itself."[108]

Laura Cházaro has argued that for Rodríguez, Flores, and many of their contemporaries, the field of specifically Mexican obstetrics required the development of a plethora of instruments and procedures adapted to the particularities of Mexican women's reproductive anatomy.[109] Among other procedures, Rodríguez promoted as a "national procedure" the injection of cold water into the uterus to dilate the cervix and provoke birth.[110] Rodríguez had also introduced a "maniobra nacional" (national maneuver) to aid in the procedure of facilitating the extraction of fetus's heads during difficult labor. His procedure recommended a modification on the method used by "foreign authors" such that assisting physicians learned to turn the fetus's head inside the uterus by depressing the occipital bone rather than by inserting their fingers into fetus's mouths, a procedure often injurious to both fetus and mother.[111] Rodríguez, too, designed his own variation of the forceps specifically for Mexican women's bodies.[112] Rodríguez was far from unique. In a work revealingly titled *La invención de la mujer* (The invention of womankind), physician and historian Roberto Uribe Elías lists twenty-two nineteenth-century physicians who developed over fifty procedures, instruments, and maneuvers specifically designed for Mexican women's gynecological and obstetrical experiences.[113]

While it is difficult to ascertain the frequency with which attending physicians actually used such instruments to assist women in childbirth in the country overall, the records of Mexico City's Casa de Maternidad reveal that physicians in that institution enthusiastically adopted surgical instruments to their obstetrical practices. An inventory of the medical instruments held in the Casa dating from 1880 lists a remarkable variety of instruments designed to aid Mexican women experiencing difficult labors. These included five different kinds of forceps; three types of cephalotribes (instruments used to crush the skull of stillborn fetuses to facilitate extraction); various types of pincers, including those designed for performing both embryotomies and craniotomies (operations involving the cutting and removal of the skull); pelvimeters (calipers used to measure the diameter of the pelvis); and a pair of articulated spoons used to detach the placenta from the walls of the uterus after birth.[114] Further details about physicians' use of such instruments are revealed in the statistics the Casa kept about the numbers of "natural" and "artificial" births and statistics concerning maternal deaths occurring there. Whereas in 1869 less than 6 percent of recorded births required interventions (from the use of forceps to turning the fetus at birth manually or with instruments), one decade later medical staff intervened in 10 percent of the births they oversaw.[115]

Such interventions, including operations designed to address Mexican women's "fatally flawed" reproductive anatomy, often did not end happily. The Supreme Court of the Federal District opened one criminal investigation in 1880, for example, into the death of Matilde Montes de Oca and her baby at the Casa de Maternidad. She had died from "nervous exhaustion" after undergoing a three-hour surgery undertaken at the hospital to correct "a narrowing of her pelvis." The fetus she was carrying had been "mutilated" by the surgery, although an autopsy revealed the fetus had died prior to the operation.[116] The court did not charge any of the hospital staff with any offense.

Physicians' use of instruments in nonroutine deliveries are also documented in the Casa's records detailing the epidemics of "puerperal fever" that punctuated the hospital's history from its establishment until its absorption into the Mexico City General Hospital in 1905. A particularly severe outbreak occurred in 1881. In the first quarter of that year, ten women who had given birth in the Casa had died: three from lung infections, one from a brain hemorrhage, one from eclampsia, and five from infections of the perineum.[117] The epidemic intensified, and in late March 1881, news of the outbreak reached the Consejo Superior de Salubridad. While debating whether to close the institution indefinitely, the

Consejo Superior conducted an investigation into the Casa's previous twenty-eight months of operation and found that between August 1877 and December 1881, 800 women had given birth in the institution. From that group, 724 were *partos eutóxicos*, or natural births, that did not require medical intervention. In the remaining seventy-six births, doctors had used forceps in thirty-eight cases, performed manual maneuvers seventeen times, extracted the placenta in twenty instances, and performed one cephalotripsy. The overall maternal mortality rate of the Casa was 5.5 percent, a rate typical of contemporary lying-in hospitals in Europe.[118] But the Casa had an unusually high rate of maternal deaths in cases of surgical intervention. A total of forty-four women had died in childbirth, twenty-eight of these from the group of natural births and sixteen who had undergone some type of intervention. The rate of maternal mortality in natural births was only 3.87 percent, while in intervention births it was 21 percent.

The women who died in the cases of the interventionist births did so as a result of the underlying conditions that had provoked intervention, from the surgery itself, or because of infections the surgery introduced; such infections were more common in women who underwent medical intervention than those who did not. Historically the most frequent cause of maternal death was puerperal fever, mainly caused by virulent bacterial infections (which spread at higher rates in conditions of nonsterile surgical intervention) and deaths from eclampsia and hemorrhage.[119] The most frequently indicated causes of maternal death indicated for seventy-three of the women who died in childbirth at the Casa between 1869 and 1887 were peritonitis (infection of the peritoneum) or metroperitonitis, puerperal fever, eclampsia, and pneumonia.[120] According to general practitioner and medical historian Irving Loudon, until the early twentieth century, "in more than 95% of normal labors or labors with only minor complications, delivery by a midwife was generally safer than delivery by a doctor, home deliveries were generally safer than hospital, and separate maternity hospitals were certainly safer than maternity units in general hospitals" because of the risk of infection.[121] In cases of complicated deliveries, which physicians and midwives responded to with greater manual or surgical intervention, the most important medical development for lowering maternal death rates was the development of systematic use by birth attendees of antiseptics and antibiotics.

The 1881 outbreak of puerperal infection in Mexico's Casa de Maternidad occurred at least four years after Joseph Lister's pioneering work on antiseptic surgery had begun circulating in Mexico. Mexican physician Jesús San Martín diffused Lister's research in his 1877 medical thesis "Heridas de las serosas tratada por el pensamiento de Lister."[122] As Roberto Uribe Elías notes, physicians Luís Muñoz, Juan María Rodríguez, and Manuel Carmona Valle had all "anticipated the antiseptic era" even before this with their recommendations to use soap and the Labarrque solution (sodium hypochlorite) prior to surgery.[123] And physician Ricardo Vertiz Berruecos, who initiated the adoption of the antiseptic method in Mexico, credited the Casa de Maternidad's director, Eduardo Liceaga (who was also the president of the National Academy of Medicine in 1879, and then again in 1906, and president of the National Medical Congress of Hygiene) as one of the chief influences on his research.[124] One physician's monthly observations about a similar epidemic of perinatal infection at the Casa in 1876 noted that he had ordered all parturient women vaginally injected with potassium permanganate, an inorganic chemical compound used as a disinfectant, a procedure that Mexico City's maternity hospital adopted fifteen years before staff at one of the leading American institutions regularly implemented such treatment.[125] For his part, Juan María Rodríguez advised in his 1878 *Guía clínica de partos* that the vaginal canal should be injected twice daily with a mixture of water, alcohol, and carbolic acid in order to reduce the risk of puerperal infection.[126]

While research on the prevention of puerperal infection was available to them, the medical staff at the Casa de Maternidad and the public health officials who investigated the outbreak seemed unable to apply their knowledge of antiseptics to the context before them. While Rodríguez detailed the steps medical staff should take to reduce puerperal infection, his recommendations mainly involved procedures aimed at sterilizing women's genitals. And while he also described the precautions physicians should take before attempting forceps deliveries, these did not include the sterilization of the instruments used in the procedures. Instead, he instructed that before introduction of the instruments into a patient's vagina "they should be gently warmed in lukewarm water and then greased."[127] The continuity of nonsterile birth procedures in nineteenth-century facilities in part reflected the normal lag time generally associated with the adoption of new standard medical procedures.[128] Yet physicians and public health officials were also hindered from correctly perceiving the source of infection in puerperal women because they were blinded by the "national question."

Physicians working in the Casa did perceive that inadequate hygiene in the institution's practices was largely responsible for the epidemic. On February 25, 1881, Doctor Ignacio Orihuela, one of the hospital's administrators, reported that the epidemic had reached such heights that the Casa had enacted all the hygienic practices available to it—"those that had been more or less successful in other epidemics, such as frequent carbolic fumigations in the birth chambers and in the rooms of the pregnant women, greater cleanliness, and the frequent changing of linens."[129] Casa director and senior physician Liceaga himself recommended the introduction of much stricter hygienic practices, including restricting access to the Casa to women in advanced stages of labor, isolating patients already infected with the fever, isolating each woman's bed linens before washing and fumigation, and discarding the linens of infected women.

Some elements of the report that the state Consejo Superior de Salubridad generated from its investigation into the epidemic supported the Casa staff's recommendations about introducing stricter hygiene standards to reduce the spread of infection, though these were limited only to remarks about the availability of clean linen rather than about the role of medical practitioners and their instruments spreading disease. Nevertheless, the central elements of the Consejo Superior's report eclipsed the statistical evidence that surgical interventions themselves had contributed to spreading infection and provoking maternal mortality, and instead located the central cause of maternal mortality, in the bodies—and natures—of the women themselves.

Dismissing the Casa's own statistics about maternal mortality, the Consejo Superior's report declared that its examination of European medical research revealed that no correlation existed between surgical interventions at childbirth and higher rates of maternal mortality. In Europe, the report asserted, "the immense majority of women who have died have died in natural childbirth."[130] The Consejo Superior concluded, without studying the issue further, that although there was something unhygienic in the material conditions of the Casa, nothing was likely amiss with the procedures or operations in which its staff engaged.

M. Gamorra y Valle, a state functionary of the Consejo de Beneficiencia, the counsel charged with regulating public hospitals, also examined the workings of the Casa to assess the causes of epidemic. He observed that since the mortality rate at the Casa for women who had experienced medical interventions was far higher than that for women who had had natural births, the "operations and the circumstances in which these occurred must be responsible."[131] Gamorra appeared here on the brink of perceiving the root causes of higher maternal mortality, but for him, too, nationalist preoccupations took center stage. He observed that the maternal death rates at the Casa were not truly unusual because "such epidemics of puerperal fever are not particular to us, but are seen developing from time to time in the best European maternity hospitals, even in those that are the best constructed and best staffed and those with the best care."[132] If puerperal fever was good enough for Europe, he implied, it was good enough for Mexico. Nevertheless, he pursued an explanation for the high rates of mortality that characterized surgical births at Mexico's Casa de Maternidad in comparison to those that occurred in Europe: "The difference depends probably not on our operators, who must be as able as the Europeans, but instead on the diverse conditions in which the operation occurs in Mexico and in Europe. If we take into account all the conditions of the phenomenon, and do not pay attention only to the simple numeric results, it will be seen that a great number of our women operated upon have been in worse condition, since in arriving at the hospital they have already been subjected to treatment that is more or less barbaric."[133]

Gamorra continued in the same vein, denouncing not the medical procedures used in operations but instead the extent to which the material conditions—poverty, malnourishment, poor housing, and alcoholism—of the Mexican "proletarian class" accounted for the higher mortality rates in maternity hospitals. Mexican women's national merits, in comparison to their ostensibly healthier, wealthier, and less alcoholic French sisters, explained the cause of death in surgical operations. Gamorra's nationalist preoccupations obliterated his ability to accurately perceive the true cause of increased rates of maternal mortality at the Casa at the very instant he appeared on the brink of apprehending them. High rates of puerperal infection continued to plague the Casa throughout its existence.[134]

We catch a glimpse of the propensity for nationalist preoccupations to obscure the ability of public health officials and physicians from perceiving Mexican women's actual experiences of childbirth in another contemporary medical episode. The long-running daily newspaper *El Siglo Diez y Nueve* published an article on July 5, 1877, describing a rare obstetrics case that had unfolded in Guadalajara's Belem Hospital. The case involved a pregnancy, "although certainty about its existence vacillated because, as we will see below, there were significant reasons to doubt the pregnancy."[135] Two doctors at the hospital, Antonio E. Naredo and Fortunato Arce, examined the woman in question and declared her pregnant in front of an auditorium of students. Naredo, pursued his diagnosis further, the paper commented, and "since he noted the existence of a small tumor in the region of her liver and wishing to verify the nature of this tumor, Dr. Naredo did not vacillate in confirming that the said tumor was none other than a foot belonging to the fetus."[136]

The woman had died shortly after the doctors reached this diagnosis. Other physicians performed an autopsy before a group of spectators, but did so too hastily to adequately explore her uterus. The news story reported that seeing that some incisions they had made produced an abundance of liquid when her uterine cavity was pressed, those performing the autopsy and their audience assumed that this was caused by some kind of tumor whose existence had been overlooked rather than by a pregnancy. When Naredo learned of this, he rushed to the site of the autopsy and "to the great surprise of the students, extracted a nine-month old fetus, perfectly developed."[137] Hospital staff then resumed the autopsy more carefully, discovering that the fetus had developed partially in the uterus and partially in the belly (*vientre*), which explained why Naredo had identified the fetus's foot in the region of the woman's liver. This was a case, the paper observed, of a uterotubal pregnancy, "one of the types of pregnancy so rarely verified that some classical authors of childbirth even deny the possibility of its existence."[138]

The article celebrated the achievements of Naredo, who had "with such precision" correctly diagnosed the woman's state: "Anyone who is not ignorant of the science of curing, will understand that the diagnosis of Sr. Naredo is not a common diagnosis, but rather one of those diagnoses that would have generated honor even in the setting of Europe [que le hubieran hecho honor hasta en Europa]."[139] For the publishers of *El Siglo Diez y Nueve*, as apparently for the students and attendant physicians at the Belem Hospital, the significance of this event was the Mexican physician's triumphant diagnosis of the unfortunate woman as pregnant. Her death and the death of the fetus she carried, rather than representing the focus of her contemporaries' sober attention, were necessary steps in the creation of a story about a Mexican physician who demonstrated himself capable of diagnostically outperforming even European doctors.

Mexican obstetricians shared the propensity for seeking to establish distinctively national traits of their citizens with many of their peers in other domains of medicine, science, and culture more broadly. Porfirian-era scientists articulated their vision of national identity through their reverential imitation of French culture, while simultaneously struggling to identify a foundation of Mexico's national distinctiveness from France.[140] As Nancy Leys Stepan has shown, late nineteenth-century eugenicists in Mexico and elsewhere adopted Lamarckian genetics rather than Mendelian genetics, the latter being more popular in contemporary Europe. In Latin America, the educated classes "wished to be white and feared they were not," so they embraced the work of Jean-Baptiste Lamarck because his model of genetics allowed for the possibility that culture and environment could alter a nation's genetic destiny.[141]

Porfirians sought both similarity to and distinctiveness from Europe, but where were they to locate that distinctiveness? In the late eighteenth century, Mexican and Peruvian creoles sometimes staked their claim to patriotic distinctiveness on a foundation of identity with the New World's indigenous past—preferably a far remote past.[142] But Porfirian elites were more likely to reject or repress all aspects of indigenous Mexico's contribution to the formulation of symbols and practices of national identity. In the field of cuisine, for example, Jeffrey Pilcher observes that in this period "wealthy Mexicans abandoned their Hispanic heritage as an unfashionable relic of the past, replacing the *mole* sauces of traditional colonial kitchens with the *timbale* pastries of French haute cuisine."[143]

Similarily, Porfirians rejected identification with indigenous health practices that persisted in most women's birth experiences. It was the very persistence of these that likely provoked the agents of institutional medicine—licensed doctors, medical schools, public health regulatory bodies—to so painstakingly manufacture another source of national medical distinctiveness, because national distinctiveness based on identification with indigenous Mexico was abhorrent. Thus, when Dolores Román, an indigenous woman and the Casa de Maternidad's first head midwife, was the first practitioner in the institution to successfully turn a fetus before birth by external manipulation of the womb, the medical press reported that she had done so "under the direction" of doctor Martínez del Río, identifying the procedure as an invention of Mexican *tocología* even though early sixteenth-century accounts record the practice as known to pre-Columbian midwives.[144] When medical staff at the Casa subsequently turned fetuses before or during labor, they preferred to frame the procedure (as did Juan María Rodríguez in his *Guía clínica del arte de los partos*) as the "Hippocratic method" rather than link the procedure to pre-Columbian precedents.[145]

The report of the inspector the Consejo de Beneficia sent to assess the causes of high maternal death rates in cases of obstetrical surgery at the Casa de Maternidad in 1881 is also revealing on this point. In his assessment, M. Gamorra y Valle decried not only the lower national health conditions of Mexican women but also the medical care they received before arriving at the Casa de Maternidad: "A large number of our women who have been operated upon have arrived at the hospital already subjected to more or less barbarous treatment. Some have been given hot chocolate with chile; others have taken zinapatle or cuernecillo de centeno; some have been struck in the hips, others have been ill-treated . . . women have even arrived at the hospital with their vaginas and uteruses ripped open."[146] We note in his comments that women in Mexico's capital who arrived at the doorstep of the country's first national maternity hospital continued to use the very same medicinal substances to provoke abortions that they had been using in the pre-Columbian period. But professional obstetricians and state health officials could not define a national obstetrical practice on such common practices derived from pre-Columbian and colonial midwifery. They instead developed a national medical practice based on such notions as Mexican women's distinctively shaped hymens and their pathologically narrow pelvises. In their fervor to establish a national practice on such foundations, however, concerns about improving the actual conditions of childbirth were, unfortunately, often obscured.

Birthing the Nation

In the period from the mid-eighteenth century to the late nineteenth, some central aspects of women's experiences of giving birth in Mexico remained constant. First, women gave birth with the same high regularity across time. Robert McCaa, the demographic historian who has most carefully studied available statistical sources for both the colonial period and the nineteenth century, observes that, across the nineteenth century, "the number and spacing of children in Mexico was more or less constant" among women in some form of conjugal union. Variation instead occurred from the proportion of women who entered such unions and from their precocity in forming them.[147] For women from a Tzeltal-speaking village in Amatenango, Chiapas, as for those of Euromestizo elites in Mexico City, birth intervals averaged three years, and average family size was 8.5 children in the late colonial period.[148]

This chapter has discussed how, across the period examined here, the health care personnel and the medicines they used likely would have remained constant for most Mexican women, although the details of many such experiences are frustratingly scarce for this period. Most women chose midwives to attend them at childbirth from the late colonial period through the late nineteenth century, and many of these women continued to use the same medicines that had been available to Mexican *parteras* even in the preconquest era. Some new medicines and birth techniques, introduced by European midwifery, including the use of the birthing stool and the application of the naturally occurring oxytocin *cuernecillo de centeno* were also widely adopted during the colonial period and persisted into later eras.

Still, there were other significant ways in which experiences of childbirth changed for Mexican women who gave birth in the era examined here. Although they represented a small minority, nationally speaking, increasing numbers of Mexican women by the late nineteenth century gave birth under the attendance of a licensed physician or midwife rather than an unlicensed midwife and did so in institutional settings rather than in the privacy of their own dwellings. In such settings they experienced a higher frequency of surgical intervention during childbirth and associated higher rates of puerperal infections and mortality than did women giving birth at home. Nevertheless, women sought admission to such establishments as Mexico City's Casa de Maternidad, and once it was constructed in 1905, the maternity ward in the city's new general hospital, no doubt because of increasing perceptions that physicians with access to medical technologies could and did facilitate the experience of childbirth, especially in complicated conditions. Such women may also have elected to give birth in new, institutional settings because they were both products and producers of a new public discourse crafted in colonial society that overturned the highly private nature of childbirth and contraception.

Conclusion

Change and Constancy in Mexico's Reproductive History

· ·

Academic historians operate in an environment in which we are often compelled to demonstrate the utility and relevance of our research to various audiences. Periodically, while writing this book, I have discussed it with representatives of granting agencies, engaged students, family members, and acquaintances who have asked me how my knowledge of Mexico's colonial and nineteenth-century reproductive history has a bearing on the lives of women and men in twenty-first-century North America. When pressed to answer why and how historical understanding in general is relevant and significant, statesmen and schoolchildren alike most frequently resort to the old adage that the importance of studying the past lies in the lessons it teaches us; we must, they say, learn from past mistakes in order to avoid repeating them.

Scholars in pursuit of historical understanding within our own particular areas of research expertise understand the worthlessness of this maxim, however. First, professional historians recognize that we live in a society that, far from truly seeking historical knowledge, specializes in forgetfulness. In our solemn but often superficial invocations of the past, we hasten its obliteration. Second, we grasp that the temporal and geographic differences between the contexts in which we live and those about which we study are often so radical that insights generated about the latter may have little bearing on populations existing in the former. The conclusions we draw about the past are often so nuanced that its elements are not transferable to present circumstances. Notwithstanding such observations, beyond underlining the main findings of this study, these concluding remarks provide an opportunity to consider what relevancy the examination of Mexico's reproductive history (and its discontents) might have for an audience broader than the group of scholars and students of Latin America's gendered history already invested in understanding this past in its own terms.

One contribution that knowledge about reproductive and childbirth practices in colonial and nineteenth-century Mexico makes to current audiences is that it serves as an antidote to our ongoing proclivity toward what Herbert Butterfield described over eighty years ago as generational whiggishness—the notion that the past has followed a progressive and inevitable line to the glorious and emancipated present in which we currently live.[1] Butterfield's subject, the British parliamentary system, is far afield from my own, but elements of his analysis apply. Our era frequently presumes that women today exist in an enlightened era in comparison to the dark ages of an oppressive past, whereas many aspects of my research challenge this presumption. By suggesting that the linear narrative of progress and emancipation simplifies more than it clarifies, I do not mean to advance the reductive argument that women who in eighteenth-century Mexico City used the contraction-inducing plants *altamisa* and *cihuapatli* to intentionally provoke miscarriages had access to the means of regulating their fertility that was equal or superior to the pharmaceutical options available to women in the present.

My point is a broader one. I contend that our era often presumes to enjoy the most liberated perception of women's rights to autonomy and self-determination and assumes that, in the present, we value women more than societies have in earlier periods. Various episodes in Mexico's history of childbirth and contraception challenge this perception. In our own era, the regulation of fertility is a matter of intense and politically divisive public concern. The notion that fertility regulation—decisions about conception's timing, occurrence, and even its endurance—should be matters left to the discretion of individual women is an idea currently rejected by a sizable proportion of North Americans. Substantial evidence suggests, however, that this was how colonial Mexicans understood pregnancy, contraception, abortion, and even infanticide. They viewed birth itself as a private matter and not one worthy or appropriate to public commentary and regulation. Second, when women in colonial Mexico terminated what colonial sources call "the products of conception," whether they did so before, during, or after birth, their contemporaries—whether family members, neighbors, or religious and state authorities—most often did not intervene.

In the course of the nineteenth century, however, larger groups of the Mexican populace began to take a more active interest in women's reproductive and contraceptive practices. Obstetrics was increasingly regulated and professionalized, and new technologies related to birth were increasingly promoted. The professionalization and nationalization of obstetrical medicine heralded childbirth's movement from the private to the public realm at the same time as the Mexican populace learned to consider contraception, abortion, and especially infanticide as matters of public concern. In the last quarter of the nineteenth century, members of the public denounced women to criminal courts for the crimes of infanticide and abortion far more frequently than they had done in earlier periods. And while there are some grounds for supposing that Mexican women might actually have been engaging in abortion and infanticide more often in this period than in earlier times, it is more likely that the rising number of cases in this period reflects a rise in rates of denunciation rather than of actual commission of the crimes. While colonial society witnessed elite preoccupations with the reproduction of whiteness, and consequently the scrutiny of the sexual virtue and reproductive practices of elite Spanish women, in the course of the nineteenth century Mexicans directed such preoccupations toward an expanding segment of the country's female population. One conclusion of my study is that the vast majority of Mexico's female population would have experienced less social scrutiny of their sexual and reproductive practices in the colonial period than did women who lived at the close of the nineteenth century.

A second important contribution to contemporary knowledge that the history of childbirth and contraception in colonial and nineteenth-century Mexico makes is its illustration of the social construction of two realms of reality—reproductive biology and maternity itself—that we often continue to see as natural, essential, and beyond history. Details about the development of reproduction and motherhood in colonial and nineteenth-century Mexico remind us that the boundaries we like to draw between "truth" and "perception" are always shifting. Past generations believed as adamantly as we do now in the truth of what we now describe as their distorted perceptions. Future generations will no doubt consider our truths in the same way. Thus we confront early modern and nineteenth-century Mexicans who did not draw as clear a distinction between the biological notions of conception and its absence, between virginity and nonvirginity, between what Martha Few calls the "inside-outside boundary" between a "fetus" inside the uterus and a "baby" outside of it, and even between the moral implications of terminating life before and after birth as we do in the present.[2]

Colonial Mexican society accepted the notion of social rather than strictly defined biological virginity, and colonial Mexicans were also more at ease than we are, for example, with the idea that various biological factors might explain the most well-known symptoms of pregnancy, including amenorrhea. They accepted the notion that it was perfectly respectable and reasonable for women to take menstrual regulators to treat such symptoms. Until the late nineteenth century, Mexican midwives and medical authorities believed there were few biological indicators that could indicate with absolute reliability whether or not women were technically virgins, though Francisco de Asis Flores y Troncoso attempted to combat the contemporary illegibility of women's bodies with his production of *El hímen en Mexico* to provide practitioners with an infallible formula by which they could gauge virginity with absolute precision.

Similarly, in the emotional realm, Mexico's reproductive and contraceptive history provides recurrent evidence about how maternity itself, a state and a set of associations whose social construction we are reluctant to acknowledge, has a changing history. In the colonial period, reproduction was a matter of intense public concern only for Spanish women of the colonial elite because their reproductive history mattered for the defense of *limpieza de sangre* and for the maintenance of this sector's concerns over the inheritance of titles and property. By the late nineteenth century, the group of women about whom Mexicans held maternal expectations had greatly expanded. Expectations of female purity extended to include a broader sector of the female population in a period that understood mothers as responsible for ensuring the health and wealth not only of the small and powerful elite but of the whole nation.

The associations Mexicans held about maternity shifted as well. In the colonial period and in the first decades of the nineteenth century, the public associated honor for the female population more broadly with ideas and practices other than motherhood. Witnesses to criminal courts and justices presiding at them associated female virtue with women who were dutiful, God-fearing, obedient, and belonging to honorable, tax-paying families. By the end of the nineteenth century, however, female virtue in such testimony became more explicitly related to the demonstration of nurturing motherhood and sexual purity. Ideas about the nurturing bonds and natural tenderness that we now so strongly associate with motherhood are notable in colonial documentation only in their absence. Until the mid-nineteenth century, where discussion of maternity sometimes emerged in infanticide and abortion trials, magistrates, *curadores*, witnesses and defendants did not engage in the polemics of moral outrage about the rupture of a sacred, natural bond that we accord such acts in our own era. They found evidence of mothers' violence toward their own offspring difficult to comprehend and generally searched for—and accepted—rational explanations for it.

In criminal cases in which maternal defendants themselves confessed to having committed or ordered infanticide, for example, *curadores* and justices explained these with reference to the lack of judgment drunkenness induced in women. In the 1819 infanticide case against María Dolores and several of her nieces in which the defendants confessed to murdering and burying a newborn, the defendants explained their actions by saying they had a "lack of knowledge greater than has any man who is totally drunk."[3] In the 1842 case against María de Jesús Torres, a woman who had killed her infant with a blow to the head, her *curador* argued before Mexico City's Tribunal Superior that the alcohol Torres had consumed prior to dashing her daughter against some rocks rendered her "incapable of delinquency." Because the law absolved from punishment "the insane, the furious, and others" (*al loco, al furioso, y a otros*) he argued her drunkenness also deprived her of her use of reason.[4] Her appellate judges, persuaded by this argument and by the fact that her numerous other children required her financial and practical support, absolved her of the crime. Such legal officials considered bonds of maternity normal; evidence of their rupture pushed them to attribute their loss to external forces that had intervened to change mothers' predictable behavior. They refrained, however, from attributing such actions to ideas about the monstrosity or unnatural sickness that in our own day we attribute to women who commit such crimes.

As well as illustrating episodes of dramatic change across time, reminding us of how changing national circumstances and preoccupations contribute to the construction of both medical knowledge and emotional ideals often considered natural and unchanging, the history of reproduction and contraception in colonial and nineteenth-century Mexico also includes elements remarkable for their endurance. Political activists on both the left and right have become highly visible in Mexico in the past decade, particularly over the issue of abortion. Polemics against abortion in particular often frame the act within the context of twentieth- and twenty-first-century pressures. However, medical practitioners in Mexico possessed knowledge about abortion and contraception since as early as the late postclassical period. Pre-Columbian midwives and those who continued to use pre-Columbian obstetrical knowledge throughout the colonial period and the nineteenth century had extensive knowledge of effective botanical medicines, including *altamisa* and *cihuapatli*, that acted as labor accelerators in pregnant women. They provided these to women early in their pregnancies to induce miscarriages, or during labor to facilitate stalled births.

Likewise, knowledge about childbirth is characterized by its consistency across time. During pregnancy and in labor, colonial and nineteenth-century midwives used millennia-old practices, including the *temazcal* and the external manipulation of fetuses to correctly position them for birth. Over the course of the nineteenth century, the increasingly regulated medical profession took an increasingly disparaging view of such medicines and the practitioners who employed them, but contrary to a historiography both within Mexico and beyond it that describes this as the era of midwifery's obliteration, little evidence supports that interpretation. Whether by choice or necessity, most Mexican women throughout the nineteenth century continued to seek counsel from midwives about conception and contraception, and also engaged midwives to attend them at childbirth. Nevertheless, the medical establishment did seek to institute new national medical procedures distinctive from widely practiced traditions.

Those smaller numbers of women whom doctors attended at childbirth underwent novel medical experiences. Along with cervical examinations during pregnancy, doctors after the midcentury increasingly introduced medical instruments, including numerous variations on the forceps, to aid women undergoing various kinds of stalled or difficult labors. Such innovations were not the result of male physicians' diabolical plans to subjugate female bodies to technologies of control. Eighteenth-century Scotch obstetrician William Smellie, a writer whose works were influential in colonial and nineteenth-century obstetrical medicine in Mexico, was the first writer to publish safe rules for the use of forceps. He provided obstetrical lecture-demonstrations to midwives and medical students in the 1740s, and his discussion of the use of forceps is careful, cautious, and modest. In his meticulously illustrated midwifery text that sought to encourage forceps' use, Smellie observed, "The Forceps were at first contrived to save the *Foetus*, and prevent, as much as possible, the use of sharp Instruments; but even to this salutary method recourse ought not be had but in Cases where the degree of force requisite to extract will not endanger by its consequences the life of the mother. For, by the imprudent use of Forceps, much more harm may be done than good."[5] Nevertheless, such technologies did induce higher rates of puerperal infection in women, and in the era before the consistent application of sterile surgical practices, higher rates of maternal mortality than in natural births.

As well as revealing change and continuity in Mexico's medical history and illuminating developments in shifting conceptualizations about ideal womanhood, this history also documents the role obstetrical developments played in Mexico's ongoing articulations about its national identity. In the late colonial period, at a time of growing creole defensiveness about the natural attributes of New World locales, Mexicans celebrated exceptional natural productions—monstrous births—in response to European perceptions of their territory and inhabitants as embodying racial degeneration. Over the course of the nineteenth century, such perceptions changed dramatically. The public more consistently reacted with revulsion and horror to reports of monstrous productions, while medical professionals working in the emergent field of teratology adopted the view that monsters were an extreme expression of biological traits discoverable within the normal range of human development.

Focusing on the intrauterine experiences of developing fetuses, these practitioners also championed the notion that explanations for the origins of monstrosity existed within women's bodies. Such views reoriented explanations for exceptional natural productions away from external, environmental factors and toward the internal scrutiny of female reproductive anatomy. This transformation coincided with other changes in late nineteenth-century obstetrical research at a time when practitioners increasingly identified obstetrics and gynecology as a nationalist field of medicine. Obstetrical practitioners and researchers in the closing decades of the nineteenth century devoted their energies to developing new technologies, procedures, and formulas specifically designed to assist Mexican women afflicted by the "fatal secret" of their flawed bodies in the all-important goal of producing a healthy national citizenry.

Appendix I

Abortion Cases, Mexican Archives, 1823–1884

#	Date	Reference	Accused	Charge/Outcome
1	1842	AHMO, Justicia, Juzgado de 1ª instancia, 1841–42, caja 27	Arcadia Martínez	Had been absolved due to insufficient evidence; appellate court upheld original ruling.
2	1861	AGN, TSJDF, 1861	María Luciana	Suspected of abortion.
3	1871	AGN, TSJDF, 1871	Francisco Luna	Suspected of abortion.
4	1874	AGN, TSJDF, 1874	Zeferino Martínez	Suspected of abortion.
5	1880	AGN, TSJDF, 1880, caja 703	Tomasa Escarcega	Suspected of abortion; case dismissed.
6	1880	AHJO, Villa Alta siglo 19, Criminal, exp. 2465	María Jiménez de Villa Hidalgo	Suspected of abortion.
7	1881	AGN, TSJDF, 1881	Francisco Rivera	Suspected of abortion.
8	1881	AGN, TSJDF, 1881	Eusebia Cabrera	Suspected of abortion.
9	1881	AGN, TSJDF, 1881	Tirso Hidalgo	Suspected of abortion.
10	1881	AGN, TSJDF, 1881	Luz Belmont	Suspected of abortion.
11	1881	AGN, TSJDF, 1881	Agustin Rico	Suspected of abortion.
12	1882	AGN, TSJDF, 1882	María Trinidad	Suspected of abortion.
13	1882	AGN, TSJDF, 1882	Aristeo Muñoz	Suspected of abortion.
14	1883	AGN, TSJDF, 1883, caja 841	Pomposa Acosta	Suspected of abortion; absolved.
15	1883	AGN, TSJDF, 1883	Prisco Montaño	Suspected of abortion.
16	1883	AGN, TSJDF, 1883	Remiga Gutiérrez	Suspected of abortion.
17	1883	AGN, TSJDF, 1883	Francisco González	Suspected of abortion.
18	1883	AGN, TSJDF, 1883	Jesús Rivas	Suspected of abortion.
19	1883	AGN, TSJDF, 1883	Santiago Ortiz	Suspected of abortion.
20	1883	AGN, TSJDF, 1883	Anuela Baez	Suspected of abortion.

(continued)

#	Date	Reference	Accused	Charge/Outcome
21	1883	AHMO, Justicia, Juzgado 1° criminal, subseries: procesos, 1883, caja 24	Juana López	Suspected of abortion; absolved.
22	1883	AGN, TSJDF, 1883	Francisca Domínguez	Suspected of abortion.
23	1884	AHMO, Justicia, Corte de Justicia 1ª sala, 1883–84, caja 7	María Reyes and María Anacleta	Suspected of abortion; court judged it was accidental.
24	1884	AGN, TSJDF, 1884	María Paz Rodríguez	Suspected of abortion.
25	1884	AGN, TSJDF, 1884	Juan Navarro	Suspected of abortion.
26	1884	AGN, TSJDF, 1884		Suspected of abortion.
27	1884	AGN, TSJDF, 1884	Luciano Zamudio	Suspected of abortion.
28	1886	AGN, TSJDF, 1886		Suspected of abortion.
29	1886	AGN, TSJDF, 1886	Pedro Cadena	Suspected of abortion.
30	1886	AGN, TSJDF, 1886		Suspected of abortion.
31	1886	AGN, TSJDF, 1886	Juan Villafana	Suspected of abortion.
32	1886	AGN, TSJDF, 1886	Mariano López	Suspected of abortion.
33	1886	AGN, TSJDF, 1886		Suspected of abortion.
34	1886	AGN, TSJDF, 1886	José Aguila	Suspected of abortion.
35	1886	AGN, TSJDF, 1886	Tomás Franco L.	Suspected of abortion.
36	1886	AGN, TSJDF, 1886	Juan Ramírez	Suspected of abortion.
37	1887	AGN, TSJDF, 1887	Virginia Domínguez	Suspected of abortion.
38	1887	AGN, TSJDF, 1887	J. Enarnación Contreras	Suspected of abortion.
39	1887	AGN, TSJDF, 1887	María Carmen Jiménez	Suspected of abortion.
40	1887	AGN, TSJDF, 1887	Nazario Reyes	Suspected of abortion.
41	1888	AGN, TSJDF, 1888	José Aguila	Suspected of abortion.
42	1888	AGN, TSJDF, 1888	Josefa Gutiérrez	Suspected of abortion.
43	1888	AGN, TSJDF, 1888	Bonifacia Gutiérrez	Suspected of abortion.
44	1888	AGN, TSJDF, 1888	José Vargas	Suspected of abortion.

#	Date	Reference	Accused	Charge/Outcome
45	1888	AGN, TSJDF, 1888		Suspected of abortion.
46	1888	AGN, TSJDF, 1888	Gregorio Vargas	Suspected of abortion.
47	1888	AGN, TSJDF, 1888	Toribio Rosas	Suspected of abortion.
48	1888	AGN, TSJDF, 1888	J. Ascención Rodríguez	Suspected of abortion.
49	1888	AGN, TSJDF, 1888	Merced Camacho	Suspected of abortion.
50	1888	AGN, TSJDF, 1888	Roque Briseño	Suspected of abortion.
51	1888	AGN, TSJDF, 1888	Francisco Gómez	Suspected of abortion.
52	1889	AGN, TSJDF, 1889	Feliciano Merino	Suspected of abortion.
53	1889	AGN, TSJDF, 1889	María Saturnina	Suspected of abortion.
54	1889	AGN, TSJDF, 1889	José Ysaac García	Suspected of abortion.
55	1889	AGN, TSJDF, 1889	Enriqueta Pelaez	Suspected of abortion.
56	1889	AGN, TSJDF, 1889	Gorgonio Rubin	Suspected of abortion.
57	1889	AGN, TSJDF, 1889	Guadalupe Alcalá	Suspected of abortion.
58	1890	AGN, TSJDF, 1890	Calixto López	Suspected of abortion.
59	1890	AGN, TSJDF, 1890	María González	Suspected of abortion.
60	1890	AGN, TSJDF, 1890	Carlos Fernández	Suspected of abortion.
61	1890	AGN, TSJDF, 1890	Felipa Ruíz	Suspected of abortion.
62	1890	AGN, TSJDF, 1890		Suspected of abortion.
63	1891	AGN, TSJDF, 1891	Jacob Padilla	Suspected of abortion.
64	1891	AGN, TSJDF, 1891		Suspected of abortion.
65	1891	AGN, TSJDF, 1891		Suspected of abortion.
66	1891	AGN, TSJDF, 1891		Suspected of abortion.
67	1893	AGN, TSJDF, 1893	Carmen de Reguera	Suspected of abortion.
68	1893	AGN, TSJDF, 1893	Perfecto Guzman	Suspected of abortion.
69	1893	AGN, TSJDF, 1893	Fernando Salas	Suspected of abortion.
70	1894	AGN, TSJDF, 1894	Pedro Ramírez	Suspected of abortion.
71	1894	AGN, TSJDF, 1894	Felipa Granados	Suspected of abortion.
72	1894	AGN, TSJDF, 1894	Fernando Salas	Suspected of abortion.
73	1896	AGN, TSJDF, 1896	Luis Maldonado	Suspected of abortion.
74	1896	AGN, TSJDF, 1896	Natalia Hosoyos	Suspected of abortion.

(continued)

#	Date	Reference	Accused	Charge/Outcome
75	1896	AGN, TSJDF, 1896	Trinidad Hernández	Suspected of abortion.
76	1897	AGN, TSJDF, 1897		Suspected of abortion.
77	1897	AGN, TSJDF, 1897	Maximinom Suarez	Suspected of abortion.
78	1897	AGN, TSJDF, 1897	Sotero Rodríguez	Suspected of abortion.
79	1898	AGN, TSJDF, 1898	Antonio Maria Pizaña	Suspected of abortion.
80	1898	AGN, TSJDF, 1898		Suspected of abortion.
81	1898	AGN, TSJDF, 1898		Suspected of abortion.
82	1898	AGN, TSJDF, 1898		Suspected of abortion.
83	1899	AGN, TSJDF, 1899	J. Jesús Castro	Suspected of abortion.
84	1899	AGN, TSJDF, 1899		Suspected of abortion.
85	1899	ACSCJ, 73859	Dr. Federico Abrego	Suspected of providing an abortion; underwent a lengthy criminal investigation, but ultimately absolved.

Sources: AHMO, Justicia; AHJO, Villa Alta, Criminal, Siglo 19; AGN, TSJDF; ACSCJ.

Note: The titles whose records do not indicate an outcome have only been located in the box list catalog of the TSJDF rather than acquired in totality.

Appendix II

Infanticide Cases, Mexican Archives, 1823–1897

#	Date	Reference	Accused	Charge/Outcome
1	1829	AGN, Justicia, vol. 113, exp. 18	Gregoria Camargo	Suspected of infanticide of the baby she was raising; acquitted.
2	1837	AHMO, Justicia, caja Juzgado de 1ª instancia, 15, 1836–37	Felipa Romero	Midwife suspected of infanticide; acquitted.
3	1837	AHJO, Teposcolula, Criminal, legajo 58, exp. 21	María Ricarda Osorio	Suspected of infanticide; acquitted.
4	1840	ACSCJ, 1815	María San José Romo de Vivar	Suspected of infanticide; acquitted.
5	1840	ACSCJ, 1816	Modesta Sanderos, Doña Socorros Díaz	Suspected of infanticide; acquitted.
6	1842	AGN, TSJDF, 1842, Juzgado de Paz de Honor	Josefa Ruiz	Suspected of infanticide.
7	1843	AGN, TSJDF, 1843, caja 180	Mariá de Jesús Torres	Convicted of infanticide; sentenced to six months' service in the kitchen of the jail.
8	1843	AGN, TSJDF, 1843, caja 180	Lorenza Castro	Convicted of infanticide by court of first instance; appellate court acquitted.
9	1845	AHJO, Teposcolula, Criminal, legajo 64, exp. 3	Tomasa Maldonado	Suspected of infanticide; acquitted.
10	1846	AGN, TSJDF, Juzgado de Paz de Milpa Alta	María Francisca	Suspected of infanticide.

(continued)

#	Date	Reference	Accused	Charge/Outcome
11	1852	AGN, TSJDF, Juzgado de Paz 2° Civil, caja 292	Petra Juárez (Torres)	Suspected of infanticide; inconclusive documentation.
12	1853	AHMO, Justicia, Juzgado de 1ª instancia 1853, caja 42	María González	Suspected of infanticide; acquitted.
13	1855	AHJO, Ejutla, Criminal, legajo 14, exp. 3	Ignacia Teodora	Suspected of committing infanticide on child she was minding; acquitted.
14	1857	AHMO, Justicia, Juzgado de 1ª instancia, 1857–61 caja 46	Anacleta Avila	Suspected of infanticide; acquitted.
15	1857	AHJO, Villa Alta, Criminal legajo 69, exp. 30	Basilio Gabriel de Salaga	Suspected of infanticide; acquitted.
16	1857	AGN, TSJDF, Sello Sesto de Oficio, caja 327	Francisca Rojas	Suspected of infanticide; acquitted.
17	1859	ACSCJ, 5988	a fourteen-year old	Suspected of infanticide; acquitted.
18	1860	ACSCJ, 6133	María Vicenta	Suspected of infanticide; acquitted.
19	1860	AGN, TSJDF, 3ª sala, caja 341	María Can	Convicted of infanticide by judge of first sentence; appellate court acquitted.
20	1860	AGN, TSJDF, 3ª sala, caja 341	Leocardia Hernández	Convicted of infanticide by judge of first sentence; appellate court acquitted.
21	1861	AGN, TSJDF, Juez de Letras de Distrito	Margarita Juárez	Suspected of infanticide.
22	1862	AGN, TSJDF, 2° criminal	Jesús Teran	Suspected of infanticide.
23	1863	ACSCJ, 6765	María Sebastiana	Suspected of infanticide; acquitted.
24	1863	ACSCJ, 6771	María Abila	Suspected of infanticide; acquitted.

#	Date	Reference	Accused	Charge/Outcome
25	1864	AGN, TSJDF, 1864, caja 391	María Guadalupe Pérez, Hilaria Vázquez	Suspected of infanticide; acquitted.
26	1864	ACSCJ, 7135	Mother-in-law of Felipa de Jesús	Suspected of infanticide; acquitted.
27	1864	ACSCJ, 7543	María Cresencia	Suspected of infanticide; acquitted.
28	1864	ACSCJ, 7164		Convicted of infanticide by court of first sentence; sentenced to two years' service in jail; appellate court acquitted.
29	1864	ACSCJ, 7589	María Lucia	Convicted of infanticide; sentenced to nine months' imprisonment.
30	1864	ACSCJ, 7603	María Dolores	Suspected of infanticide; inconclusive documentation.
31	1864	AGN, TSJDF, Superior tribunal de justicia.	Manuel Sierra y socio	Suspected of infanticide.
32	1864	AGN, TSJDF, Juzgado menor de Tacubaya	Q.R.R.	Suspected of infanticide.
33	1864	AGN, TSJDF, 2ª sala	José Santos Sigales	Suspected of infanticide.
34	1864	AGN, TSJDF, 2ª sala	María Guadalupe Pérez y otra	Suspected of infanticide.
35	1865	ACSCJ, 7775		Suspected of infanticide; acquitted.
36	1865	ACSCJ, 7970	Marcelino Jiménez	Suspected of infanticide; acquitted.
37	1865	ACSCJ, 7913	Felix Hernández, María Soledad	Suspected of infanticide; inconclusive documentation.

(*continued*)

#	Date	Reference	Accused	Charge/Outcome
38	1865	ACSCJ, 7842	María Trinidad	Suspected of infanticide; inconclusive documentation.
39	1865	ACSCJ, 7864		Suspected of infanticide; convicted.
40	186?	AHMO, Justicia, Alcalde 1 constitucional, 1868–81, caja 6	María Sabina	Suspected of infanticide; inconclusive documentation.
41	1865	AGN, TSJDF	María Guadalupe López	Suspected of infanticide.
42	1865	AGN, TSJDF, 5º criminal	Josefa Avila	Suspected of infanticide.
43	1865	AGN, TSJDF, 3ª sala	María de la Luz	Suspected of infanticide.
44	1865	AGN, TSJDF, 2ª clase de oficio	Petra Morales	Suspected of infanticide.
45	1870	AGN, TSJDF	Agustina Lara	Suspected of infanticide.
46	1870	AGN, TSJDF	Miguel Larralde	Suspected of infanticide.
47	1870	AGN, TSJDF, 6º criminal	Luz Bernal	Suspected of infanticide.
48	1870	AGN, TSJDF, 6º criminal	Miguel Serralde	Suspected of infanticide.
49	1870	AHMO, Justicia, Juzgado 3ª de letras, 1869–70, caja 4	Agustina Sánchez	Midwife convicted of infanticide; sentenced to time already served during the trial.
50	1871	AGN, TSJDF, 3º criminal	Epitacia Yáñnez	Suspected of infanticide.
51	1871	AGN, TSJDF, 2º clase de oficio	Juana Paula	Suspected of infanticide.
52	1872	AGN, TSJDF	Fernanda Pimentel	Suspected of infanticide.
53	1872	AGN, TSJDF, Sello 6º de oficio	Rosenda Nava	Suspected of infanticide.
54	1874	AGN, TSJDF, Juzgado de alcaldía		Suspected of infanticide.

#	Date	Reference	Accused	Charge/Outcome
55	1874	AGN, TSJDF	Antonio Cruz	Suspected of infanticide.
56	1876	AGN, TSJDF, Juzgado 2° de letras criminal	Antonio Rosas	Suspected of infanticide.
57	1876	AGN, TSJDF, Juzgado 2° de letras criminal	Vicente Mata Pastrana	Suspected of infanticide.
58	1876	AGN, TSJDF, Juzgado 5° criminal	Petra Acosta	Suspected of infanticide.
59	1878	AGN, TSJDF, Juzgado 6° de instrucción	Q.R.R.	Suspected of infanticide.
60	1879	AGN, TSJDF		Suspected of infanticide.
61	1880	AHMO, Corte de Justicia 1ª sala, 1879–80, caja 4; AHMO, Justicia, Juzgado 2° criminal, 1880–81, caja 12	María Natividad de los Santos	Convicted of infanticide; sentenced to two years' reclusion in a *recogimiento* from which she escaped.
62	1880	AGN, TSJDF, 1880, caja 681; AGN, TSJDF, 1880, caja 687	María Concepción Mejía	Midwife convicted of infanticide.
63	1880	AGN, TSJDF, 1880, caja 703	Dolores García	Midwife suspected of infanticide; acquitted.
64	1880	AGN, TSJDF, 1880, caja 703	Tomasa Montiel	Convicted of infanticide; sentenced to one year, four months' imprisonment.
65	1880	AGN, TSJDF 1880, caja 703	Lorenza Rodríguez	Suspected of infanticide; acquitted.
66	1880	AGN, TSJDF, 1880, caja 703	Midwife and doctor at the Casa de Maternidad	Suspected of infanticide; acquitted.
67	1880	AGN, TSJDF, 1880, caja 703	Apolina Mayor	Suspected of infanticide; acquitted.
68	1880	AGN, TSJDF, 1880, caja 703	Dolores Ortiz	Midwife suspected of infanticide; acquitted.
69	1880	AGN, TSJDF, 1ª instancia	Ponciano Vazquez	Suspected of infanticide.

(*continued*)

#	Date	Reference	Accused	Charge/Outcome
70	1880	AGN, TSJDF, 1° criminal	Patricia Uribe	Suspected of infanticide.
71	1881	AHJO, Ejutla, Criminal, legajo 79, exp. 25	María Martínez	Suspected of infanticide; inconclusive documentation.
72	1881	AHMO, Justicia, Juzgado 2° criminal, 1880–81, caja 12; AHMO, Corte de Justicia, 1ª sala, caja 4, 1879–80	María Natividad de los Santos	Suspected of infanticide.
73	1881	AGN, TSJDF, 1ª instancia del Partido sur de B.C.	Domingo González	Suspected of infanticide.
74	1881	AGN, TSJDF, Juzgado 4° correccional AGN, TSJDF, 2ª sala Juez 4° correccional	Placida Chavero	Suspected of infanticide.
75	1881	AGN, TSJDF, de Letras de Tlalpan	Guadalupe y Domingo Ybañez	Suspected of infanticide.
76	1881	AGN, TSJDF, 2° de letras correccional; AGN, TSJDF, Juzgado 4° correccional	María Soledad Nava, Ignacio Avila	Suspected of infanticide.
77	1881	AGN, TSJDF, 4° correccional	Bernarda Cortes	Suspected of infanticide.
78	1881	AGN, TSJDF, 1° correccional	Manuel Andrade	Suspected of infanticide.
79	1882	AGN, TSJDF	Mariano Hernández	Suspected of infanticide.
80	1882	AGN, TSJDF, 1ª instancia del partido de Tlalpan	María Petra	Suspected of infanticide.
81	1882	AGN, TSJDF, 1ª instancia del partido de Tlalpan	María Eulalia	Suspected of infanticide.
82	1882	AGN, TSJDF, 3° criminal	Juan Rodríguez y otro	Suspected of infanticide.

#	Date	Reference	Accused	Charge/Outcome
83	1883	AHMO, Corte de Justicia 1ª sala, 1882–83, caja 6	María Getrudis Gregoria	Convicted of infanticide; sentenced to five years' reclusion.
84	1883	AGN, TSJDF, Juzgado 2° criminal	Margarita Corona	Suspected of infanticide.
85	1883	AGN, TSJDF, 3° criminal	Feliciano Pérez	Suspected of infanticide.
86	1883	AGN, TSJDF, 1° criminal	Patricia Uribe	Suspected of infanticide.
87	1883	AGN, TSJDF, 4° correccional	Josefa Armas y otro	Suspected of infanticide.
88	1883	AGN, TSJDF, 4° correccional		Suspected of infanticide.
89	1883	AGN, TSJDF, 4° correccional	Q.R.R.	Suspected of infanticide.
90	1883	AGN, TSJDF, 4° correccional		Suspected of infanticide.
91	1883	AGN, TSJDF, 4° correccional	Librada Martínez	Suspected of infanticide.
92	1883	AGN, TSJDF, 4° correccional	Guadalupe Carbajal	Suspected of infanticide.
93	1883	AGN, TSJDF	Antonia Salgado	Suspected of infanticide.
94	1884	AHJO, Ejutla, Criminal, 90/25	Juana María	Suspected of infanticide; acquitted.
95	1884	AHMO, Justicia, Corte de Justicia 1ª sala, 1883–84, caja 7	María del Carmen	Convicted of infanticide; sentenced to two years, eight months; Supreme Court raised it to four years.
96	1884	AHMO, Justicia, Corte de Justicia 1ª sala, 1883–84, caja 7	Merced López	Convicted of infanticide; sentenced to eighteen months' service in the Hospital General.
97	1884	AHMO, Justicia, Juzgado 2° criminal, 1884, caja 20	Pilar Ramírez	Suspected of infanticide; acquitted.

(continued)

#	Date	Reference	Accused	Charge/Outcome
98	1884	AGN, TSJDF, 1ª instancia	María Paz Rodríguez	Suspected of infanticide.
99	1885	AGN, TSJDF, 1885, caja 939	Josefa Vázquez	Midwife suspected of infanticide; acquitted.
100	1885	AGN, TSJDF, 1885, caja 940	María Magdalena	Suspected of infanticide; acquitted.
101	1885	AHMO, Justicia, Corte de justicia 2ª sala, 1884–85, caja 7	Dionicia Mota, Epigeminia, Micaela y Zenon Mota, Miguel Paz	Convicted of infanticide; court of first instance sentenced to three years' imprisonment; appellate court reduced sentence to one year.
102	1885	AHMO, Justicia, Corte de justicia 1ª sala, 1884–85, caja 8	Santiago Antonio, Ignacia Juana	She is acquitted; he is convicted of infanticide and sentenced to eight years' imprisonment.
103	1885	AHMO, Justicia, Corte de Justicia 1ª sala, 1884–85, caja 8	Juana Jiménez	Convicted of infanticide; sentenced to two years' imprisonment and a one-hundred-peso fine, deprivation of *patria potestad* for three years.
104	1885	AHMO, Justicia, Corte de Justicia, 2ª sala, 1884–85, caja 7	María de Petrocinio García	Convicted of infanticide; sentenced to six years, six months' imprisonment in the *carcel de mujeres*.
105	1885	AHMO, Justicia, caja 29	Margarita Morales	Suspected of infanticide; inconclusive documentation.
106	1885	AGN, TSJDF, 1ª instancia de Tlalpam	Santiago Miranda	Suspected of infanticide.
107	1885	AGN, TSJDF, 3º correccional	Ramona Torres	Suspected of infanticide.
108	1886	AHMO, Justicia, Corte de Justicia, 2ª sala, 1885–87, caja 8	Toribio Vargas	Convicted of infanticide; sentenced to two years, 190 days (later reduced slightly), five-peso fine, suspension of *patria potestad* for two years.

#	Date	Reference	Accused	Charge/Outcome
109	1886	AGN, TSJDF, 4º correccional	José Sotero García y otro	Suspected of infanticide.
110	1887	AGN, TSJDF, 4º correccional		Suspected of infanticide;
111	1888	AHMO, Justicia, Juzgado 1º criminal, 1888, subserie: procesos, caja 42	Felicitas Cruz	Suspected of infanticide; dies before judgment rendered, but likely would have been acquitted.
112	1888	AGN, TSJDF, 1888 caja 1092	Pascuala Chávez	Suspected of infanticide; indication is that she was acquitted.
113	1888	AHMO, Justicia, Juzgado 2º criminal, 1888, caja 64	Guadalupe García	Suspected of infanticide; acquitted.
114	1888	AGN, TSJDF, 2ª sala	Casmira Montes de Oca	Suspected of infanticide.
115	1889	AHMO, Justicia, 2ª sala, 1889–90, caja 10	Antonia María	Convicted of infanticide; sentenced to three years' reclusion and fined.
116	1889	AHMO, Justicia, Juzgado 2º de lo criminal, 1889, caja 72	Micaela Velasco, Francisca y Sixta Pérez	Suspected of infanticide; acquitted.
117	1889	AGN, TSJDF, 2ª sala	Juana Morales	Suspected of infanticide.
118	1889	AGN, TSJDF, 3º criminal	Trinidad Espindola	Suspected of infanticide.
119	1889	AGN, TSJDF, 4º criminal	María Sostenes Benitez	Suspected of infanticide.
120	1889	AGN, TSJDF, 1º criminal	Guadalupe Rosas	Suspected of infanticide.
121	1889	AGN, TSJDF, Juzgado 1ª instancia del partido de Tlalpam	Gerónima Dávila	Suspected of infanticide.
122	1889	AGN, TSJDF, 4º correccional	María Ysabel González	Suspected of infanticide.

(continued)

#	Date	Reference	Accused	Charge/Outcome
123	1890	ACSCJ, 48418	Luz Morales	Convicted of infanticide; sentenced to service in a hospital.
124	1890	AGN, TSJDF, 5° criminal		Suspected of infanticide.
125	1890	AGN, TSJDF, 1° criminal	Q.R.R.	Suspected of infanticide.
126	1890	AGN, TSJDF		Suspected of infanticide.
127	1890	AGN, TSJDF, 1ª instancia de Tlalpam	María Teodora Ybañez	Suspected of infanticide.
128	1890	AGN, TSJDF, 4° criminal	Eligio Cortes	Suspected of infanticide.
129	1891	AHMO, Justicia, Juzgado 2° Criminal, 1891, caja 79	Marciala Lotarriba	Suspected of infanticide; acquitted.
130	1891	AHMO, Justicia, Juzgado 2° de lo criminal, 1891, caja 79	Mauricia García	Convicted of infanticide by court of first sentence; appellate court acquitted.
131	1891	AGN, TSJDF, 2ª sala	Petra Moreno	Suspected of infanticide.
132	1891	AGN, TSJDF		Suspected of infanticide.
133	1891	AGN, TSJDF, 1ª instancia del partido de Tlalpam	Manuel Zavala	Suspected of infanticide.
134	1891	AGN, TSJDF, 3° criminal	Marciana Martínez	Suspected of infanticide.
135	1894	AGN, TSJDF, 5° criminal	María Dolores Valenzuela	Suspected of infanticide.
136	1894	AGN, TSJDF, 5° criminal	Pedro Chavarria y otro	Suspected of infanticide.
137	1894	AGN, TSJDF, 5° criminal		Suspected of infanticide.
138	1895	AGN, TSJDF, 5° criminal	Q.R.R.	Suspected of infanticide.
139	1895	AGN, TSJDF	Rosario Wilkes	Suspected of infanticide.
140	1895	AGN, TSJDF, 5° criminal		Suspected of infanticide.

#	Date	Reference	Accused	Charge/Outcome
141	1896	AGN, TSJDF, 5° criminal	Severiana Santillan	Suspected of infanticide.
142	1896	AGN, TSJDF, 1° criminal	QRR	Suspected of infanticide.
143	1897	AHMO, Justicia, Corte de justicia 2ª sala, 1897–98, caja 17; AHMO, Justicia, Juzgado 2° criminal, 1896–97, caja 102	Paula López	Convicted of infanticide; sentenced to three years, one month in city prison.
144	1897	AGN, TSJDF, Juzgado 1° criminal	QRR	Suspected of infanticide.
145	1898	AGN, TSJDF, 1ª instancia de Tlalpam y Xochilmil	Los que resulten responsables	Suspected of infanticide.
146	1898	AGN, TSJDF, Juzgado de Tlalpam y Xochimilco	Felipa Telles	Suspected of infanticide.
147	1898	AGN, TSJDF, 3° correccional	Marcelino Cortes	Suspected of infanticide.
148	1898	AGN, TSJDF, Juzgaco 1ª instancia del partido de Tlalpam y Xochilmilco	Julia Velázquez	Suspected of infanticide.
149	1899	AGN, TSJDF, Juzgado 3° correccional		Suspected of infanticide.

Sources: AGN, Justicia, TSJDF; AHJO, Criminal, Teposcolula, Villa Alta, Ejutla; ACSCJ.

Notes: Excluded were 176 cases recorded in the AGN's Tribunal Superior del Distrito Federal. Fonds caja list inventory described as instances in which officials or members of the public discovered newborn or fetal corpses but in which the court had no suspects to pursue; neither are cases of abandoned, exposed, or the accidental killing of children or fetuses included here. The titles whose records do not indicate an outcome have only been located in the caja list catalog of the TSJDF rather than acquired in totality.

Glossary

aborto   abortion; miscarriage

alcalde   first instance judge and municipal official

alcalde mayor   magistrate and district administrator

altamisa   artemisia

boticario   pharmacist

botico   pharmacy

buenas costumbres   moral habits

calidad   quality or status

casta   person of mixed racial ancestry

castiza/o   person with one indigenous and three Spanish grandparents

cátedra   professorship; formal curriculum of study

cihuapatli   aster flower

cirujano   surgeon

comadre   midwife; godmother; gossip

criolla/o   creole; a person of Spanish descent born in the Spanish America

cuernecillo de centeno   ergot, a fungus grown on rye that acted as a labor accelerator

curandera   healer

curador   court-appointed legal defender

depósito   supervised custody

estupro   deflowering

falcultativo   accredited physician

hechicería   spell making, witchcraft

limpieza de sangre   blood purity

matrona   midwife

médico   physician

palabra de casamiento   promise of matrimony

partera/o   midwife

parto   birth

protomédico   head of the medical board

Protomedicato   medical board

recogimiento   reformatory institution for wayward women

soltera   single woman reputed to not be a virgin

temazcal   Mesoamerican steam bath

teniente   deputy of a municipal council officer

tenedora/o   birth assistant responsible for physically restraining women in labor

teratología   the study of birth abnormalities

ticitl   Nahua healers

tlaquatzin   dried tail of an opossum; believed to have expulsive properties

tocología   obstetrics

zaguán   breezeway

Notes

All translations are the author's own unless indicated otherwise. A glossary of Spanish terms appears prior to the notes.

Preface

1. Vela, "Current Abortion Regulation," 11–13.

2. Acero, "Más de 700 mujeres criminalizadas."

3. García Vázquez, Moncayo Cuagliotti, and Sánchez Trocino, "El parto en México," 820.

4. Scheper-Hughes's important study *Death without Weeping* was one of the earliest books to critically examine the topic of mothering in contemporary Latin America. Foucault's *The History of Sexuality* is the classic work introducing the notion of the constructed nature of what had previously been considered a topic that had no history. Laqueur's *Making Sex* is also foundational in this regard. See also McClive's historicization of reproductive biology, *Menstruation and Procreation*.

Introduction

1. AHJO, Teposcolula, Criminal, 1845, legajo 64, exp. 3.

2. Dore, "One Step Forward, Two Steps Back." Like Dore, I take a more pessimistic view of the implications of liberalism on family law and social expectations than did Arrom in "Changes in Mexican Family Law in the Nineteenth Century."

3. Briggs, "Introduction," 3. Blum, Tamera, Puerto, and Warren present an excellent introduction to the links between reproduction and nation-building in *Women, Ethnicity, and Medical Authority*. In the Mexican context, Lipsett-Rivera examines the emergence of a more explicit discourse of motherhood in the late colonial and early republican periods in legal disputes concerning child custody and property law in "Marriage and Family Relations in Mexico."

4. Birn and Necochea López, "Footprints in the Future," 505.

5. The Protomedicato was a board usually composed of three *protomédicos*, licensed medical examiners. New Spain acquired its first *protomédico* in 1527, but the position was not regularized until the era of Philip II in 1570. A *Real Cédula* of 1646 dictated that the head professor of medicine at Mexico's Royal University would simultaneously serve as the head of the board. On the history of this body, see Lanning, *The Royal Protomedicato*.

6. The heyday of the Mexican eugenicist movement was in the postrevolutionary era. However, the science of *puériculture* and the celebration of public health campaigns promoting and regulation reproduction of the national citizenry originated in the Porfirian period. Schell, "Eugenics Policy and Practice," 485; Stern, "Responsible Mothers."

7. Stepan, *"The Hour of Eugenics,"* 110.

8. For an introduction to these positions, see Duffin, *History of Medicine*, 276–310.

9. Flores y Troncoso, *Historia de la Medicina en México*, 3:621.

10. Arney reproduces Cianfrani's chart of obstetrical progress in *Power and the Profession of Obstetrics*, 4. Uribe Elías, *La invención de la mujer*.

11. Brodsky, *The Control of Childbirth*, 5.

12. Carillo, "Nacimiento y muerte de una profesión," 167.

13. Hernández Sáenz, *Learning to Heal*, 205.

14. Díaz Robles and Oropeza Sandoval, "Las parteras de Guadalajara."

15. McLaren, *A History of Contraception*, 152.

16. Murphy-Lawless, *Reading Birth and Death*; Jordanova, *Sexual Visions*; Duden, *The Woman beneath the Skin*.

17. Murphy-Lawless, *Reading Birth and Death*, 33.

18. Brodsky, *The Control of Childbirth*, 49.

19. Mary Daly, quoted in Duffin, *History of Medicine*, 278. Such presentations are predominant in much writing about the history of obstetrics, particularly in the United States. See Borst, *Catching Babies*, and McGregor, *From Midwives to Medicine*.

20. See Numbers, *Medicine in the New World*, 7.

21. For a discussion of past approaches and current challenges to this view of "traditional" indigenous medical practice, see Palmer, *From Popular Medicine to Medical Populism*, 1–10.

22. Lanning, *The Royal Protomedicato*, 303.

23. Marland, "Introduction," 1, 8.

24. Fields, *Pestilence and Headcolds*, is an illuminating example of a work embodying Goodman's insistence, in "Science, Medicine, and Technology," that histories of science and medicine in Latin America followed more complex development than mere "transmission from Europe, from cultural center to periphery" (25).

25. Díaz Robles and Oropeza Sandoval, "Las parteras de Guadalajara," 238.

26. Sesia, "'Women Come Here on Their Own,'" 121–22. See also Carillo, "Nacimiento y muerte de una profesión," 189.

27. Miguel Jiménez, "Temascales," *El Siglo Diez y Nueve*, August 20, 1874, 2.

28. León, *La obstetricia en México*, 143.

29. Ibid., 159.

30. Ventura Pastor, *Preceptos generales*, 1:324–29.

31. Penyak's insightful essays "Midwives and Legal medicine in México" and "Obstetrics and the Emergence of Women" were influential on my development of this reading of Mexican midwives.

32. This is a reading of the relationship between official and popular medicine supported by Palmer's research of medicine in the context of modern Costa Rica. See *From Popular Medicine to Medical Populism*.

33. Few, "Medical *Mestizaje*," 133.

34. Few, *For All of Humanity*, 14.

35. Holler, "Hybrid Births," 6.

36. Few, *Women Who Live Evil Lives*, 95.

37. Of sixteen such denunciations made to the Mexican Holy Office from the mid-seventeenth to the mid-eighteenth century that I located, the court only pursued five cases past the denunciation phase.

38. Sahagún, quoted in Flores y Troncoso, *Historia de la Medicina en México*, 1:292.

39. Few discusses the merging of pre-Columbian understandings of supernatural illnesses involving birth and colonial suspicions of indigenous sorcery in "Medical *Mestizaje*," 138–39.

40. Flores y Troncoso, *Historia de la Medicina en México*, 3:620–21.

41. Such views are presented in Carillo, "Nacimiento y muerte de una profesión"; Hernández Sáenz, *Learning to Heal*; Díaz Robles and Oropeza Sandoval, "Las parteras de Guadalajara"; and McClain, "Reinterpreting Women in Healing Roles."

42. Few, *Women Who Live Evil Lives*, 5.

43. Díaz Robles and Oropeza Sandoval, "Las parteras de Guadalajara," 260.

44. Cueto and Palmer, *Medicine and Public Health*, 6.

45. Very little research exists on the topics of childbirth and contraception in the colonial period, although both Lanning, *The Royal Protomedicato*, and Hernández Sáenz, *Learning to Heal*, treat obstetrics in their general medical histories of New Spain, and Few, "Atlantic World Monsters," and "Medical *Mestizaje*," and Holler "Hybrid Births" have both produced research on colonial midwifery and obstetrical developments. A developing literature on nineteenth-century Mexican midwifery does exist to which Penyak and Carillo, in particular, have contributed important works. Most nineteenth-century scholarship, particularly the excellent work of Speckman Guerra, "Morir a manos de una mujer," and Cházaro, "Mexican Women's Pelves," focus exclusively on the era of the Porfiriato. Gorbach's *El monstruo* is an interesting introduction to the nineteenth-century development of teratology, the study of birth abnormalities, in Mexico. There is an older and more developed historiography of childbirth, contraception, and obstetrics in both the United States and Western Europe. Classic works in theses contexts include Arney, *Power and the Profession of Obstetrics*; Marland, ed., *The Art of Midwifery*; Wertz and Wertz, *Lying-In*; and Wilson, *The Making of Man-Midwifery*.

46. One such study is Wrigley, Davies, Oeppen, and Schofield, *English Population History*.

47. Pilbean, ed., *Themes in Modern European History*, 185.

48. Reina Aoyama, *Caminos de luz y sombra*, 42.

49. Cook and Borah, *Essays in Population History*, 2:289.

50. Ibid., 297.

51. McLaren, *A History of Contraception*, 142, 145.

52. Brodsky, *The Control of Childbirth*, 62.

53. Shorter, *A History of Women's Bodies*, 98.

54. Tanck de Estrada, "Muerte Precoz," 216. See also Newson, "The Demographic Impact of Colonization," 170.

55. Hernández Sáenz, *Learning to Heal*, 208.

56. On the underreporting of neonatal mortality in eighteenth-century Mexico, see Rabell Romero, "Evaluación del subregistro de defunciones infantiles."

57. McCaa, "The Peopling of Nineteenth-Century Mexico," 605–7.

58. Ibid., 620.

59. Ibid.

60. In Mexico City, I used the following archives: The Archivo General de la Nación de México, the Archivo Histórico del Distrito Federal (sometimes called the ex-Ayuntamiento Archives), the Archivo Histórico de la Secretaría de Salud, the Archivo Central de la Supreme Corte de Justicia de la Nación, the Archivo Histórico de la Facultad de Medicina, and the Biblioteca Nicolás León. In Oaxaca, I used the Archivo Histórico Judicial del Estado de Oaxaca, the Archivo Histórico Municipal de la Ciudad de Oaxaca, and the Biblioteca Francisco de Burgoa.

61. Taylor, *Drinking, Homicide, and Rebellion*; Stern, *The Secret History of Gender*.

62. Overmyer-Velázquez and Yannakakis, "The Renaissance of Oaxaca City's Historical Archives."

63. Jaffary, *False Mystics*.

64. Archivo Histórico del Arzobispado de México, Base de Pelagio Antonio de Labistida y Dávalos, caja 155, exp. 47, Sección: Secretaría Arzobispal, Serie: Parroquias. Año 1883. Milpa Alta. El Párroco sobre un caso de aborto. Fs. 3.

65. Publications searched in the database include the *El Diario de México*, *El Monitor Republicano*, *La Patria*, *El Universal*, and *El Siglo Diez y Nueve*. I am grateful to Campos's *Home Grown* for alerting me to the existence of the database and to Concordia University's history librarian, Geoffrey Little, for arranging my access to it.

Chapter One

1. Powers, *Women in the Crucible of Conquest*, 53, 55.

2. Kellogg, *Weaving the Past*, 73. Twinam discovered elites engaging in similar practices in eighteenth-century Mexico; see "Honor, Sexuality, and Illegitimacy," 129.

3. López Austin, "La sexualidad entre los antiguos nahuas," 160; Quezada, "Creencias tradicionales sobre embarazo y parto"; Schlegel, "Status, Property and the Value on Virginity," 723.

4. Lavrin, "Introduction," 10.

5. Vives's work was first published in Latin in 1523 and printed in Spanish in 1528. He dedicated his tract to Catherine of Aragon, daughter of Queen Isabella I of Castile and the first wife of Henry VIII. Vives designed the work to be a model for the education of Catherine's daughter, Mary Tudor.

6. This quotation comes from Franciscan theologian Arbiol y Diez's 1731 *Explicacion breve de todo el sagrado texto de la doctrina christiana*, 17. However, Arbiol's precise articulation dates to a 1555 decree issued by Pope Paul V. Sixteenth-century Spanish American catechisms declared that Jesus Christ "was born from the virginal womb of the Holy Virgin Mary, who was herself a Virgin before the birth, during the birth and after the birth"; see "Acuerdo de los prelados del III Concilio limense," 172. The concept of Mary's perpetual virginity dates back to the fourth century. Haffner, *The Mystery of Mary*, 164–65.

7. Catholic Church, *Catecismo para uso de los párrocos*, 41.

8. Ibid., 44.

9. León records these and other prayers circulating in the colonial era in *La obstetricia en México*, 146.

10. AGN, Inquisición, vol. 873, exp. 12, fol. 415; emphasis in the original.

11. Ibid.

12. AGN, Inquisición, vol. 1445, exp. 30, fol. 143; emphasis in the original.

13. Ibid., fol. 151v.

14. Ibid., fol. 167v.

15. These included devotions to the thirteenth-century saint Ramón Nonato, who had apparently been extracted from his mother by caesarean section. Nonato's novenario for pregnant women was published in New Spain in 1780 and reprinted in 1848. Rodríguez, "Costumbres y tradiciones en torno al embarazo y al parto," 506.

16. León, *La obstetricia en México*, 147, 170.

17. On race and sexual honor in the colonial era, see Martínez, *Genealogical Fictions*; and Twinam, *Public Lives, Private Secrets*.

18. Pérez Duarte y Noroña, "Los alimentos en la historia del México independiente," 875.

19. Seed, *To Love, Honor, and Obey*.

20. Jaffary, "Incest, Sexual Virtue and Social Mobility," 96.

21. Don Joseph Antonio Barrango, quoted in Jaffary, "Incest, Sexual Virtue and Social Mobility," 100.

22. The classic work on the connection between female honor as sexual virtue in colonial society is Gutiérrez, *When Jesus Came, the Corn Mothers Went Away*.

23. Lavrin, "Introduction," 10.

24. Erauso, *Lieutenant Nun*.

25. Urban's quote is contained in the 1653 pamphlets titled *Relaciones* that recounted Erauso's story. These documents, in turn, were reproduced in Cumplido, *La ilustración Mexicana*, 3:630.

26. Boyer, "Catarina María Complains." For more information on such suits, see Twinam, "The Negotiation of Honor"; and Seed, *To Love, Honor, and Obey*.

27. Boyer, "Catarina María Complains," 156, 160.

28. Socolow, *The Women of Colonial Latin America*, 152–53. See also Socolow, "Women and Crime."

29. Socolow, *The Women of Colonial Latin America*, 153.

30. Medina, *Cartilla nueva util y necesaria*, chap. 2, n.p.

31. Ibid.

32. Torres mentions in his prologue that Medina's work was still commonly consulted in his day. Torres, *Manual de partos*, iv.

33. León, *La obstetricia en México*, 217; Izquierdo, *Raudón*, 162.

34. Mauriceau, *Traité des maladies des femmes grosses*, 28.

35. Baudelocque, *Principes sur l'art des accouchements*, 59; emphasis in the original.

36. Other contemporaries concurred. Levret wrote that a woman could become pregnant although her hymen might still be intact. Levret, *Tratado de partos*, 23.

37. *Cartilla de partos*, 7.

38. Torres, *Manual de partos*, 34.

39. Huacuja, *Tratado práctico de partos*, 13.

40. In 1576, the *alcalde* of Teposcolula, Oaxaca, called upon two midwives to examine a plaintiff in order to determine whether or not she was a virgin. AHJO, Teposcolula, Criminal, legajo 1, exp. 54.

41. Penyak, "Midwives and Legal Medicine in Mexico," 258.

42. AHJO, Teposcolula, Criminal, legajo 18, exp. 34.

43. Ibid., fol. 4.

44. Ibid., fol. 4v.

45. Ibid., fol. 20.

46. AHJO, Ejutla, Criminal, legajo 34, exp. 18, fol. 3.

47. Hernández Sáenz, *Learning to Heal*, 207.

48. Penyak, "Midwives and Legal Medicine in Mexico," 262.

49. AGN, Criminal, vol. 705, exp. 2, fol. 2v.

50. Ibid., fol. 27.

51. Ibid., fol. 28v. Midwives provided similar testimony judging that the victim had not been raped. AGN, Criminal, vol. 585, exp. 9.

52. Penyak, "Midwives and Legal Medicine in Mexico," 260.

53. AHJO, Ejutla, Criminal, legajo 21, exp. 27, fols. 7, 11.

54. Ibid., legajo 70, exp. 5.

55. Ibid., fol. 3v.

56. Ibid., fol. 5.

57. Ibid., legajo 105, exp. 9. When describing her status in her daughter's case in 1879, Pacheco declared her she was a "widow, mature in age, y de ejericio analogo," which I interpret to mean that she performed work normally expected of women of her position.

58. AHJO, Ejutla, Criminal, legajo 105, exp. 9, fol. 3v.

59. In, for instance, AGN, Criminal, vol. 705, exp. 2, fol. 2v; AGN, Criminal, vol. 670, exp. 2; AHJO, Teposcolula, Criminal, legao 18, exp. 34; and AHJO, Ejutla, Criminal, legajo 21, exp. 27, fol. 11.

60. AGN, Criminal, vol. 624, exp. 1.

61. Ibid., fols. 7–7v.

62. Twinam, *Public Lives, Private Secrets*, 11. Baptismal records from Mexico City's cathedral show a rate of 33 percent illegitimacy for Spanish women over the last sixty years of the seventeenth century. Blum, "Public Welfare and Child Circulation," 242.

63. For further discussion, see Lavrin, "Sexuality in Colonial Mexico."

64. Columbia University Libraries, Special Collections, Mexico—Historical Manuscripts, 1649–1886, no. 654, n.p.

65. Similar cases are represented in Columbia University Libraries, Special Collections, Mexico—Historical Manuscripts, 1649–1886, nos. 668 and 719.

66. Ibid., no. 762.

67. Lavrin, "Sexuality in Colonial Mexico," 64; Twinam, "Honor, Sexuality and Illegitimacy"; Lipsett-Rivera, "A Slap in the Face of Honor," 191–94.

68. AGN, Inquisición, vol. 561, exp. 6, fol. 557v.

69. Esteyneffer, *Florilegio medicinal*, 324.

70. Juan Manuel Venegas, quoted in León, *La obstetricia en México*, 132. Other works that discuss the "detention of the menses" include Farfán, *Tractado breve de medicina* and Vigarous, *Curso elemental de las enfermedades*.

71. Venegas, *Compendio de la medicina*, 241–43.

72. Riddle, *Contraception and Abortion*, 27.

73. For further discussion of menstrual regulators in the European context, see McClive, *Menstruation and Procreation*, 125–26.

74. AGN, Inquisición, vol. 561, exp. 6, fol. 557v.

75. Twinam, "Honor, Sexuality, and Legitimacy," 124–46.

76. See Twinam, "The Negotiation of Honor"; and Nazzari, "An Urgent Need to Conceal."

77. Apan was a plains territory in the southeast of what is now the state of Hidalgo.

78. Columbia University Libraries, Special Collections, Mexico—Historical Manuscripts, 1649–1886, no. 716, n.p.

79. Similar cases can be found in the Columbia University Libraries, Special Collections, Mexico—Historical Manuscripts, 1649–1886, nos. 661, 658, 718, 723.

80. Lipsett-Rivera, *Gender and the Negotiation of Daily Life*, 81–103.

81. Ibid., 94.

82. Ibid.

83. Ibid., 102.

84. Sloan, *Runaway Daughters*.

85. Ibid., 4.

86. Ibid., 152.

87. Ibid., 174.

88. Dirección general de estadísticas, *Estadísticas sociales del Porfiriato*, 19, 21.

89. Blum, *Domestic Economies*, 30.

90. Milanich, who notes that the association between poverty and illegitimacy seems to have strengthened in the late nineteenth century, might be more sympathetic to my claim. See Milanich, "Historical Perspectives on Illegitimacy and Illegitimates," 74.

91. AGN, Bandos, vol. 24, exp. 55; *El Siglo Diez y Nueve*, June 9, 1851, 3.

92. *El Siglo Diez y Nueve*, July 1, 1869, 1.

93. For further discussion, see Rivera-Garza, "The Criminalization of the Syphilitic Body."

94. Tenorio-Trillo, *Mexico at the World's Fairs*, 149.

95. Flores y Troncoso, *El hímen en México*, 16.

96. Ibid., 55.

97. Ibid., 57.

98. Ibid., 33.

99. "Remitido," *El Siglo Diez y Nueve*, June 8, 1886, 2.

100. Flores y Troncoso, *El hímen en México*, 50.

101. Ibid., 56.

102. Ibid., 65.

103. Ibid., 33, 51, 70.

104. Tenorio-Trillo, *Mexico at the World's Fairs,* 150.

105. Flores y Troncoso, *El hímen en México*, 16.

106. Ibid., 20.

107. Ibid., 22, 28.

Chapter Two

1. McClive, "The Hidden Truths of the Belly."

2. Quezada, "Creencias tradicionales sobre embarazo y parto," 307. In *For All of Humanity*, Few demonstrates that the incorporation of indigenous medical expertise continued to characterize the development of medical practice in Guatemala in the era of the Enlightenment.

3. See Quiñones Keber, ed. *Representing Aztec Ritual*, and León-Portilla, *Bernardino de Sahagún*.

4. Fields, *Pestilence and Headcolds*, 45.

5. *Sahagún*, quoted in Fields, *Pestilence and Headcolds*, 47.

6. Flores y Troncoso, *Historia de la medicina en México*, 1:112.

7. Rodríguez, "Costumbres y tradiciones," 502.

8. Sahagún, quoted in Quezada, "Creencias tradicionales sobre parto y embarazo," 309.

9. Flores y Troncoso, *Historia de la medicina en México*, 1:288–89. See also Burkhart, "Mexica Women on the Home Front," 49.

10. Alcina Franch, "Procreación, amor y sexo entre los mexica," 64.

11. Quezada, "Métodos anticonceptivos y abortivos tradicionales," 226, 227; Alcina Franch, "Procreación, amor y sexo," 67.

12. Sahagún, *Historia general de las cosas de Nueva España*, 2:592–98.

13. Ibid., 605–6.

14. Ibid., 606.

15. Flores y Troncoso, *Historia de la medicina en México*, 3:646.

16. Ibid., 1:297.

17. Rodríguez, "La medicina científica y su difusión," 186.

18. Quezada, "Creencias tradicionales sobre embarazo y parto."

19. Flores y Troncoso, *Historia de la medicina en México*, 1:229–31.

20. Ibid., 146; Quezada, "Métodos anticonceptivos y abortivos tradicionales," 231.

21. Lanning, *The Royal Protomedicato*, 307.

22. Arechederreta, "Manuscrito al M.I. y Rl. Tribunal del Proto-Medicato de México," Wellcome Library, WMS Amer. 19, fol. 9.

23. León, *Historia de la obstetricia*, 199.

24. Flores y Troncoso, *Historia de la medicina en México*, 2:301.

25. *Gazeta de México*, vol. 4, 1790.

26. Archivo Histórico del Distrito Federal, Ayumtamiento Gobierno del DF, Sección Policia Salubridad, vol. 3668, exp. 14, fol. 2.

27. Flores y Troncoso, *Historia de la medicina en México*, 2:395.

28. Lanning, *The Royal Protomedicato*, 44.

29. Hernández Sáenz, *Learning to Heal*, 206.

30. Astruc, *The Art of Midwifery*, 3.

31. For an overview of the history of obstetrics and gynecology, see Duffin, *History of Medicine*, 276–310.

32. Hobby, "Introduction," xv.

33. Medina, *Cartilla nueva util y necesaria*, n.p. Medina's text was originally published in Madrid in 1750 at the direction of the Royal Protomedicato when it passed legislation requiring the licensing of midwives. The text was to serve as a handbook for preparing midwives for the Protomedicato's examination of their professional knowledge and skills.

34. AGN, Inquisición, vol. 798, exp. 8, fol. 161v.

35. Penyak, "Midwives and Legal Medicine in México," 256.

36. AGI, Indiferente, vol. 2051, n. 32, fol. 1.

37. Ibid., fols. 6, 15.

38. Ibid., fol. 1.

39. Ibid., fol. 6.

40. Díaz Robles and Oropeza Sandoval, "Las parteras de Guadalajara," 238.

41. AHJO, Ejutla, Criminal, legajo 79, exp. 25, fol. 3.

42. AGN, Inquisición, vol. 561, exp. 6, fol. 537.

43. Arrom, *The Women of Mexico City*, 198.

44. AGN, Inquisición, vol. 791, exp. 16, fols. 353–63.

45. Ibid., fol. 164.

46. AGN, Inquisición, vol. 561, exp. 6, fols. 541v, 555, 565. A an earlier case from 1614 also records a mulata woman using peyote, a cactus known to pre-Columbian indigenous healers for its hallucinogenic properties, to determine if she was pregnant. AGN, Inquisición, vol. 302, exp. 8.

47. AGN, Inquisición, vol. 599, exp. 15, fol. 541.

48. Ibid., vol. 1028, exp. 7.

49. Cook and Borah, *Essays in Population History*, 2:198.

50. Aguirre Beltrán, *La población negra de México*, 225.

51. Florescano and Sánchez, "La época de las reformas borbónicas," 520.

52. Gonzales, *Mexicanos*, 116.

53. Díaz Robles and Oropeza Sandoval, "Las parteras de Guadalajara," 239; Lanning, *The Royal Protomedicato*, 305.

54. AHFM, Protomedicato, legao 12, exp. 15, fol. 4.

55. AHMO, Justicia, Juzgada de 1ª instancia, 1836–37, caja 15, "Contra Felipa Romero partera, acusada de infanticidio," fol. 17.

56. León, *Apuntes para la historia de la obstetricia*, 2.

57. AGN, Inquisición, vol. 1313, exp. 12, fol. 2. Although most often female, men occasionally acted as *tenedoros*. AHMO, Justicia, Juzgado de 1ª instancia, 1836–37, caja 15, "Contra Felipa Romero, de oficio partera, acusada de infanticidio," fol. 13; AHJO, Ejutla, Penal, legajo 79, esp. 25, 1881, fol. 2v.

58. AGN, Inquisición, vol. 1313, exp. 12, fol. 2.

59. Ibid., fol. 3.

60. *Gazeta de México*, February 8, 1785, 267.

61. *Gazeta de México*, March 8, 1792, 84; *Gazeta de México*, December 30, 1793, 709; *Gazeta de México*, November 13, 1794, 638.

62. AGN, Inquisición, vol. 302, exp. 8, fol. 128.

63. Epps, *Peyote vs. The State*, 54.

64. These include AGN, Inquisición, vol. 513, exp. 31 (1665); vol. 561, exp. 6 (1652); vol. 599, exp. 15 (1664); vol. 952, exp. 3 (1705); vol. 723, exp. 3 (1708); vol. 753, fol. 396 (1713); vol. 872, exp. 31 (1736); and vol. 992, exp. 10 (1754).

65. AGN, Indiferente Virreinal, vol. 6271, exp. 26, fol. 3v.

66. AHMO, Justicia, Juzgado de 1ª instancia, 1857–61, caja 46, "Contra Anacleta Avila, por el infanticidio que cometió con su niña recién nacida," fol. 8.

67. AGN, TSJDF, 1883, caja 841, "Contra Pomposa Acosta por aborto provocado," fol. 8.

68. AGN, Criminal, vol. 626, exp. 1, fol. 1v.

69. AHJO, Teposcolula, Criminal, legajo 58, exp. 21, fol. 5v.

70. ACSCJ, (1840), 1815, "Toca á la causa instruida á María San José Romo por infanticidio," fols. 7–12.

71. Hernández Sáenz, *Learning to Heal*, 211.

72. León, *La obstetricia en México*, 221.

73. Lanning, *The Royal Protomedicato*, 50.

74. Ibid., 299.

75. Doctor Luis José Montaña was a key advocate of the founding of the Royal Botanical Gardens, which he saw as essential to developing physicians' practical knowledge of botany and natural remedies. Montaña was also instrumental in the establishment of a clinic of practical medicine at the Royal Pontifical University in 1806. Rodríguez, "La medicina científica," 183.

76. Ignacio Bartolache, "Avisos acerca del mal hysterico, que llaman *latido*," *Mercurio Volante* 6 (1772): 48.

77. Ibid. Spain's Real Colegio de Cirugía published the *Compendio de el arte de partear compuesto para el uso de los reales colegios de cirugía* in 1765. León, *La obstetricia en México*, 218, notes that the work circulated in Mexico.

78. AGI, México, vol. 1880, fols., 1, 3, 3v, 4.

79. Díaz Robles and Oropeza Sandoval, "Las parteras de Guadalajara," 240. Nueva Galicia was a territory northwest of the capital, encompassing the present-day states of Aguascalientes, Colima, Jalisco, Nayarit, and Zacatecas.

80. Voekel, *Alone before God*, 173.

81. Muñoz, *Recopilación de las leyes*, 309. I have encountered one document suggesting that formal examinations of Mexican parteras may have preceded the 1750 decree. In 1709, the Protomedicato registered a formal request with a colonial judicial officer for the payment of interest for services rendered in administering exams for doctors, *boticarios*, surgeons, barbers, and midwives. AGN, Indiferente Virreinal, caja 5481, exp. 81.

82. See also, for example, Ventura Pastor, *Preceptos generales*, 1:3.

83. AHFM, Protomedicato, legajo 4, exp. 24, fol. 6v.

84. Ortiz, "From Hegemony to Subordination," 98.

85. The Royal College of Surgery, quoted in Izquierdo, *Raudón*, 161.

86. Izquierdo, *Raudón*, 161.

87. Carillo, "Nacimiento y muerte de una profesión," 178.

88. Miguel Moreno y Peña, quoted in Fields, *Pestilence and Headcolds*, 66.

89. AHFM, Protomedicato, legajo 10, exp. 12; and legajo 12, exp. 15. Hernández Sáenz located a third midwife licensed in the colonial era; see *Learning to Heal*, 206.

90. Flores y Troncoso, *Historia de la medicina en México*, 2:399.

91. Hernández Sáenz, *Learning to Heal*, 207.

92. AGN, Indiferente Virreinal, caja 574, exp. 2.

93. Díaz Robles and Oropeza Sandoval, "Las parteras de Guadalajara," 240.

94. Hernández Sáenz, *Learning to Heal*, 210.

95. AGN, Protomedicato, legajo 3, exp. 16, fol. 333v.

96. Carillo, "Nacimiento y muerte de una profesión, 170–71.

97. Karchmer Krivitsky, "La ginecología y la obstetricia," 285.

98. Maygrier, *Nuevo metodo para operar en los partos*.

99. León, *Historia de la obstetricia*, 217; Izquierdo, *Raudón*, 162. Other important European works include Alcalá Martínez, *Disertación Médico-quirúrgica, sobre una operación cesárea ejectuada en muger y feto vivos, en la ciudad de Valencia* (1753) and Virgili, *Compendio de el arte de partear* (1765).

100. León, *Historia de la obstetricia*, 221; Izquierdo, *Raudón*, 161, 163.

101. AGN, Indiferente Virreinal, caja 2325, exp. 28, fol. 1.

102. Levret, *Tratado de partos*, 56. As late as 1857, the explanation of how the "fertile principal journeyed to the egg" remained a mystery. Huacuja, *Tratado práctico de partos*, 21.

103. Vidart, *El discípulo instruido*, 20.

104. Ventura Pastor, *Preceptos generales*, 1:66–67.

105. Huacuja, *Tratado práctico de partos*, 20.

106. Medina, *Cartilla util y necesaria*, chap. 3, n.p.

107. *Cartilla de partos*, 14. On the medial ambiguity surrounding amenorrhea, see McClive, *Menstruation and Procreation*, 137–65.

108. Medina, *Cartilla util y necesaria*, chap. 3, n.p.

109. Vidart, *El discípulo instruido*, 30. Izquierdo, *Raudón*, 161, notes that Vidart's text was considered "one of the most instructive and indispensable" in the late colonial era.

110. Ventura Pastor, *Preceptos generales*, 1:125–27.

111. Esteyneffer, *Florilegio medicinal*, 341.

112. Ibid., 342.

113. "Prontuario o método fácil en donde se contienen las más eficaces medicinas," Wellcome Library, MS Amer. 18, fols. 42, 56, 63.

114. Ibid., fol. 86.

115. Torres, *Manual de partos*, 81–85.

116. Rodríguez, *Guía clínica del arte de los partos*, 32.

117. *El Siglo Diez y Nueve*, June 17, 1862, 4.

118. *El Siglo Diez y Nueve*, February 3, 1870, 4.

119. *El Siglo Diez y Nueve*, May 25, 1874, 4.

120. Neither does one of the most comprehensive midwifery tracts from the English context, Sharp's *The Midwives Book*, published in 1671, contain any discussion of cervical exams except during child delivery.

121. Lindemann, *Medicine and Society*, 269.

122. Ventura Pastor, *Preceptos generales*, 1:109–10. chap. 2, article 7.

123. Torres, *Manual de partos*, 88.

124. Rodríguez, *Guía clínica*, 1.

125. Ibid., 6.

126. Arechederreta, "Manuscrito al M.I. y Rl," fol. 9v.

127. Ventura Pastor, *Preceptos generales*, 1:183.

128. Ibid.

129. The texts of Maygrier circulated in late colonial Mexico. One of his tracts, *Nuevo metodo para operar en los partos*, was published in Mexico in 1821.

130. AGN, Inquisición, vol. 953, exp. 41, fol. 310.

131. Ibid.

132. Ibid.

133. Ibid.

134. AGN, Inquisición, vol. 1378, exp. 10, fol. 194; emphasis in the original.

135. Ibid., fols. 194–94v.

136. Ventura Pastor, *Preceptos generales*, 1:343. He describes other such cases on 311, 354, and 365.

137. Flores y Troncoso, *Historia de la medicina en México*, 3:676.

138. "Lección 3 (núm. 264) el parto," *El Diario de México*, July 3, 1806, 258.

139. "Concluye la 2. Carta sobre la preñez," *El Diario de México*, July 22, 1806, 213.

140. Carrillo, "Nacimiento y muerte de una profesión," 174.

141. Ibid.

Chapter Three

1. Calvo, "The Warmth of the Hearth," 292.

2. Arrom, *The Women of Mexico City*, 318n49. McCaa, "The Peopling of Nineteenth-Century Mexico," 620, notes that breast-feeding would have been the only effective contraceptive available to Tzeltal speakers in the highly fertile community of eighteenth-century Amatenango, Chiapas, and that women there did not even recognize it as such.

3. AHSS, Beneficiencia Pública, Establecimiento Hospitalarios, Hospital de Maternidad y de Infancia, legajo 4, "Estado que manifiesta el movimiento general de Enfermos habidas en los tres Departamentos del expresado desde el 1° de Julio de 1886 hasta el 30 de Junio de 1888."

4. Quezada, "Métodos anticonceptivos y abortivos tradicionales," 229. The closely related term *ayoxochquilitl* has also been translated as "pumpkin flower."

5. Rodríguez-Shadow, *La mujer azteca*, 121.

6. Quezada, "Métodos anticonceptivos y abortivos tradicionales," 230.

7. Gonzalo Fernández de Oviedo, quoted in Few, "Medical *Mestizaje*," 134.

8. Quezada, "Métodos anticonceptivos y abortivos tradicionales," 232.

9. Flores y Troncoso, *Historia de la medicina en México*, 1:342–43. Their use of *tlaquatzin* is surprising given that this was also a substance pre-Columbian midwives administered to encourage fertility. Quezada, "Métodos anticonceptivos y abortivos tradicionales," 226.

10. Quezada, "Métodos anticonceptivos y abortivos tradicionales," 232.

11. Ibid., 233; Flores y Troncoso, *Historia de la medicina en México*, 1:343.

12. Mexico would not be unique in this regard. Eccles, *Obstetrics and Gynaecology in Tudor and Stuart England*, 71, notes that evidence exists that women used both the contraceptive sponge and the condom in seventeenth-century England. Although both devices are mentioned in contemporary poetic works, neither are discussed in contemporary medical tracts.

13. Segura, *Avisos saludables a las parteras*, 15.

14. Medina, *Cartilla nueva util y necesaria*, n.p.

15. Fray Bartolomé de Alva, quoted in Zeb Tortorici, "Women at the Margins of the Unnatural," 8.

16. AGN, Inquisición, vol. 561, exp. 6, fol. 566.

17. Ibid.

18. Ibid., vol. 180, exp. 2, fol. 215; vol. 522, exp. 2, fol. 104; vol. 1246, exp. 5, fol. 130; and vol. 1231, exp. 1, fol. 152. For an excerpt of one such seventeenth-century Inquisition trial, see Rodríguez and Calvo, "Sobre la práctica del aborto en el Occidente de México."

19. Huntington Library, HM 4297, "Medicina Mexicana," fol. 56.

20. Ibid., fols. 5, 70.

21. Venegas, *Compendio de la medicina*, 241.

22. Jütte, *Contraception: A History*, 39, 75. One late nineteenth-century authority on American medicinal plants, Charles Millspaugh, noted that pennyroyal, "will often bring on the menses nicely; and if combined with a gill of brewer's yeast, it frequently acts well as an abortivant, should the intender be not too late with her prescription." Millspaugh, quoted in Brodie, *Contraception and Abortion in Nineteenth-Century America*, 44. Anthropological research from the 1970s revealed that many of the same substances described in sixteenth-century medical texts, including *manzanilla*, *zopatle* (*cihuapatli*), the tail of the *tlacuache*, and *altamisa*, continued to be popularly used by Mexican women seeking to regulate pregnancies through provoked miscarriages. Quezada, "Metodos anticonceptivos y abortivos tradicionales," 235–38. Current medical research demonstrates *altamisa*'s abortive properties. See Hijazi and Salhab, "Effects of Artemisia."

23. "Mexico, 18th Century: Compendium of Remedies," Wellcome Library, WMS Amer. 58, fol. 26.

24. "Supplemento á la Gazeta de México del viernes 18 de septiembre de 1795," 418, 422, 423, *Gazeta de México*.

25. "Prontuario o método fácil en donde se contienen las más eficaces medicinas," Wellcome Library, WMS Amer. 18, fol. 14.

26. Ibid., fol. 41.

27. Vásquez, "Florilegio medicinal," Wellcome Library, WMS Amer. 26, fol. 20v.

28. "Mexico, 18th Century: Compendium of Remedies," Wellcome Library, WMS Amer. 58, fol. 10.

29. AGN, Indiferente Virreinal, caja 6271, exp. 26, fol. 4.

30. Alexander von Humboldt, quoted in Arrom, *The Women of Mexico City*, 124.

31. Arrom, *The Women of Mexico City*, 125.

32. Morin, "Age at Marriage and Female Employment in Colonial Mexico," note 6.

33. Nieto de Piña, *Instruccion medica*, 7. The undated edition I viewed in the Wellcome Library was published in Madrid, but another edition was also published in Seville in 1783.

34. Ventura Pastor, *Preceptos generales*, 1:314.

35. Espejo y Cienfuegos, "Lecciones de obstetricia," Wellcome Library, WMS Amer. 122, fol. 15v.

36. Ibid., fol. 18v.

37. Ibid., fols. 20v–21.

38. Huacuja, *Tratado práctico de partos*, 129.

39. Ibid., 153, 154, 158.

40. Flores y Troncoso, *Historia de la medicina en México*, 3:621, 675; see also 618.

41. AHSS, Beneficiencia Pública, Establecimiento Hospitalarios, Hospital de Maternidad y de Infancia, legajo 6, exp. 16.

42. Ibid., legajo 2, exp. 29. Another condemnation of a midwife's criminal administration of *cihuaptali* to induce an abortion appears in "Contra María Concepcion Mejia por infanticidio," fol. 8, AGN, TSJDF, 1880, caja 681.

43. Ortega, "Obstetricia. Entuertos," *Gaceta Médica de México* 3, no. 8 (1867): 123.

44. León, *Apuntes para la historia de la obstetricia*, 4–5.

45. *El Siglo Diez y Nueve*, June 7, 1844, 4.

46. "Mexico: Casa de Maternidad," Wellcome Library, WMS Amer. 121.

47. Ibid.

48. Garza has comprehensively covered this trial in *The Imagined Underworld*, 139–54.

49. Garza, *The Imagined Underworld*, 143.

50. Ibid., 146.

51. Quezada, "Métodos anticonceptivos y abortivos tradicionales," 232.

52. Haslip-Viera, *Crime and Punishment in Late Colonial Mexico City*, 37.

53. Cutter, "The Administration of Law," 102.

54. Landers, "Female Conflict and Its Resolution," 572n44.

55. Parsons Scott, trans., *Las Siete Partidas*, 5:xxii.

56. Segura, *Avisos saludables a las parteras*, 16. Similarly, Medina's *Cartilla nueva util y necesaria*, chap. 3, n.p. warned that midwives needed, under pain of the death penalty, to resist all entreaties to perform abortions or advise women on how to obtain them.

57. Noonan, *Contraception: A History*, 362–64.

58. Riddle, *Eve's Herbs*, 158.

59. Jaffary, *False Mystics*, 130; "Inventory of the Casos reservados sinodales en la Diocesis de Mexico, y privilegios de los Indios en esta materia," University of Arizona Library Special Collections, MS 130.

60. Rodríguez, "Costumbres y tradiciones," 509.

61. Speckman Guerra, "Justicia, revolución y proceso," 190.

62. Escriche, *Diccionario razonado*, 112, 224.

63. Valdés, *Diccionario de Jurisprudencia Criminal Mexicana*, 9.

64. Ibid., 9, 179.

65. See *Código Penal para el Distrito Federal y Territorio de la Baja California*.

66. Buffington, *Criminal and Citizen*, 28–35.

67. Speckman Guerra, "Los jueces, el honor y la muerte," 1419.

68. Antonio Martínez de Castro, quoted in Buffington, "Looking Forward, Looking Back," 21.

69. Buffington, "Looking Forward, Looking Back," 22.

70. On gender and honor in the colonial period, see Twinam, *Public Lives, Private Secrets*; and Johnson and Lipsett-Rivera, *The Faces of Honor*.

71. Piccato, *The Tyranny of Opinion*, 3.

72. Sloan, "The Penal Code of 1871," 307; Reyes García Márkina, "*De jure* and *de facto*," 274. Infanticide and abortion were not represented in this section of the Code, but instead were classified as "Crimes against people committed by individuals."

73. Reyes García Márkina, "*De jure* and *de facto*," 275.

74. *Código Penal para el Distrito Federal y Territorio de la Baja California*, chap. 2, art. 35:8.

75. Speckman Guerra, "Morir a manos de una mujer," 300.

76. *Código Penal para el Distrito Federal y Territorio de la Baja California*, chap. 9, art. 570. This provision, however, obviously had earlier precedents. Arnold, "When Not Even Safe in Her Own Home," discusses an 1850 infanticide trial in which the court prosecutor declared that mothers were justified in committing the act in order to save their own lives.

77. *Código Penal para el Distrito Federal y Territorio de la Baja California*, chap. 9, art. 572.

78. Ibid., chap. 9, art. 573. These conditions reducing sentences for women who have maintained honorable reputations endure in current abortion legislation in the states of Campeche, Jalisco, Nayarit, Oaxaca, Puebla, Tamaulipas, Zacatecas, and Yucatán, as well as in the Distrito Federal. Vela, "Current Abortion Regulation," 13.

79. These represent my findings from the AGN, the AHJO, the Oaxaca municipal archives, and the Mexico City municipal archives. Not included in this analysis are an additional nineteen cases I found in these archives pertaining to what we would now classify as miscarriages, which are also termed *abortos* in catalogs and indexes when documentation indicates that they involved miscarriages induced when parties physically harmed women who were pregnant.

80. In these cases, abortions are often one of many religious crimes for which the accused are denounced.

81. AGN, Inquisición, vol. 757, exp. 5, fol. 81; vol. 1328, exp. 4, fols. 400–401.

82. Ibid., vol. 826, exp. 54, fol. 532v.

83. Ibid., vol. 1246, exp. 5, fol. 124. See also his appearance before the court, fol. 129.

84. Ibid., fol. 155v.

85. Ibid., fol. 130.

86. Such was the case in the trials of María Manuela Sanabria, who was alleged to have had three abortions "of animated fetuses," AGN, Inquisición, vol., 1364,

exp. 3; Isabel Hernández, AGN, Inquisición, vol. 561, exp. 6; María Marta de la Encarnación, AGN, Inquisición, vol. 788, exp. 24; and Barbara de Echagaray, who confessed to having procured three abortions, AGN, Inquisición, vol. 1231, exp. 1.

87. AGN, Indiferente Virreinal, caja 5969, exp. 19.

88. AGN, Indiferente Virreinal, caja 6473, exp. 29. My thanks to Zeb Tortorici for alerting me to the existence of this case.

89. AGN, Bienes Nacionales, vol. 731, exp. 4, fol. 8. I am grateful to Eddie Wright-Rios for drawing my attention to this case.

90. Ibid., fol. 12v.

91. AGN, Indiferente Virreinal, caja 6271, exp. 26. This is a reading Tortorici develops in "Women at the Margins of the Unnatural," 10.

92. The same description also applies to the municipal archives of the city of Oaxaca's judicial collection, which are currently organized by type of tribunal and by year, but which have no means of correlating to an existent index documenting the criminal cases according to an earlier classification system by type of crime.

93. I have located only 7 percent of the cases (six of the eighty-five indicated records).

94. As for the colonial period, I have not included cases of what appear to have been unintentional miscarriages.

95. McCaa, "The Peopling of Mexico from Origins to Revolution," 279.

96. Foucault, "Illegalities and Delinquency," 226–33.

97. Chambers, "Crime and Citizenship," 25.

98. There are none, at least, that are indicated in the finding aids for the fonds housed at the AGN.

99. The index for this fond is available only in the reference room of the AGN. The index contains over a thousand references to the crime of *lesions* (injuries).

100. Jackson, "The Trial of Harriet Vooght," 5–6.

101. AGN, TSJDF, 1883, caja 841, "Contra Pomposa Acosta por aborto provocado," fol. 2.

102. Ibid., fol. 7.

103. Ibid., fol. 5.

104. Ibid., fol. 6.

105. Ibid., fol. 2v.

106. AGN, TSJDF, 1880, caja 70, "En averiguación de la muerte de un feto. Sospechas de aborto provocado," fol. 1.

107. Ibid., fol. 6.

108. *Cartilla de partos*, 35. Espejo y Cienfuegos asserted the same in his 1854 obstetrical lectures, "Lecciones de obstetricia," fol. 18v.

109. "Testimonio de la Sentencia pronunciada contra la reo Arcadia Martínez de esta villa por haber habortado voluntariamente," AHMO, Justicia, Juzgado de 1ª instancia, 1841–42, caja 27.

110. Ibid., fol. 1v.

Chapter Four

1. AGN, Criminal, vol. 251, exp. 10, fol. 278.

2. Birth and death concealment were frequently linked to newborn child murder. In England between 1624 and 1803, the concealment of an illegitimate child's death was punishable with execution. Jackson, "The Trial of Harriet Vooght," 5–6.

3. In the other 29 percent of the cases, defendants were unlicensed and licensed midwives, a doctor, other family members (including fathers), unrelated strangers, and caregivers to infants.

4. Speckman Guerra, "Las flores del mal," 189n8.

5. I am grateful to Zeb Tortorici for sharing a reference to a case in the AHET with me. All of the cases Lipsett-Rivera examined in her study "A Slap in the Face of Honor" are treated in the following discussion.

6. An enormous number of documents, for instance, are known to have been burned in the Mexico City riot of 1692.

7. Uribe-Uran suggests this might have been the case with regard to mid-eighteenth-century homicide records in the Guadalajara's Audiencia de la Nueva Galicia. See "Innocent Infants or Abusive Patriarchs?"

8. My preliminary searching of infanticide and abortion cases in regional archives has not turned up many more cases. I discovered no infanticide cases dating from the colonial era in the judicial collection of the AHMO, and only three cases in the state of Oaxaca's judicial holdings from the colonial period. In his paper "Women at the Margins of the Unnatural," Zeb Tortorici similarly has found small numbers of cases in regional archives in Oaxaca and Puebla in the colonial period (one abortion case from Puebla, one infanticide case from Tlaxcala, and one from Oaxaca).

9. Ávila Espinosa, "Los niños abandonados de la casa de niños expósitos," 270. The literature on foundling homes provides extensive discussion of the frequency of child abandonment throughout colonial Latin America. See Gonzalbo Aizpuru, "La Casa de Niños Expósitos de la cuidad de México"; González, "Consuming Interests"; Twinam, "The Church, the State, and the Abandoned"; and Twinam, *Public Lives, Private Secrets.*

10. For example, England's County Chester had a population roughly the same size as that of the Mexican capital in the eighteenth century. In the period between 1700 and 1800, forty-nine cases of infanticide from Chester were opened before the Court of Great Sessions; Dickinson and Sharpe, "Infanticide in Early Modern England," 38. Nearly two hundred women were tried for the crime between 1720 and 1800 in the northern circuit courts of Cumberland, Northumberland, Westmoreland, and Yorkshire; Jackson, *New-Born Child Murder,* 3.

11. Jackson, "The trial of Harriet Vooght," 5.

12. Aguirre and Salvatore, "Introduction," 3. Arnold studied an 1850 infanticide trial in which the prosecutor cited an eighth century Visigothic Fuero Juzgo,

a royal edict of 1788, and Escriche's *Diccionario razonado de legislación y juris-prudencia*; see Arnold, "When Not Even Safe in Her Own Home," 89.

13. Parsons Scott, trans., *Las Siete Partidas*, 5:xxii, 1344. Although justifica-tion for the death penalty may have existed in legal theory, I have found no case in which colonial magistrates sentenced those convicted with this penalty.

14. Nieto de Piña, *Instruccion medica*, 24.

15. AGN, Bandos, vol. 19, exp. 78–79, fol. 1797.

16. Such preoccupations dated back much earlier. In the Ordenanzas for the government of the Indies in 1546, Charles V had attempted to ban the practice of Indian women resisting Spanish domination through the killing of their mixed-race offspring. Rodríguez and Calvo, "Sobre la práctica del aborto en el Occidente de México," 33. Rodríguez and Calvo believe such practice continued to signifi-cantly reduce New Spain's population into the seventeenth century.

17. AGN, Bandos, vol. 24, exp. 55, fol. 143.

18. AGN, Indiferente Virreinal, caja 3503, exp. 1.

19. AGN, Criminal, vol. 68, exp. 7, fol. 235.

20. AHMO, Justicia, Juzgado de 1ª instancia, 1836–37, caja 15, "Contra Felipa Romero partera, acusada de infanticidio," fol. 17. Despite this statement, Romero's was the only infanticide trial I located in this archive for the period 1820–40.

21. AHJO, Ejutla, Criminal, legajo 79, exp. 25, fols. 1–3v.

22. AHJO, Teposcolula, Criminal, legajo 64, exp. 3, fol. 4v.

23. AHMO, Justicia, Juzgado 2º criminal, 1896–97, caja 102, "Contra Paula N., por el delito de infanticidio," fols. 9–10. Witnesses who lived with or routinely saw defendants made similar claims in AHJO, Teposcolula, Criminal, legajo 58, exp. 21, fol. 5; AHMO, Justicia, Juzgado de 1ª instancia, 1857–61, caja 46, "Contra Anacleta Avila, por el infanticidio que cometió con su niña recién nacida," fol. 1; and AHMO, Justicia, Juzgado 2º criminal, 1891, caja 79, "Contra Mauricia García por infanticidio," fol. 5v.

24. AHJO, Villa Alta, Criminal, legajo 10, exp. 8.

25. Ibid., legajo 6, exp. 8, fol. 2.

26. Premo, *Children of the Father King*, 97, 99; Blum, "Reproductive Health in Latin American Transitions," 82.

27. AHJO, Villa Alta, Criminal, legajo 6, exp. 8, fol. 11. *Casas de depósito* were houses of "good reputation" where courts might order morally suspect women to reside during or at the outcome of judiciary proceedings. See Penyak, "Safe Harbors and Compulsory Custody."

28. In one case, the accused, charged with having thrown her newborn down a well, managed to escape apprehension and could not be investigated. Tortorici, "Women at the Margins of the Unnatural," 16. María del Carmen Gusman's 1802 infanticide trial also ended ambiguously; AGN, Criminal, vol. 626, exp. 1. The court had no suspects to investigate in the 1818 cases from Popotla; AGN, Indiferente Virreinal, caja 3503, exp. 1. The court's judgment is

not indicated in Juan de los Santos's 1800 trial; AGN, Indiferente Virreinal, caja 1829, exp. 1.

29. AGN, Criminal, vol. 98, exp. 9, fol. 234.

30. Ibid., vol. 98, exp. 9, fol. 246.

31. Ibid., vol. 52, exp. 12, fol. 495.

32. Ibid., vol. 68, exp. 7, fol. 223v.

33. Ibid., fol. 224v.

34. Ibid., fol. 234v.

35. Ibid., fol. 226.

36. Ibid., fol. 250.

37. Similar cases are found in AGN, Criminal, vol. 98, exp. 16, fols. 412–26; and AHJO, Teposcolula, Criminal, legajo 49, exp. 32.

38. Soman, "Anatomy of an Infanticide Trial," 248.

39. Dickinson and Sharpe, "Infanticide in Early Modern England," 38.

40. Langer, "Infanticide: A Historical Survey," 356.

41. Most received sentences of three to six years' imprisonment; see Ruggiero, "Honor, Maternity, and the Disciplining of Women." Landers, "'On Consideration of Her Enormous Crime,'" has also discussed the crime in Spanish Florida in the context of African slavery. In the case Landers examined, a black slave was sentenced to two hundred lashes and to wearing an iron collar for killing her two children.

42. Haslip-Viera, *Crime and Punishment in Late Colonial Mexico City*, 103.

43. Newson, "The Demographic Impact of Colonization," 170.

44. AGN, Criminal, vol. 251, exp. 10, fols. 286–88.

45. Rabin believes such tendencies explain the fall in conviction rates for infanticide in eighteenth-century England, where juries adopted sympathetic views of unwed mothers and legal authorities grew uncomfortable with the harshness of the infanticide statute of 1624. See Rabin, "Bodies of Evidence, States of Mind."

46. Haslip-Viera, *Crime and Punishment in Late Colonial Mexico City*, 102–3; Uribe-Urban, "Innocent Infants or Abusive Patriarchs?" 811.

47. Nieto de Piña, *Instruccion medica*, 14. Medical experts used this method in several nineteenth-century infanticide trials, as can be found in AGN, TSJDF, 1843, caja 2, and 1880, caja 681; AHMO, Justicia, Juzgado 2° criminal, 1884, caja 20, "En averiguación del infanticidio de que es acusada Pilar Ramírez"; AHMO, Justicia, Juzgado 1° criminal, 1888, subseries: procesos, caja 42, "Contra Felicitas Cruz acusada de infanticidio."

48. Premo, *Children of the Father King*, 104.

49. Ávila Espinosa, "Los niños abandonados," 293.

50. Twinam, "The Church, the State, and the Abandoned," 171.

51. AGN, Criminal, vol. 98, exp. 16, fol. 414.

52. Ibid., fol. 421.

53. Ibid., fol. 425.

54. Difficult material conditions tied to agrarian economic cycles lie at the heart of Malvido's explanation for rates of child abandonment in seventeenth- and eighteenth-century Tula. See Malvido, "El abandono de los hijos."

55. AHJO, Teposcolula, Criminal, legajo 49, exp. 32.

56. AGN, Criminal, vol. 52, exp. 12, fol. 482.

57. Ibid., vol. 98, exp. 9, fol. 232.

58. Ibid., vol. 52, exp. 12, fol. 483.

59. Premo, *Children of the Father King*, 137–78.

60. Lipsett-Rivera, "Marriage and Family Relations in Mexico," 138.

61. Arrom, *The Women of Mexico City*, 15.

62. Ibid., 20.

63. Schell, "Nationalizing Children through Schools and Hygiene."

64. AGN, Indiferente Virreinal, caja 3503, exp. 1, fol. 17v.

65. AHJO, Villa Alta, Criminal, legajo 6, exp. 8, fol.11.

66. AGN, Criminal, vol. 251, exp. 10, fols. 288v, 290.

67. AGN, TSJDF, 1843, caja 2, "Toca á la causa contra M.a de Jesús Torres por infanticidio."

68. In two other infanticide cases, witnesses and justices treated inebriation as legitimate grounds for absolving women of responsibility for the crimes. AGN, Justicia, vol. 113, exp. 18, fol. 97; AHMO, Justicia, Alcalde 1º constitucional, 1868–81, caja 6, "Ignacio García del pueblo de S. Sebastián ante V. con el respecto debido expongo . . ."

69. AHJO, Ejutla, Criminal, legajo 14, exp. 3l, fol. 7.

70. Ibid., fols. 5v, 9, 14v, 25v.

71. Ibid., fols. 18–19.

72. Ibid, fols. 21–23.

73. Ibid., fol. 67.

74. Shelton discovered similar patterns characterizing infanticide trials in the northern borderland region of Sonora, where the numbers of infanticide, abortion, and abandonment cases rose dramatically after 1850 and where justices most often exercised considerable leniency in convicting and sentencing defendants. See Shelton, "'Al parecer de buena conducta.'"

75. Statistics published in the *Anuario estadístico de la República Mexicana* from the late nineteenth century indicated sixty-eight women investigated for abortion and infanticide in 1891, fifty-four in 1892, forty-four in 1893, and forty-six in 1894, after which the numbers start to decline; Speckman Guerra, "Las flores del mal," 229.

76. This was also the case in AHJO, Teposcolula, Criminal, legajo 58, exp. 21 (1837); ACSCJ, (1840), 1815 "Toca á la causa instruida á María San José Romo por infanticidio"; AGN, TSJDF, 1843, caja 180, "Toca á la causa contra Lorenza Castro por infanticidio é incesto"; AHMO, Justicia, Juzgado de 1ª instancia, 1853, caja 42, "En averiguación del delito de infanticidio de que a acusado María Gonzáles"; AHJO, Ejutla, Criminal, legajo 14, exp. 3 (1855); AGN, TSJDF, 1857, caja 327,

"Averiguación formada contra María Francisca Rojas por descuido que esta tubo de su hijo haberse ahogado. Sospecho de infanticidio"; AHJO, Villa Alta, Criminal, legajo 69, exp. 30 (1857); AHMO, Justicia, Juzgado de 1ª instancia, 1857–61, caja 46, "Contra Anacleta Avila, por infanticidio que cometió contra su niña recién nacida" (1857); ACSCJ, (1859) 5988, "Toca á la causa instruida contra [blank] por infanticidio"; and AGN, TSJDF, 1860, caja 341, "Toca á la causa instruida por el juez 5º de lo criminal, contra Leocadia Hernández por infanticidio."

77. AGN, TSJDF, 1852, Juzgado de la Paz Segundo de lo Civil, caja 292, "Por delito de infanticidio cometido por Petra Torres el dia 9 del presente."

78. This was also the case in ACSCJ, (1840) 1815, "Toca á la causa instruida á María San José Romo por infanticidio"; AHMO, Justicia, Juzgado de 1ª instancia, 1841–42, caja 27, "Testimonio de la Sentencia pronunciada contra la reo Arcadia Martínez de esta villa por haber habortado voluntariamente"; AGN, TSJDF, 1843, caja 180, "Toca á la causa contra Lorenza Castro por infanticidio é incesto"; AHMO, Justicia, Juzgado de 1ª instancia, 1853, caja 42, "En averiguación del delito de infanticidio de que a acusado María Gonzáles"; AHJO, Ejutla, Criminal, legajo 14, exp. 3 (1855); AGN, TSJDF, 1857, caja 327, "Averiguación formada contra María Francisca Rojas por descuido que esta tubo de su hijo haberse ahogado. Sospecho de infanticidio"; AHJO, Villa Alta, Criminal, legajo 69, exp. 30 (1857); AHMO Justicia, Juzgado de 1º instancia, 1857–61, caja 46, "Contra Anacleta Avila, por infanticidio que cometió contra su niña recién nacida" (1857); ACSCJ, (1859), 5988, "Toca á la causa instruida contra [blank] por infanticidio"; and AGN, TSJDF, 1860, box 341, "Toca á la causa instruida por el juez 5º de lo criminal, contra Leocadia Hernández por infanticidio."

79. AGN, TSJDF, 1880, caja 703, "Contra Lorenza Rodríguez por infanticidio," fol. 1. Similar examples are also found in AGN, TSJDF, 1880, box 703, "En Averiguación de la muerte de un feto. Sospechas de aborto provocado"; AGN, TSJDF, 1888, caja 1092, "Contra Pascuala Chávez por infanticidio"; AHMO, Justicia, Juzgado 1º criminal, 1888, subseries: procesos, caja 42, "Contra Felicitas Cruz acusada de infanticidio"; AHMO, Justicia, Juzgado 2º criminal, 1889, caja 72, "En Averiguación de la muerte del niño Margarita Bazan"; AHMO, Justicia, Juzgado 2º criminal, 1896–97, caja 102, "Contra Paula N., por el delito de infanticidio."

80. Arnold, "Why Pablo Parra Wasn't Executed," 2, 5.

81. Arnold, "When Not Even Safe in Her Own Home," 79. In 1828, the state of Oaxaca produced the first postindependence civil code in all of Latin America. Veracruz enacted the first penal code in the nation in 1835. Oaxaca must have produced at least earlier individual criminal statutes on the subject, because one 1857 trial cites presumably a state law, article 33, chapter 11 of September 15, 1825, defining the act of infanticide. AHMO, Justicia, Juzgado de 1ª instancia, 1857–61, caja 46, "Contra Anacleta Avila, por infanticidio que cometió contra su niña recién nacida," fol. 9v.

82. Escriche, *Diccionario razonado de legislación y jurisprudencia*, 112, 224; Valdés, *Diccionario de Jurisprudencia Criminal Mexicana*, 9, 179.

83. *Código Penal para el Distrito Federal*, chapter 10, article 584. Ruggiero, "Not Guilty: Abortion and Infanticide in Nineteenth-Century Argentina," 157, notes that identical provisions characterized Argentina's late nineteenth-century infanticide legislation.

84. AGN, TSJDF, 1880, caja 703, "Contra Tomasa Montiel por conato de infanticidio."

85. Ibid.

86. Chambers, "Crime and Citizenship," generates an analysis of crime rates in Arequipa, Peru, and finds a dramatic increase in criminal prosecutions in the 1820s and 1830s. She concludes that judicial and administrative reforms were partially responsible for the rise in cases, but that it was also likely that there had been a real rise in crime.

87. Speckman Guerra, "Disorder and Control," 372, uses statistics from Herrera, *Estadística del ramo criminal en la República Mexicana* to show criminal conviction rates overall of 61.15 percent in 1877 and 63.38 percent in 1886, and a slightly lower 55.99 percent in 1887. Haslip-Viera's analysis of late eighteenth-century conviction rates in the Sala de Crimen in Mexico City revealed overall conviction rates of 68 percent, and his analysis of early nineteenth-century statistics from the court of Mexico City's Cuartel No. 7 shows rates of 64 percent. Haslip-Viera, *Crime and Punishment in Late Colonial Mexico City*, 103.

88. Speckman Guerra, "Disorder and Control," 384. Speckman Guerra also found that when justices did find women guilty of these crimes, they sentenced them less harshly than according to the penalties dictated by the 1871 penal code; Speckman Guerra, "Morir a manos de una mujer," 302, 304. Arnold did locate one infanticide trial from Mexico City, dating from 1850, in which the defendant was found guilty and sentenced to ten years of hard labor by an appellate court judge; see Arnold, "When Not Even Safe in Her Own Home," 91.

89. AHMO, Justicia, Juzgado de 1ª instancia, 1853, caja 42, "En averiguación del delito de infanticidio de que a acusada María González," fol. 24v. Similar judgments were found in AHJO, Teposcolula, Criminal, file 58, exp. 21; AHJO, Teposcolua, Criminal, file 64, exp. 3; AHMO, Justicia, Juzgado de 1ª instancia, 1857–61, caja 46, "Contra Anacleta Avila, por el infanticidio que cometió contra su niña recién nacida"; AHJO, Ejutla, Criminal, file 90, exp. 25; AHMO, Justicia, Juzgado 2° criminal, 1884, caja 20, "En averiguación del infanticidio de que es acusada Pilar Ramírez."

90. AHMO, Justicia, Juzgado 2° criminal, 1888, caja 64, "En averiguación de la causa de la muerte del niño Wilfrido Saldas contra Guadalupe García por infanticidio," fol. 31v.

91. Examples include AHMO, Justicia, Juzgado de 1ª instancia, 1841–42, caja 27, "Testimonio de la sentencia pronunciada contra Arcadia Martínez por haber abortado voluntariamente"; AHMO, Justicia, Corte de Justicia 2ª sala, 1884–85,

box 7, "Dionicia Mota sentenciada a tres años de prisión contada desde el 1 de mayo de 1885"; AHMO, Justicia, Corte de Justicia Serie 2ª, 1885–87, caja 8, "Sentencia contra Toribio Vargas por el delito de infanticidio."

92. The demographic research presented in McCaa, "The Peopling of Nineteenth-Century Mexico," 603, suggests that nineteenth-century population growth rates were in fact much higher than earlier research had suggested, and that Mexico effectively tripled its population from five to fifteen million in the century after independence. But even these more dramatic growth figures are far out of line with the skyrocketing rates of infanticide and abortion cases in the nineteenth century. Therefore, regular increases per capita do not offer a satisfactory explanation. Chambers has suggested that transformations in record keeping might have increased the number of archived criminal cases in postindependence Arequipa, Peru, but she does not consider this a major factor in explaining the change. Chambers, "Crime and Citizenship," 24.

93. Cook and Borah, *Essays in Population History: Mexico and the Caribbean,* 1:63–65.

94. I am grateful to Sarah Chambers for drawing this point to my attention. For further discussion, see Pérez Duarte y Noroña, "Los alimentos en la historia de México independiente"; García Peña, "Madres solteras, pobres y abandonadas"; and Chambers, "Private Crimes, Public Order."

95. Milanich, *Children of Fate,* 68.

96. Blum, *Domestic Economies,* 49.

97. López-Alonso, "Growth with Inequality," 83.

98. Chassen López, *From Liberal to Revolutionary Oaxaca,* 18, 81.

99. Shelton, "'*Al parecer de buena conducta,*'" 10.

100. AHMO, Justicia, Juzgado 3° de letras, 1869–70, caja 4, "Contra Agustina Sánchez de oficio partera, por el fallecimiento de un recién nacido, Oaxaca, 1870," fols. 4v, 10. Malvido, "El abandono de los hijos," finds a strong correlation between periods of economic duress and higher rates of child abandonment in seventeenth- and eighteenth-century Mexico. Blum, *Domestic Economies,* xv, notes that by the eve of the Mexican Revolution, poverty had more often become a motivator for abandoning children than honor, which she believes characterized the chief preoccupation of an earlier era.

101. AHMO, Justicia, Juzgado 2° criminal, 1888, caja 64, "Contra Joaquina Chávez por exposición de su hija Pilar Pompoza," fol. 23.

102. AHMO, Justicia, Juzgado 2° criminal, 1891, caja 79, "Contra Mauricia García por infanticidio," fol. 7v.

103. Ibid., fol. 18.

104. Ibid., fol. 34v.

105. AHMO, Justicia, Juzgado 2° criminal, 1888, caja 64, "Averiguación de la muerte del niño Wilfrido Sadot," fols. 4, 12, 12v.

106. Such language is also invoked in AHMO, Justicia, Juzgado 2° criminal, 1888, caja 64, "Contra Joaquina Chávez por exposición de su hija Pilar

Pompoza"; AHMO, Justicia, Corte de Justicia 1ª sala, 1883–84, caja 7, "María del Carmen"; AHMO, Justicia, Corte de Justicia 1ª sala, 1883–84, caja 7, "Merced López sentenciada a diez y ocho meses de servicio en el Hospital general contados desde el 2 de abril de 1884"; AHMO, Justicia, Corte de Justicia 2ª sala, 1884–85, caja 7, "Dionisia Mota sentenciada a tres años de prisión contada desde el 1 de mayo de 1885." *Curadores* also frequently made the same claims about women who had hidden their pregnancies; indeed, this reasoning long preceded the 1871 penal code. María Ricardo Osorio's *curador* used it to defend her in her 1837 trial. AGHO, Teposcolula, Criminal, legajo 58, exp. 21, fol. 21.

107. This occurred, for instance, in two separate trials found in AHMO, Justicia, Corte de Justicia 1ª sala, 1883–84, caja 7, "Mercedes López sentenciada a diez y ocho meses de servicio en el Hospital general contados desde el 2 de abril de 1884" and "Maria del Carmen." It can be found as well in AHMO, Justicia, Corte de Justicia 2ª sala, 1884–85, caja 7, "Dionisio Mota y socios sentenciada a tres años de prisión contada desde el 5 de mayo de 1885"; and two cases in AHMO, Justicia, Corte de Justicia 1ª sala, 1884–5, caja 8, "Testimonio de la sentencia pronunciada contra Santiago Antonio e Ignacio Juna, por el delito de infanticidio. Tuxtepec," and "Testimonio de la sentencia pronunciada contra Juana Jiménez, por el delito de exposición de parto."

108. AHJO, Teposcolula, Criminal, legajo 58, exp. 21, fol. 16.

109. Ibid., fol. 16v.

110. ACSCJ, (1840), 1815 "Toca á la causa instruida á María San José Romo por infanticidio," fol. 10.

111. Shelton, *For Tranquility and Order*, 10–11, 48–49.

112. *El Siglo Diez y Nueve*, June 7, 1851, 3.

113. AGN, TSJDF, 1883, caja 841, "Contra Pomposa Acosta por aborto provocado," fol. 13.

114. Ibid., fols. 4–5.

115. The timing of the late nineteenth-century naturalization of maternity is consistent with Nari's findings in the context of Argentina; see Nari, *Políticas de maternidad*.

116. AHMO, Justicia, Juzgado de 1ª instancia, 1853, caja 42, "En averiguación del delito de infanticidio de que a acusada a María González," fol. 25.

117. AHMO, Justicia, Corte de Justicia 2ª sala, 1884–85, caja 7, "Testimonio de la sentencia pronunciada contra María Petrocinio García por infanticidio. Teposcolula, 1885," fol. 1. In Piccato, *The Tyranny of Opinion*, argues that the Porfirian state undertook a novel and vigorous defense of individuals' public reputations.

118. Buffington, *Criminal and Citizen*, 64.

119. Garza, *The Imagined Underworld*, 3. See also Rivera-Garza, "The Criminalization of the Syphilitic Body."

120. Two exceptions are Lipsett-Rivera, *Gender and the Negotiation of Daily Life*, which discusses the pronounced issue of public scrutiny of community members' honorable and dishonorable practices, and the examination of gossip and

public scrutiny in *rapto* cases in nineteenth-century Oaxaca City in Sloan, *Runaway Daughters*, 106–20.

121. Such instances also occurred in AHJO, Ejutla, Criminal, legajo 90, exp. 25; AHMO, Justicia, Juzgado 1° criminal, subseries: procesos, 1883, caja 24, "En averiguación por la causa en que nació sin vida un niña dado a luz por Juana López"; and AHMO, Justicia, Juzgado 2° criminal, 1880–81, caja 12, "Contra María Natividad de los Santos por quebrantamiento de condenado."

122. AHJO, Ejutla, Criminal, legajo 79, exp. 25, 1881. Shelton, "'*Al parecer de buena conducta*,'" 14–18, also notes strong indications of the community members' heightened scrutiny of women's sexual and social conduct in the nineteenth-century cases examined in Sonora.

123. AHJO, Teposcolula, Criminal, legajo 58, exp. 21, fols. 2–3v. Similar circumstances characterized the infanticide trials found in AHMO, Justicia, Juzgado de 1ª instancia, 1853, caja 42, "En averiguación del delito de infanticidio de que a acusada María González"; AHJO, Ejutla, Criminal, legajo 14 exp. 3; and AHMO, Justicia, Juzgado de 1ª instancia, 1857–61, caja 46, "Contra Anacleta Avila, por el infanticidio que cometió contra su niña recién nacida."

124. Speckman Guerra, "Las flores del mal," 213.

125. Racial identifiers are not used in nineteenth-century cases, but in the second half of the nineteenth century, Oaxaca City was between 77 and 87 percent indigenous. Sloan, *Runaway Daughters*, 5.

126. Speckman Guerra, "Morir a manos de una mujer," 310, actually characterizes nineteenth-century criminologists of the liberal and Porfirian era, with the notable exception of Julio Guererro, to be markedly disinterested in women's violent crimes, including infanticide.

127. On race and sexual honor in the colonial era, see Martínez, *Genealogical Fictions*; and Twinam, *Public Lives, Private Secrets*.

128. Sloan, *Runaway Daughters*, 170–77.

129. Overmyer-Velázquez, *Visions of the Emerald City*, 127.

130. French, "Prostitutes and Guardian Angels."

131. Buffington, *Criminal and Citizen*, 29.

132. Arnold, "When Not Even Safe in Her Own Home, 71.

133. Arnold, "Why Pablo Parra Wasn't Executed," 1.

134. The archivists at the Oaxaca municipal archives informed me that the same photographic studio, and presumably the same backdrops, were used for inmates' portraits as were used by the general public. They also explained that the state housed the small children of imprisoned women at a separate institution near the city's prison. For further discussions of such photography in nineteenth-century Oaxaca, see Overmyer-Velázquez, "Portraits of a Lady"; and Poole, "An Image of 'Our Indian.'"

135. Garza, *The Imagined Underworld*, 3.

Chapter Five

1. The topic of monstrous births has been largely untouched in the context of colonial Latin America, although it is one Few addresses in her current research on Guatemala. See Few, "Atlantic World Monsters" and "'That Monster of Nature.'" Announcements of unusual births in Mexican papers are briefly treated in Adank, "Accommodation and Innovation," 222–30, 240–47; and Guedea, "La medicina en las gacetas de México." The only scholarly work I have encountered on nineteenth-century monstrous productions in Mexico is Gorbach, *El monstruo, objeto imposible.*

2. *Gazeta de México*, March 22, 1785, 267.

3. "Horroroso fenómeno," *El Siglo Diez y Nueve*, March 24, 1893, 3.

4. For discussions of creole patriotism and the generation of narratives of Mexican history, see Florescano, *National Narratives in Mexico*, 220–60; and Cañizares-Esguerra, *How to Write the History of the New World*, 204–65. On the issue of colonial science and creole patriotism, see Cañizares-Esguerra, "New World, New Stars"; and Cowie, "Peripheral Vision."

5. For further discussion of this issue, see Blum et al., *Women, Ethnicity and Medical Authority.*

6. Tavera Alfaro, "Documentos para la historia del periodismo Mexicano," 340. Tavera has collected here a number of sources treating the periodical found in the AGN, Historia, vol. 399.

7. Adank, "Accommodation and Innovation," 135.

8. Marley, "Introducción," ii.

9. Tavera Alfaro, "Documentos para la historia del periodismo Mexicano," 331.

10. Manuel Antonio Valdés, quoted in Ruiz Castañeda, "La tercera gaceta de la Nueva España," 142.

11. Ruiz Castañeda, "La tercera gaceta de la Nueva España," 144.

12. Adank, "Accommodation and Innovation," 158–60.

13. *Gazeta de México*, February 11, 1784, 20.

14. *Gazeta de México*, October 23, 1787, 417.

15. *Gazeta de México*, February 25, 1784, 28.

16. *Gazeta de México*, February 24, 1789, 253.

17. Adank, "Accommodation and Innovation," 96.

18. Ibid., 166.

19. See Guedea, "La medicina en las gacetas de México"; and Cowie, "Peripheral Vision."

20. See Jaffary, Osowski, and Porter, eds., *Mexican History*, 185–87. On the Catholic foundations of the Mexican Enlightenment, see Voekel, *Alone before God.*

21. Brading, *The First America*, 275.

22. *Gazeta de México*, January 28, 1784, 12–13.

23. The mortality rates in these unusual births were high. At the time of the announcements' publication (generally a few weeks after birth), offspring survived in

thirteen out of twenty-four of the instances of multiple births and only three out of the twenty "monstrous" births.

24. *Gazeta de México*, December 30, 1793, 709–10.

25. Premo, *Children of the Father King*, 99–100.

26. This is discussed further in chapter 6.

27. Gruzinsky, *Images at War*, 165.

28. Ximénez, *Coleccion de estampas*, plate 52.

29. Few, "Atlantic World Monsters," 211.

30. Few, "That Monster of Nature," 170–71.

31. Knoppers and Landes, "Introduction," 8.

32. Crawford, *Marvelous Protestantism*, 9.

33. Spinks, "Wondrous Monsters," 81. For similar characterizations, see Brammall, "Monstrous Metamorphosis."

34. Daston and Park, *Wonders and the Order of Nature*, 175–90.

35. Burke, "Frontiers of the Monstrous," 28.

36. Ibid., 37.

37. Von Sneidern, "Joined at the Hip," 214.

38. Ibid.

39. Daston and Park, *Wonders and the Order of Nature*, 190–201.

40. Ibid., 13, 192; see also Daston and Park, "Unnatural Conceptions," 23.

41. Adank, "Accommodation and Innovation," 222–23, 240–41.

42. Ibid., 241.

43. AGN, General de Parte, 1799, vol. 76, exp. 208, fol. 153. This is possibly the same "monstrous" child as the one discussed below and pictured in figure 8, for the body's construction is the same, and the geographic and temporal details are not inconsistent with those in the image. The boy's father in the earlier *Gazeta* notice is recorded as "Antonio Ramón."

44. Daston and Park, *Wonders and the Order of Nature*, 201–9.

45. Leclerc, *Natural History, General and Particular*, 2:416.

46. Daston and Park*, Wonders and the Order of Nature*, 172. Similar observations are included in Pender, " 'No Monsters at the Resurrection.' "

47. For example, the 1780 *Diccionario de la lengua castellana compuesto por la Real Academia Español* defines "monster" as something produced against nature, but also as anything "excessively large or extraordinary in any line."

48. *Gazeta de México*, February 8, 1785, 241.

49. *Gazeta de México*, February 25, 1784, 28.

50. *Gazeta de México*, July 12, 1785, 349. A similar announcement originating in Chilapa ran a few months later; see *Gazeta de México*, November 22, 1785, 441.

51. There is a community called Santa Catarina Quiane just south of Oaxaca City. Penélope Orozco Sánchez, the curator of the library's exhibits, informed me that the library had no means of further tracing the larger manuscript from which this page is extracted, or its author.

52. These multiple meanings are found in several eighteenth-century editions of the *Diccionario de la lengua castellana*, published by the Real Academia de la Lengua Española.

53. This connotation of perfection continued in some notices about monstrous births from the first half of the nineteenth century. For example, an announcement published in *El Siglo Diez y Nueve* reported that the mining town of Tlalpujagua, Michoacán, had witnessed a "very unusual phenomenon of nature" wherein a woman had given birth to twins "united without any deformity, from the chest to the belly." *El Siglo Diez y Nueve*, July 19, 1845, 2–3.

54. *Gazeta de México*, February 8, 1785, 267.

55. *Gazeta de México*, May 19, 1789, 306.

56. *Gazeta de México*, December 30, 1793, 709–10.

57. *Gazeta de México*, December 23, 1794, 709.

58. Besides the "perfectly formed and organized" infant's body noted above, the *Gazeta* also described the birth of one girl born with only one eye, all of "whose members were perfect and complete below the neck"; *Gazeta de México*, August 18, 1802, 121. And one baby born "with a monstrous face" and several other irregularities nevertheless possessed a "perfect" right arm; *Gazeta de México*, November 17, 1784, 185. One notice described an eight-year-old boy born without arms and only one leg who managed to move about "with the most perfection"; *Gazeta de México*, June 19, 1787, 370. Two other such sets of fetuses are similarly described in *Gazeta de México*, August 21, 1787, 395, and June 17, 1788, 74. Few, "Atlantic World Monsters," 213, notes a similar case of conjoined twins in Guatemala in 1675, "born with two distinctly perfect bodies" despite their possession of three legs.

59. *Gazeta de México*, September 28, 1803, 365.

60. *Gazeta de México*, November 13, 1794, 638.

61. *Gazeta de México*, July 11, 1786.

62. AGN, Indiferente Virreinal, caja 3280, exp. 42.

63. *Gazeta de México*, April 19, 1806, 257.

64. *Gazeta de México*, October 20, 1784, 169.

65. *Gazeta de México*, February 8, 1785, 267.

66. *Gazeta de México*, November 22, 1785, 440.

67. AGN, Inquisición, vol. 1378, exp. 10, fol. 194v.

68. *Gazeta de México*, November 13, 1794, 638.

69. *Gazeta de México*, December 30, 1793, 709. Other medical procedures are detailed in *Gazeta de México*, May 8, 1792, 84; February 8, 1785, 267; April 19, 1785, 282; and May 8, 1792, 84.

70. Gorbach, *El monstruo, objeto imposible*, 73, indicates that Joseph María de la Vega executed the drawing.

71. AGI, MP-México, 1426.

72. AGI, MP-México, 420BIS/26-02-1789/Criatura deforme. New Spain's viceroy sent another similar notice to the King of Spain with an accompanying

image in 1817. AGI, Estado, 31, 57/31-05-1817. Few discovered that the cadaver of the 1675 monstrous child was displayed in the homes of Santiago's elite citizens; see Few, "Atlantic World Monsters," 214.

73. AGI, Mapas y Planos, Filipinas, 105.

74. Premo, *Children of the Father King*, 137.

75. Brading, *The First America*, is the standard treatment of creole patriotism.

76. For a discussion of the origins of the idea of American degeneration, see Bauer and Mazzotti, "Introduction." For a discussion of emergent seventeenth-century creole nationalism in the Peruvian context, see Mazzotti, "El Dorado, Paradise, and Supreme Sanctity."

77. Cornelius de Pauw, quoted in Brading, *The First America*, 429.

78. Creole patriotism in historical writings are dealt with in Florescano, *National Narratives in Mexico*; and Cañizares-Esguerra, *How to Write the History of the New World*. On creole patriotism and scientific writing, see Cañizares-Esguerra, "New World, New Stars"; Cowie, "Peripheral Vision"; and Goodman, "Science, Medicine, and Technology in Colonial Spanish America."

79. Georges-Louis Leclerc, Comte de Buffon, quoted in Brading, *The First America*, 429.

80. Brading, *The First America*, 430.

81. Leclerc, *The Natural History of Animals, Vegetables, and Minerals*, 270.

82. Ibid., 275, 286.

83. *Gazeta de México*, March 10, 1784, 45.

84. Von Sneidern, "Joined at the Hip," 213–31, addresses the history of their reception.

85. *Gazeta de México*, December 30, 1793, 710.

86. The *Gazeta* again compared New Spain's ability to produce exceptional fetuses with Europe's in a 1786 announcement when it likened a girl born in Guanajuato with her heart outside her body to "the boy who the celebrated physician Martin Martínez in the Imperial Court of Madrid observed in the year 1706." *Gazeta de México*, June 27, 1786, 143.

87. Clavijero, *Historia antigua de México*, 455. For further discussion of Clavijero's writings, see Brading, *The First America*, 450–64.

88. Clavijero, *Historia antigua de México*, 511.

89. Adank, "Accommodation and Innovation," 208; Cowie, "Peripheral Vision," 150; Goodman, "Science, Medicine, and Technology," 27. For more extensive treatments of Alzate and his relationship to the notion of creole patriotism, see Clark, " 'Read All About It' "; and Cañizares-Esguerra, *How to Write the History of the New World*, 281–300.

90. I have located twenty announcements of monsters in Mexican papers in this period, all but four of them from *El Siglo Diez y Nueve*.

91. Galindo y Villa, *Breve noticia histórico-descriptiva del Museo Nacional de México*, 13. The Museo Nacional de México was originally founded in 1825, but

reinvigorated after 1876 when the state charged it with the mandate to exhibit objects and promote research on the official history of the country. Rico Mansard, *Exhibir para educar*, 68, 190.

92. Ramírez, *Catálogo de las anomalías coleccionadas en el museo nacional*.

93. Juan Nepomuceno Bolaños, "Un fenómeno raro nacido en el departamento de Oajaca," *El Museo Mexicano*, 3 (1844): 346; emphasis in the original.

94. "El Antecristo," *El Siglo Diez y Nueve*, July 6, 1887, 3.

95. "El fin del Mundo," *El Siglo Diez y Nueve*, March 27, 1895, 2.

96. "Fenómeno," *El Siglo Diez y Nueve*, March 22, 1854, 4.

97. Juan María Rodríguez, "Descripción de un monstruo humano cuádruple, nacido en Durango el año de 1868," *Gaceta Médica de México* 5 (1870): 18.

98. Ibid., 42. Similar calls for preserving and displaying monstrous corpses in museums are found in "Un ciclope," *El Siglo Diez y Nueve*, March 26, 1862, 2; "Un fenómeno," *El Siglo Diez y Nueve*, March 26, 1881, 3; and "Un fenómeno," *El Siglo Diez y Nueve*, November 5, 1892, 3.

99. Juan María Rodríguez, "Tocología y Teratología," *Gaceta Médica de México* 7 (1872): 256.

100. "Fenómeno," *El Monitor Republicano*, August 20, 1885, 3.

101. "Nacimiento de un monstruo," *El Monitor Republicano*, May 13, 1887, 3. One article announcing the monstrous birth of an "Egyptian mommy" declared that the creature's horrendousness had also caused its mother's death. "Un fenómeno," *El Siglo Diez y Nueve*, November 5, 1892, 3.

102. José Guadalupe Posada, "Importante noticia de rarísimo fenómeno dado á luz en la Villa de Guadalupe," Mexican Broadsides Collection, University of New Mexico. http://econtent.unm.edu/cdm/singleitem/collection/joseguad/id /385.

103. For an excellent treatment of the evolution of French perceptions of monstrosity in the eighteenth and nineteenth century, see Gill, *Eccentricity and the Cultural Imagination in Nineteenth-Century Paris*.

104. "Monstruosidad," *El Universal*, August 23, 1853, 4.

105. "Nacimiento de un monstruo," *El Monitor Republicano*, May 13, 1887, 3.

106. "Monstruosidades," *El Museo Mexicano* 3 (1844): 20. Definitions of these terms are taken from Dunglison, *Medical Lexicon*, 26, 320, 522.

107. Ibid., 20.

108. Bolaños, "Un fenómeno raro nacido en el departamento de Oajaca," 346–48.

109. Gill, *Eccentricity and the Cultural Imagination*, 224.

110. Ibid.

111. Bolaños, "Un fenómeno raro nacido en el departamento de Oajaca," 350.

112. Gorbach, *El Monstruo*, 40.

113. Juan María Rodriguez, "Teratología. Descripción de un monstruo humano diplogenésico, monocéfalo, autositario, onfalósito, no viable," *Gaceta*

Médica de México 4 (1869): 165. Cephalotripsy was a medical procedure by which the head of a fetus was crushed in order to effect delivery.

114. Juan María Rodríguez, "Teratología," *Gaceta Médica de México* 7 (1872): 130–32.

115. Rodríguez, "Teratología" (1869), 145–55.

116. Gill, *Eccentricity*, 225.

117. Ibid.

118. Ibid., 228.

119. Étienne Geoffroy Saint-Hilaire, quoted in Gill, *Eccentricity*, 226, 230.

120. Stepan, *The Hour of Eugenics*, 45.

121. Rodríguez, "Teratología" (1872), 382.

122. "Mexico: Casa de Maternidad," Wellcome Library, WMS Amer. 121, n.p.

123. Ramírez, *Catálogo de las anomalías*, v.

124. Gorbach, *El monstruo*, 153.

125. Ibid., 183–93.

126. Ramírez, *Catálogo de anomalías*, vi.

Chapter Six

1. Colonial Latin Americanists can only read with envy the comparably rich sources treating these topics available to our northern colleagues and used to such effect in such works as Ulrich, *A Midwife's Tale*; Brodie, *Contraception and Abortion in Nineteenth-Century America*; and Klepp, *Revolutionary Conceptions*.

2. AGN, Bandos, vol. 19, exp. 15, fol. 26.

3. AGN, TSJDF, 1880, caja 703, "Tomasa Montiel por conato de infanticidio," fols. 2–7v.

4. AHJO, Villa Alta, Civil, legajo 21, exp. 19, fol. 2.

5. *Gazeta de México*, August 18, 1794, 421.

6. AHJO, Teposcolula, Civil, legajo 19, exp. 4, fol. 8.

7. Sahagún, *Historia general de las cosas de Nueva España*, 2:606–7.

8. Ibid., 611.

9. Fields, *Pestilence and Headcolds*, 48.

10. Sahagún, *Historia general de las cosas de Nueva España*, 2:615–16.

11. León, *La Obstetricia en México*, 123–27.

12. Van Patten, "Obstetrics in Mexico Prior to 1600," 210.

13. León, *La obstetricia en México*, 142–43.

14. Vásquez, "Florilegio Medicinal," Wellcome Library, WMS Amer. 26, fol. 54.

15. Flores y Troncoso, *Historia de la medicina en México*, 2:407. The *Botica general* of Cadíz, republished in Puebla in 1797, also endorsed this remedy; see Rodríguez, "Costumbres y tradiciones en torno al embarazo y al parto," 511.

16. Segura, *Avisos saludables a las parteras*, 18.

17. Medina, *Cartilla nueva util y necesaria*, chap. 4, n.p.

18. We again see evidence in later eras of the persistence of pre-Columbian custom. In her 1652 Inquisition trial, the *partera* Isabel Hernández had to be fetched to the court from a baptism she had been attending. AGN, Inquisición, vol. 652, exp. 6, fol. 534.

19. Sahagún, *Historia general de las cosas de Nueva España*, 2:462.

20. Berdan and Anawalt, *The Essential Codex Mendoza*, Part 3, 118.

21. León, *La obstetricia en México*, 92.

22. Fernández de Lizardi, *The Mangy Parrot*, 13; emphasis in the original.

23. The items Fernández de Lizardi mocks here as superstitious relics (*faja de dijes, ojos de venado, maintas de azabache, colmillos de caiman*) are still common protections against the folk illnesses of wind (*aire*), anger (*coraje* or *rabia*), and evil eye (*mal de ojo*) in many Mexican communities. *Ojo de venado* is the eyelike seed of the plant known in English as cowage; *azabache* is jet, a black mineral that can be carved into the shape of charms. Fernández de Lizardi, *The Mangy Parrot*, 13n5.

24. Pérez Salas, *Costumbrismo y litografía en México*, 249.

25. Lizardi, *The Mangy Parrot*, 13. Lizardi makes no reference to the object in his text, but the cloth might be an Augustine belt, which women placed upon their wombs to pray for success in childbirth (see chapter 1).

26. *El Diario de México*, July 25, 1806, 298, 351.

27. León, *La obstetricia en México*, 92.

28. *El Diario de México*, November 24, 1805, 230.

29. *El Diario de Mexico*, March 1, 1806, 238.

30. AGN, Inquisición, vol. 561, exp. 6, fols. 565–565v.

31. Ibid., vol. 360, exp. 55, fols. 159–61, 169.

32. Ibid., vol. 878, exp. 40, fol. 368. Another similar case involved charges of witchcraft against the eighteenth-century mulata *partera* Agustina Carrasco; AGN, Inquisición, vol. 1378, exp. 10.

33. Dozens of midwives were denounced for witchcraft in the colonial era. Examples include AGN, Inquisición, vol. 561, exp. 6; vol. 599, exp. 15; vol. 952, exp. 3; vol. 723, exp. 3; vol. 733, exp. 10; vol. 765, exp. 10; vol. 791, exp. 16; vol. 798, exp. 8; vol. 872, exp. 31; vol. 826, exp. 54; vol. 953, exp. 41; vol. 992, exp. 10; vol. 1313, exp. 12; and vol. 1378, exp. 10.

34. Segura, *Avisos saludables a las parteras*, 17.

35. See chapter 2.

36. AHMO, Justicia, Juzgado de 1ª instancia, 1836–37, caja 15, "Contra Felipa Romero, de oficio partera, acusada de infanticidio," fol. 8.

37. AGN, Inquisición, vol. 878, exp. 40; and vol. 1181, exp. 10. The objection in the second case is somewhat curious. Segura, *Avisos saludables a las parteras*, 12, 13, specified that the water midwives were to use in baptism might be rainwater or water from oceans, pools, or *pilas* (troughs or fonts), and that it was not necessary to add salt to it.

38. Ruiz Guadalajara, "'Con la sangre de todo un Dios,'" 207.

39. This edition was subsequently reissued in both 1773 and 1799. Rodríguez's translation is reproduced in "'Con la sangre de todo un Dios.'"

40. Segura, *Avisos saludables a las parteras*, 4.

41. Ibid., 5–6.

42. *Gazeta de México*, May 29, 1779, quoted in León, *Historia de la obstetricia*, 207–8.

43. *Gazeta de México*, June 20, 1795, 298. *El Diario de México* reported another instance of a missionary performing a caesarean section on a dead Indian woman in Huamantla, Puebla, in 1807. The woman had died three hours before the priest arrived to perform the operation; the infant survived for only fifteen minutes after the extraction. *El Diario de México*, June 28, 1807, 133.

44. Cited in Léon, *Historia de la obstetricia*, 208.

45. Flores y Troncoso, *Historia de la medicina en México*, 3:656.

46. Uribe Elías, *La invención de la mujer*, 77, 78.

47. *Gaceta Médica de México* 2 (1866): 391; *Gaceta Médica de México* 3 (1867): 81–84.

48. *El Siglo Diez y Nueve*, November 6, 1853, 3; *El Siglo Diez y Nueve*, November 7, 1853, 1.

49. This information is taken from the *Biblioteca Digital de la Medicina Tradicional Mexicana*, prepared by the Universidad Autónoma Nacional de Mexico: http://www.medicinatradicionalmexicana.unam.mx/monografia.php?l=3&t =&id=7433.

50. Esteyneffer, *Florilegio medicinal*, 347.

51. "Medicamentos experimentados y provechosas para las enfermedades siguientes," Wellcome Library, WMS Amer. 7, fol. 2.

52. The effectiveness of this plant as a sedative, anxiolytic, and analgesic has been substantiated in recent pharmacological research. Herrera-Ruiz, "Flavonoids from *Tilia americana*," and Martínez et al., "Antinociceptive Activity of *Tilia americana*."

53. "Mexico: Casa de Maternidad," Wellcome Library, WMS Amer. 121, n.p. I am grateful to Ryan Amir Kashanipour for his reading of this document and sharing his knowledge that these medicines were used by pre-Columbian healers.

54. *Gaceta Médica de México* 3, no. 8 (1867): 122.

55. Ibid.

56. Rodríguez, *Guía clínica del arte de los partos*, 41.

57. Esteyneffer, *Florilegio medicinal*, 344.

58. Medina, *Cartilla util y necesaria*, chap. 4, n.p.

59. In 1854 physician José Ferrer Espejo y Cienfuegos was still advocating the efficacy of bleeding women suffering from protracted labor in the obstetrical lectures he offered at the Escuela de Medicina. Espejo y Cienfuegos, "Lecciones de obstetricia, dadas oralmente para curso de segundo año," Wellcome Library, WMS Amer. 122, fol. 5.

60. Ventura Pastor, *Preceptos generales*, 1:192.

61. Duffin, *History of Medicine*, 289.

62. Vidart, *El discípulo instruido*, 48.

63. Venegas, *Compendio de la medicina*, 289–90.

64. Ventura Pastor, *Preceptos generales*, 1:328–29. Ventura includes descriptions of several similar instances in his text.

65. Karchmer Krivitsky, "La ginecología y la obstetricia," 283.

66. AGN, Indiferente Virreinal, caja 574, exp. 2, fol. 2.

67. AHFM, Protomedicato, legajo 4, exp. 24, fols. 7–8.

68. The Establecimiento de Ciencias Médicas replaced the Escuela Nacional de Cirugía, which in turn had changed its name in 1822 from the Real Escuela de Cirugía. The Consejo Superior de Salubridad, which operated from 1841 to 1917, replaced the brief postindependence body, the *Facultad Médica del Distrito Federal*.

69. At the time of its creation in 1833, the Establecimiento de Ciencias Médicas created a course on obstetrics and operations, and shortly thereafter, a course for midwives.

70. Carillo, "Nacimiento y muerte de una profesión," 170; AGN, Segundo Imperio, vol. 59, exp. 17, fol. 1.

71. *El Siglo Diez y Nueve*, March 30, 1855, 4. The paper published three additional ads for similar French midwives in the 1840s and 1850s.

72. *El Siglo Diez y Nueve*, December 11, 1845, 1.

73. Radkau, "Los médicos (se) crean una imagen," 140.

74. "Reglamento para el ejercicio de las parteras, espedido en cumplimiento del artículo tercero de la ley de 2 marzo de 1852," article 2.2, reproduced in Huacuja, *Tratado práctico de partos*, appendix.

75. Radkau, "Los médicos (se) crean una imagen," 140.

76. Carillo, "Nacimiento y muerte de una profesión," 178.

77. "Política Interior," *El Hijo del Ahuizote*, May 15, 1892, 6. President Porfirio Díaz had then been in power for sixteen years, arriving in office by virtue of the rebellion at Tuxtepec.

78. "Acuerdo de los prelados del III Concilio límense," 172.

79. AHMO, Justicia, Juzgada de 1ª Instancia, 1836–37, caja 15, "Contra Felipa Romero partera, acusada de infanticidio," fols. 2–6.

80. Ibid., fol. 8v.

81. Ibid., fols. 16–16v.

82. Ibid., fols. 6–7.

83. AHJO, Ejutla, Criminal, legajo 69, exp. 31.

84. Ibid., fol. 3.

85. Ibid., fol. 8.

86. Ibid., fol. 8v. Riojano was undoubtedly a professor of obstetrics; by the last quarter of the nineteenth century, women began securing such titles. Díaz

and Oropeza, "Las parteras de Guadalajara," 251, mention another woman who obtained such a title in Guadalajara in 1879.

87. AHJO, Ejutla, Criminal, legajo 79, exp. 25.

88. *El Siglo Diez y Nueve*, August 10, 1894, 2.

89. Cházaro and Kersey, "Mexican Women's Pelves and Obstetrical Procedures," 101.

90. Radkau, "Los médicos (se) crean una imagen," 128.

91. Carbajal, "Tocologia," Wellcome Library, WMS Amer. 127, fol. 1.

92. Klepp comments how in British America before the War of Independence, both childbirth and reproduction were publicly celebrated; colonial Americans of all class welcomed children because they were understood to produce wealth for families and nations. Colonial Americans described women who reproduced in terms of "flourishing" and "breeding" or as "teeming" and "fruitful." Klepp, *Revolutionary Conceptions*, 3–4, 61–64. Wertz and Wertz, *Lying-In*, 1–28, 77–108, emphasizes the "social" nature of childbirth in the colonial period to its movement toward privacy in the nineteenth and early twentieth century and discusses how, in the nineteenth century, the discourse of childbirth became shameful and private rather than public and celebrated. Volo and Volo, *Family Life in Nineteenth-Century America*, 196–97, describes how, in nineteenth-century America, discussion of anything related to sex—including conception, pregnancy, and birth—was private; pregnant women were expected to retreat entirely from public view. The U.S. context also presents other contrasts to Mexico in that in America, starting in the last third of the eighteenth century, women began to more systematically limit birth than they had in earlier periods. Through the course of the nineteenth century, information about abortifacients and contraception was published broadly in the popular American press. See Klepp, *Revolutionary Conceptions*, 6, 54, 277. See also Leavitt, *Brought to Bed*, 19; and Brodie, *Contraception and Abortion in Nineteenth-Century America*, 4, 5.

93. I located fifteen articles on the Casa de Maternidad in *El Monitor Republicano, El Siglo Diez y Nueve, La Patria*, and *La Voz de México* for the period 1851–90; I located a further sixty-three notices treating obstetrical medicine and ads directed toward pregnant women between 1842 and 1897 in *El Imparcial, El Monitor Republicano, El Siglo Diez y Nueve, El Universal, La Patria*, and *La Voz de México*; nearly half these were published in the 1880s and 1890s.

94. *El Universal*, July 10, 1855, 4.

95. *El Siglo Diez y Nueve*, December 12, 1891.

96. *El Siglo Diez y Nueve*, June 24, 1870, 2.

97. Ibid.

98. "Mexico: Casa de Maternidad," n.p.

99. Flores, *Ligeros apuntes de pelvimetría comparada*.

100. Ibid., 9.

101. Ibid., 10, 55.

102. Ibid., 56.

103. Cházaro and Kersey, "Mexican Women's Pelves," 110.

104. Rodrígezl, "Tocologia"; *Gaceta Médica de México* 7 (1872): 54.

105. Ibid., 111.

106. Flores y Troncoso, *Historia de la medicina en México*, 3:625–26.

107. Ibid., 622.

108. Manuel Ramos, quoted in Radkau, "Los médicos (se) crean una imagen," 128.

109. Cházaro and Kersey, "Mexican Women's Pelves," 113.

110. Radkau, "Los médicos (se) crean una imagen," 142.

111. Flores y Troncoso, *Historia la medicina en México*, 3:655.

112. Uribe Elías, "Mexican Obstetrical-Gynecological Surgery in the 19th Century," 108.

113. Uribe Elías, *La invención de la mujer*, 80–82.

114. AHSS, Beneficiencia Pública, Establecimiento Hospitalarios, Hospital de Maternidad y de Infancia, legajo 2, exp. 17.

115. "Mexico: Casa de Maternidad," n.p.; AHSS, Beneficiencia Pública, Establecimiento Hospitalarios, Hospital de Maternidad y de Infancia, legajo 2, exp. 23.

116. AGN, TSJDF, 1880, caja 703, "En averiguación de la muerte de Matilda Montes de Oca y de su hijo."

117. AHSS, Beneficiencia Pública, Establecimiento Hospitalarios, Hospital de Maternidad y de Infancia, caja 2, exp. 23.

118. Annual death rates per one thousand live births in England and Wales between 1850 and 1900 fluctuated between forty and sixty-five; Chamberlain, "British Maternal Mortality," 560. In Sweden, maternal mortality rates in lying-in hospitals in 1861 were 5.67 percent; Högberg, Wall, and Brostrom, "The Impact of Early Medical Technology on Maternal Mortality," 251.

119. Loudon, "The Transformation of Maternal Mortality," 1559.

120. "Mexico: Casa de Maternidad," n.p.; AHSS, Beneficiencia Pública, Establecimiento Hospitalarios, Hospital de Maternidad y de Infancia, legajo 2, exp. 23. The records only indicate statistics for 1869, 1876, four months of 1877, three months of 1881, and July 1886–June 1888. In addition, the Casa's records show one woman died for each of the following: vaginal gangrene, phlegmasia alba dolens (an inflammation related to deep vein thrombosis), acute diarrhea, complications caused by prolonged application of the forceps, an unspecified infection, and cerebral hemorrhage.

121. Loudon, "The Transformation of Maternal Mortality," 1559.

122. Ibid.

123. Uribe Elías, "Mexican Obstetrical-Gynecological Surgery in the 19th Century," 139.

124. Ibid.

125. "Mexico: Casa de Maternidad," n.p. It was another fifteen years before medical staff at Johns Hopkins University Hospital regularly adopted such a treatment. *New York Journal of Gynaecology and Obstetrics*, November 1891, 120.

126. Rodríguez, *Guía clínica del arte de los partos*, 122.

127. Ibid., 70.

128. Morris, Wooding, and Grant, "The Answer Is 17 Years," documents that the current lag time between the publishing of medical research and its implementation is nearly two decades.

129. AHSS, Beneficiencia Pública, Establecimiento Hospitalarios, Hospital de Maternidad y de Infancia, legajo 2, exp. 27.

130. Ibid, exp. 29.

131. Ibid.

132. Ibid.

133. Ibid.

134. AHSS, Beneficiencia Pública, Establecimiento Hospitalarios, Hospital de Maternidad y de Infancia, legajo 7, exp. 33.

135. *El Siglo Diez y Nueve*, July 5, 1877, 2.

136. Ibid.

137. Ibid.

138. Ibid.

139. Ibid.

140. Tenorio-Trillo, *Mexico at the World's Fairs*, 20–27; Priego, "Symbolism, Solitude, and Modernity."

141. Stepan, *The Hour of Eugenics*, 45.

142. Cañizares-Esguerra discusses this phenomenon in *How to Write the History of the New World*.

143. Pilcher, "Tamales or Timbales," 196. Recently, Aviles-Galan has questioned the idea of the Porfirian era's total rejection of indigenous influences on national identity in his study of the indigenous population's embodiment of the historical and biological base for Mexican nationality in the writings of the prominent nineteenth-century historian Vicente Riva Palacio. See Aviles-Galan, "Measuring Skulls."

144. Carillo, "Nacimiento y muerte de una profesión," 174.

145. "Mexico: Casa de Maternidad," n.p.; Rodríguez, *Guía clínica del arte de los partos*, 81.

146. AHSS, Beneficiencia Pública, Establecimiento Hospitalarios, Hospital de Maternidad y de Infancia, legajo 2, exp. 27.

147. McCaa, "The Peopling of Nineteenth-Century Mexico," 622.

148. Ibid., 620.

Conclusion

1. Butterfield, *The Whig Interpretation of History.*

2. Few discusses the "inside-outside" distinction in *For All of Humanity,* 98–99.

3. AGN, Criminal, vol. 68, exp. 7, fol. 243.

4. AGN, TSJDF, 1843, caja 2, "Toca á la causa contra María de Jesús Torres por infanticidio," fol. 5v.

5. Smellie, *A set of anatomical tables with explanations,* thirty-seventh table.

Bibliography

Archival Collections

Archivo Central de la Suprema Corte de Justicia de la Nación, Mexico City
Archivo General de Indias, Seville, Spain
  Estado
  Indiferente
  Mapas y planos
  México
  MP-ESTAMPAS
  MP-MÉXICO
Archivo General de la Nación, Mexico City
  Bandos
  Bienes Nacionales
  Criminal
  General de Parte
  Historia
  Indiferente General
  Indiferente Virreinal
  Inquisición
  Segundo Imperio
  Tribunal Superior de Justicia del Distrito Federal
Archivo Histórico del Arzobispado de México, Mexico City
  Base de Pelagio Antonio de Labistida y Dávalos
Archivo Histórico del Distrito Federal, Mexico City
  Ayuntamiento Gobierno del DF
Archivo Histórico del Estado de Tlaxcala, Tlaxcala City
Archivo Histórico de la Facultad de Medicina, Mexico City
  Protomedicato
Archivo Histórico Judicial del Estado de Oaxaca, Oaxaca City
  Material in this archive is catalogued, interchangeably, under the categories
      "Penal" and "Criminal" but I have referred to all such material as
      "Criminal."
  Ejutla, Penal
  Teposcolula, Penal
  Villa Alta, Penal

Archivo Histórico Municipal de la Ciudad de Oaxaca, Oaxaca City
    Justicia
Archivo Histórico de la Secretaría de Salud, Mexico City
    Beneficiencia Pública
Biblioteca Francisco de Burgoa de la Universidad Autónoma Benito Juárez de
    Oaxaca, Oaxaca City
Biblioteca Nicolás León, Mexico City
Columbia University Libraries, Special Collections, New York City
    Mexico—Historical Manuscripts, 1649–1886
Huntington Library, Pasadena, California
    HM 4297, "Medicina Mexicana"
University of Arizona Library Special Collections, Tucson
    "Inventory of the Casos reservados sinodales en la Diocesis de Mexico,
        y privilegios de los Indios en esta materia." MS 130.
University of New Mexico, Albuquerque
    Mexican Broadsides Collection
        José Guadalupe Posada, "Importante noticia de rarísimo fenómeno dado
        á luz en la Villa de Guadalupe."
Wellcome Library, London
    Arechederreta, Juan Bautista. "Manuscrito al M.I. y Rl. Tribunal del
        Proto-Medicato de México." WMS Amer. 19.
    Carbajal, Antonio J. "Tocologia." WMS Amer. 127.
    Espejo y Cienfuegos, José Ferrer. "Lecciones de obstetricia, dadas oralmente
        para curso de segundo año." WMS Amer. 122.
    "Medicamentos experimentados y provechosas para las enfermedades
        siguientes," WMS Amer. 7.
    "Mexico: Casa de Maternidad." WMS Amer. 121.
    "Mexico, 18th Century: Compendium of Remedies." WMS Amer. 58.
    "Prontuario o método fácil en donde se contienen las más eficaces
        medicinas." WMS Amer. 18.
    Vásquez, Lucas. "Florilegio medicinal para los misioneros entre las naciones
        bárbaras de México," WMS Amer. 26.

Periodicals

El Diario de México
El Hijo del Ahuizote
El Imparcial
El Monitor Republicano
El Mosaico Mexicano, ó, Colección de Amenidades Curiosas é Instructivas
*El Museo Mexicano, ó, Miscelánea Pintoresca de Amenidades Curiosas é
    Instructivas*
El País

El Siglo Diez y Nueve
El Universal
Gaceta Médica de México
Gazeta de México
La Patria
La Voz de México
Mercurio Volante
New York Journal of Gynaecology and Obstetrics

Published Primary Sources

"Acuerdo de los prelados del III Concilio límense, sobre el catecismo único en castellano y en las lenguas de las diversas regiones." In *La conquista espiritual de la América Española. Doscientos documentos del siglo XVI*, edited by Paulo Suess, 171–79. Quito, Ecuador: Abya-Yala, 2002.

Alcalá Martínez, Jaime. *Disertación Médico-quirúrgica, sobre una operación cesárea ejecutada en muger y feto vivos, en la ciudad de Valencia.* Valencia: Viuda de Gerónimo Conejos, 1753.

Arbiol y Diez, Antonio. *Explicacion breve de todo el sagrado texto de la doctrina christiana para consuelo y aprovechamiento fundamental de las personas espirtuales.* Mexico City: J. B. de Hogal, 1731.

Astruc, Jean. *The Art of Midwifery Reduced to Principles.* London: J. Nourse, 1767.

Baudelocque, J.-L. *Principes sur l'art des accouchements par demandes et réponses en faveur des élèves sages-femmes.* Paris: Germer Baillière, 1830.

Berdan, Frances, and Patricia Rieff Anawalt. *The Essential Codex Mendoza.* Berkeley: University of California Press, 1997.

Boyer, Richard. "Catarina María Complains That Juan Teoioa Forcibly Deflowered Her." In *Colonial Lives: Documents on Latin American History, 1550-1850*, edited by Richard Boyer and Geoffrey Spurling, 155–65. Oxford: Oxford University Press, 2000.

Cartilla de partos escrita esclusivamente para que sirva de testo en el curso que debe darse a las parteras en el Instituto del Estado. Oaxaca City, Mexico: Imprenta del Instituto del Estado, 1863.

Catholic Church. *Catecismo para uso de los párrocos: hecho por el IV Concilio Provincial Mexicano celebrado año de M.DCC. LXXI.* Mexico City: Imprenta de el Lic. D. Josef de Jaúregui, 1772.

Clavijero, Francisco Javier. *Historia antigua de México.* Mexico City: Editorial Porrúa, 1991.

Código Penal para el Distrito Federal y Territorio de la Baja California sobre Delitos del Fuero Común y para toda la República sobre Delitos contra la Federación. Veracruz, Mexico: Imprenta del "Progreso" de Ramon Lainé, 1873.

Cumplido, Ignacio. *La ilustración Mexicana*, vol. 3. Mexico City: Ignacio Cumplido, 1852.

Dirección General de Estadísticas. *Estadísticas sociales del Porfiriato 1877–1910.* Mexico City: Talleres gráficos de la nación, 1956.

Dunglison, Robert. *Medical Lexicon: A Dictionary of Medical Science.* 9th ed. Philadelphia: Blanchard and Lea, 1853.

Erauso, Catalina de. *Lieutenant Nun: Memoir of a Basque Transvestite in the New World.* Translated by Michele Stepto and Gabriel Stepto. Boston: Beacon Press, 1996.

Escriche, Joaquin. *Diccionario razonado de legislación y jurisprudencia.* Madrid: Imprenta de Eduardo Cuesta, 1874.

Esteyneffer, Juan de. *Florilegio medicinal: ó, Breve epitome de las medicinas y cirujia.* Mexico City: Litografía y Encuadernación de Ireneo Paz, 1887.

Farfán, Agustín. *Tractado brebe de medicina, y de todas las enfermedades.* Mexico City: Pedro de Ocharte, 1592.

Fernández de Lizardi, José Joaquín. *The Mangy Parrot: The Life and Times of Periquillo Sarniento, Written by Himself for His Children.* Translated by David Frye. Indianapolis: Hackett, 2004.

Flores, Florencio. *Ligeros apuntes de pelvimetría comparada.* Cuernavaca, Mexico: Imprenta del Gobierno del Estado, 1881.

Flores y Troncoso, Francisco de Asis. *El hímen en México.* Mexico City: Oficina Tipografía de la Secretaría de Fomento, 1885.

———. *Historia de la medicina en México desde la época de los indios hasta la presente,* vols. 1–4. Mexico City: Instituto Mexicano del Seguro Social, 1982.

Galindo y Villa, Jesús. *Breve noticia histórico-descriptiva del Museo Nacional de México.* Mexico City: Imprenta del Museo Nacional, 1896. Universidad Autónoma de Nuevo León, Colección Digital. http://cdigital.dgb.uanl.mx/la /1020134345/1020134345_003.pdf, accessed June 14, 2014.

Hernández, Francisco, and Francisco Jiménez. *Plantas, animales y minerales de Nueva España, usados en la Medicina, 1615.* Morelia, Mexico: José R. Bravo, 1888.

Herrera, Guillermo. *Estadística del ramo criminal en la República Mexicana que comprende un periodo de quince años, de 1871 á 1885.* Mexico City: Secretaría de Fomento, 1890.

Huacuja, Francisco F. *Tratado práctico de partos: que comprende las nociones más precisas sobre los accidentes y obstáculos que presentan y el reglamento de que habla la ley de 2 de marzo de 1852: aprobado por el supremo gobierno del estado y por la Facultad Médica para uso de las matronas.* Morelia, Mexico: Imprenta de O. Ortiz, 1857.

Leclerc, George Louis, Comte de Buffon. *The Natural History of Animals, Vegetables, and Minerals with the Theory of the Earth in General.* Translated from the French of Count De Buffon. Intendant of the Royal Gardens in France; Member of the French Academy, of the Academy of Sciences, and of the Royal Societies of London Berlin, & C. By W. Kenrick, L.L.D. and J. Murdoch. London: T. Bell, 1775.

———. *Natural history, general and particular, by the Count de Buffon, translated into English. Illustrated with above 260 copper-plates, and occasional notes and observations by the translator*, vol. 2. Edinburgh: William Creech, 1780.

León, Nicolás. *Apuntes para la historia de la obstetricia en Michoacán desde los tiempos pre-Colombianos hasta el año 1875.* Morelia, Mexico: D. J. Rosario Bravo, 1887.

———. *La obstetricia en México. Notas bibliográficas, etnicas, históricas, documentarias y críticas, de los orígenes históricos hasta el año 1910.* Mexico City: Viuda de Diaz de Leon, 1910.

Levret, Andrés. *Tratado de partos demonstrado por principios de phisica y mecanica*, vol. 1. Madrid: Pedro Marin, 1778.

Mauriceau, François. *Traité des maladies des femmes grosses et de celles qui sont nouvellement accouchées.* Paris: 1682.

Maygrier, Jacques Pierre. *Nouvelles demonstrations d'acchouchements.* Brussels: Wahlen, 1825.

———. *Nuevo método para operar en los partos.* Mexico City: M. Ontiveros, 1821.

Medina, Antonio. *Cartilla nueva util y necesaria para instruirse las Matronas que vulgarmente se llaman Comadres, en el oficio de partear.* Mexico City: Doña Maria Fernandez de Jauregui, 1806.

Muñoz, Miguel Eugenio. *Recopilación de las leyes, pragmáticas reales, decretos, y acuerdos del Real Proto-Medicato.* Valencia, Spain: Imprenta de la Viuda de Antonio Bordaza, 1751.

Nieto de Piña, Cristóbal. *Instruccion medica para discernir, si el feto muerto, lo ha sido dentro, o fuera de el utero.* Madrid: Don Manuel Nicolas Vazques, n.d.

Ortega, Ancieto. "Obstetricia. Entuertos." *Gaceta Médica de México* 3: no. 8 (1867), 115–126.

Parsons Scott, Samuel, trans. *Las Siete Partidas*, vol. 5: *Underworlds: The Dead, the Criminal, and the Marginalized.* Edited by Robert I. Burns, SJ. Philadelphia: University of Pennsylvania Press, 2001.

Ramírez, Román. *Catálogo de las anomalías coleccionadas en el museo nacional, precedido de unas nociones de teratología.* Mexico City: Imprenta del Museo Nacional, 1896.

Rodríguez, Juan María. *Guía clínica del arte de los partos.* Mexico City: Imprenta de Ignacio Escalante, 1878.

———. "Tocología." *Gaceta Médica de México* 7 (1872), 47–58.

Ruiz Guadalajara, Juan Carlos. " 'Con la sangre de todo un Dios.' La caridad del sacerdote para con los niños encerrados en el vientre de sus madres difuntas, y notas sobre la operación cesárea post mortem en el periodo novohispano tardío." *Relaciones* 24, no. 94 (2003): 201–48.

Sahagún, Bernardino de. *Historia general de las cosas de Nueva España*, vol. 2. Mexico City: Conaculta, 1988.

Segura, Ignacio. *Avisos saludables a las parteras para el cumplimiento de su obligación. Sacados de la "Embriología Sacra" del Sr. Dr. D. Francisco Manuel*

Cangiamila, y puestos en castellano por el Dr. D. Ignacio Segura, Médico de esta corte. Mexico City: F. de Zúñiga y Ontiveros, 1775.

Sharp, Jane. *The Midwives Book: Or the Whole Art of Midwifry Discovered.* Translated by Elaine Hobby. New York: Oxford University Press, 1999.

Smellie, William. *A set of anatomical tables with explanations and an abridgement of the practice of midwifery; with a view to illustrate a treatise on that subject, and collection of cases.* 2nd ed. Germany: s.n., 19—. [Facsimile of: 2nd ed., corr. London: [s.n.], 1761.

Torres, Ignacio. *Manual de partos dedicado especialmente a las parteras por el catedrático de Obstetricia en el colegio de Medicina de México.* Mexico City: Imprenta de Manuel Castro, 1858.

Valdés, Ramón Francisco. *Diccionario de Jurisprudencia Criminal Mexicana.* Mexico City: Tipografía de V.G. Torres, 1850.

Venegas, Juan Manuel. *Compendio de la medicina; ó Medicina practica, en que se declara laconicamente lo mas util de ella, que el Autor tiene observado en estas regiones de Nueva España, para casi todas las Enfermedades que acometen al cuerpo humano: dispuesto en forma alfabetica.* Mexico City: Felipe de Zúñiga y Ontiveros, 1788.

Ventura Pastor, José. *Preceptos generales sobre las operaciones de los partos,* vol.1. Madrid: Joseph Herrera, 1789.

Vidart, Pedro. *El discípulo instruido en el arte de partear.* Madrid: Imprenta Real, 1785.

Vigarous, José María Joaquin. *Curso elemental de las enfermedades de las mujeres, o, Ensayo sobre un nuevo método para clasificar y estudiar las enfermedades de este sexô.* Madrid: Imprenta de Don Juan de Brugada, 1807.

Virgili, Pedro. *Compendio de el arte de partear. Compuesto para el uso de los reales colegios de cirugía.* Barcelona: Thomas Piferrer, 1765.

Ximénez, Matteo. *Colección de estampas que representan los principales pasos, hechos y prodigios del Beato Frai Sebastian de Aparizio.* Rome: Inciser Pedro Bombelli, 1789.

Secondary Sources

Acero, Itzel. "Más de 700 mujeres criminalizadas en México por aborto." *La jornada Aguascalientes,* 8 September 2014. http://www.lja.mx/2014/09/mas -de-700-mujeres-criminalizadas-en-mexico-por-aborto, accessed November 10, 2014.

Adank, Patricia Ann Drwall. "Accommodation and Innovation: The Gazeta de México, 1784 to 1810." PhD diss., Arizona State University, 1980.

Aguirre, Carlos, and Ricardo D. Salvatore, "Introduction: Writing the History of Law, Crime, and Punishment in Latin America." In *Crime and Punishment in Latin America,* edited by Ricardo D. Salvatore, Carlos Aguirre, and Gilbert M. Joseph, 1–32. Durham, N.C.: Duke University Press, 2001.

Aguirre Beltrán, Gonzalo. *La población negra de México, 1519–1810; estudio etno-histórico*. Mexico City: Fondo de Cultura Económica, 1946.

Alcina Franch, José. "Procreación, amor y sexo entre los mexica." *Estudios de Cultura Náhuatl*, 21 (1991): 59–82.

Arney, William Ray. *Power and the Profession of Obstetrics*. Chicago: University of Chicago Press, 1982.

Arnold, Linda. "When Not Even Safe in Her Own Home: Adjudicating Violence against Children in 19th Century Mexico City." *Ars Iuris* 28 (2002): 71–98.

———. "Why Pablo Parra Wasn't Executed: Courts and the Death Penalty in Mexico, 1797–1929." Paper presented at the conference "The Death Penalty and Mexico-U.S. Relations: Historical Continuities, Present Dilemmas, An International Symposium," University of Texas at Austin, April 14, 2004.

Arrom, Silvia M. "Changes in Mexican Family Law in the Nineteenth Century: The Civil Codes of 1870 and 1884." *Journal of Family History* 10, no. 3 (1985): 305–17.

———. *The Women of Mexico City, 1790–1857*. Stanford, Calif.: Stanford University Press, 1985.

Ávila Espinosa, Felipe Arturo. "Los niños abandonados de la casa de niños expósitos de la ciudad de México: 1767–1821." In *La familia en el mundo iberoamericano*, edited by Pilar Gonzalbo Aizpuru and Cecilia Rabell, 265–310. Mexico City: Instituto de Investigaciones Sociales, Universidad Nacional Autónoma de México, 1994.

Aviles-Galan, Miguel Angel. "Measuring Skulls: Race and Science in Vicente Riva Palacio's *México a través de los siglos*." *Bulletin of Latin American Research* 29, no. 1 (2010): 85–102.

Bauer, Ralph, and José Antonio Mazzotti. "Introduction: Creole Subjects in the Colonial Americas." In *Creole Subjects in the Colonial Americas: Empires, Texts, Identities*, edited by Ralph Bauer and José Antonio Mazzotti, 1–57. Chapel Hill: University of North Carolina Press, 2009.

Birn, Anne-Emanuelle, and Raúl Necochea López. "Footprints in the Future: Looking Forward to the History of Health and Medicine in Latin America in the Twenty-First Century." *Hispanic American Historical Review* 91, no. 3 (2011): 503–27.

Bleichmar, Daniela, Paula De Vos, Kristin Huffine, and Kevin Sheehan, eds. *Science in the Spanish and Portuguese Empires, 1500–1800*. Stanford, Calif.: Stanford University Press, 2008.

Blum, Ann S. *Domestic Economies: Family, Work and Welfare in Mexico City, 1884–1942*. Lincoln: University of Nebraska Press, 2009.

———. "Public Welfare and Child Circulation, Mexico City, 1877 to 1925." *Journal of Family History* 23, no. 240 (1998): 240–71.

———. "Reproductive Health in Latin American Transitions: Late Colonialism, Abolition, and Revolution." In *Women, Ethnicity, and Medical Authority: Historical Case Studies in Reproductive Health in Latin America*, edited by Tamera Marko and Adam Warren, 79–93. San Diego: Center for Iberian and

Latin American Studies, University of California–San Diego, 2004. http://
escholarship.org/uc/item/8q4485r0, accessed September 23, 2014.

Borst, Charlotte G. *Catching Babies: The Professionalization of Childbirth,
1870–1920*. Cambridge, Mass.: Harvard University Press, 1995.

Brading, D. A. *The First America: The Spanish Monarchy, Creole Patriots, and the
Liberal State, 1492–1867*. Cambridge: Cambridge University Press, 1991.

Brammall, Kathryn M. "Monstrous Metamorphosis: Nature, Morality, and the
Rhetoric of Monstrosity in Tudor England." *Sixteenth Century Journal* 27, no.
1 (1996): 3–21.

Briggs, Charles L. "Introduction." In *Women, Ethnicity, and Medical Authority:
Historical Perspectives on Reproductive Health in Latin America*, edited by
Tamera Marko and Adam Warren, 1–4. San Diego: Center for Iberian and
Latin American Studies, University of California–San Diego, 2004. http://
escholarship.org/uc/item/8q4485r0, accessed September 23, 2014.

Brodie, Janet Farrell. *Contraception and Abortion in Nineteenth-Century
America*. Ithaca, N.Y.: Cornell University Press, 1994.

Brodsky, Phyllis L. *The Control of Childbirth: Women Versus Medicine through
the Ages*. Jefferson, N.C.: McFarland, 2008.

Buffington, Robert M. *Criminal and Citizen in Modern Mexico*. Lincoln:
University of Nebraska Press, 2000.

——. "Looking Forward, Looking Back: Judicial Discretion and State Legitimation
in Modern Mexico." *Crime, Histoire et Sociétés* 2, no. 2 (1998): 15–34.

Burke, Peter. "Frontiers of the Monstrous: Perceiving National Characters in
Early Modern Europe." In *Monstrous Bodies/Political Monstrosities*, edited by
Laura Lunger Knoppers and Joan B. Landes, 25–39. Ithaca, N.Y.: Cornell
University Press, 2004.

Burkhart, Louise M. "Mexica Women on the Home Front: Housework and
Religion in Aztec Mexico." In *Indian Women of Early Mexico*, edited by Susan
Schroeder, Stephanie Wood, and Robert Haskett, 25–54. Norman: University
of Oklahoma Press, 1997.

Butterfield, Herbert. *The Whig Interpretation of History*. New York: W. W. Norton,
1931.

Calvo, Thomas. "The Warmth of the Hearth: Seventeenth-Century Guadalajara
Families." In *Sexuality and Marriage in Colonial Latin America*, edited by
Asunción Lavrin, 287–312. Lincoln: University of Nebraska Press, 1989.

Campos, Isaac. *Home Grown: Marijuana and the Origins of Mexico's War on
Drugs*. Chapel Hill: University of North Carolina Press, 2012.

Cañizares-Esguerra, Jorge. *How to Write the History of the New World: Histories,
Epistemologies, and Identities in the Eighteenth-Century Atlantic World*.
Stanford, Calif.: Stanford University Press, 2001.

——. "New World, New Stars: Patriotic Astrology and the Invention of Indian
and Creole Bodies in Colonial Spanish America, 1600–1650." *American
Historical Review* 104, no. 1 (1999): 33–68.

Carillo, Ana María. "Nacimiento y muerte de una profesión. Las parteras tituladas en México." *Dynamis* 19 (1999): 167–90.

Chamberlain, Geoffrey. "British Maternal Mortality in the 19th and Early 20th Centuries." *Journal of the Royal Society of Medicine* 99, no. 1 (2006): 559–63.

Chambers, Sarah C. "Crime and Citizenship: Judicial Practice in Arequipa, Peru, during the Transition from Colony to Republic." In *Reconstructing Criminality in Latin America*, edited by Carlos A. Aguirre and Robert Buffington, 19–40. Wilmington, Del.: Scholarly Resources, 2000.

——. "Private Crimes, Public Order: Honor, Gender, and the Law in Early Republican Peru." In *Honor, Status and Law in Modern Latin America*, edited by Sueann Caulfield, Sarah C. Chambers, and Lara Putnam, 27–49. Durham, N.C.: Duke University Press, 2005.

Chassen López, Francie R. *From Liberal to Revolutionary Oaxaca: The View from the South, Mexico 1867–1911*. University Park: Pennsylvania State University Press, 2004.

Cházaro, Laura. "Mexican Women's Pelves and Obstetrical Procedures: Interventions with Forceps in Late 19th-Century Medicine." Translated by Paul Kersey. *Feminist Review* 70 (2005): 100–115.

Clark, Fiona. " 'Read All About It': Science, Translation, Adaptation, and Confrontation in the *Gazeta de Literatura de México*, 1788–1795." In *Science in the Spanish and Portuguese Empires, 1500–1800*, edited by Daniela Bleichmar, Paula De Vos, Kristin Huffine, and Kevin Sheehan, 147–77. Stanford, Calif.: Stanford University Press, 2008.

Cook, Sherburne F., and Woodrow Borah. *Essays in Population History: Mexico and the Caribbean*, vols. 1–2. Berkeley: University of California Press, 1971, 1974.

Cowie, Helen. "Peripheral Vision: Science and Creole Patriotism in Eighteenth-Century Spanish America." *Studies in History and Philosophy of Biological and Biomedical Sciences* 40 (2009): 143–55.

Crawford, Julie. *Marvelous Protestantism: Monstrous Births in Post-Reformation England*. Baltimore: Johns Hopkins University Press, 2005.

Cueto, Marcos, and Steven Palmer. *Medicine and Public Health in Latin America*. Cambridge: Cambridge University Press, 2015.

Cutter, Charles R. "The Administration of Law in Colonial New Mexico." *Journal of the Early* Republic 18, no. 1 (1998): 99–115.

Daston, Lorraine, and Katharine Park. "Unnatural Conceptions: The Study of Monsters in Sixteenth- and Seventeenth-Century France and England." *Past and Present* 92 (1981): 20–54.

——. *Wonders and the Order of Nature: 1150–1750*. New York: Zone Books, 1998.

Díaz Robles, Laura Catalina, and Luciano Oropeza Sandoval. "Las parteras de Guadalajara (México) en el siglo XIX: el despojo de su arte." *Dynamis* 27 (2007): 237–61.

Dickinson, J. R., and J. A. Sharpe. "Infanticide in Early Modern England: The Court of Great Sessions at Chester, 1650–1800." In *Infanticide: Historical Perspectives on Child Murder and Concealment, 1550–2000*, edited by Mark Jackson, 35–51. Aldershot, England: Ashgate, 2002.

Dore, Elizabeth. "One Step Forward, Two Steps Back: Gender and the State in the Long Nineteenth Century." In *Hidden Histories of Gender and the State in Latin America*, edited by Elizabeth Dore and Maxine Molyneux, 3–32. Durham, N.C.: Duke University Press, 2000.

Duden, Barbara. *The Woman beneath the Skin: A Doctor's Patients in Eighteenth-Century Germany*. Cambridge, Mass.: Harvard University Press, 1991.

Duffin, Jacalyn. *History of Medicine: A Scandalously Short Introduction*, 2nd ed. Toronto: University of Toronto Press, 2010.

Eccles, Audrey. *Obstetrics and Gynaecology in Tudor and Stuart England*. Kent, Ohio: Kent State University Press, 1982.

Epps, Garrett. *Peyote vs. The State: Religious Freedom on Trial*. Norman: University of Oklahoma Press, 2009.

Few, Martha. "Atlantic World Monsters: Monstrous Births and the Politics of Pregnancy in Colonial Guatemala." In *Women, Religion, and the Atlantic World (1600–1800)*, edited by Daniella Kostroun and Lisa Vollendorf, 205–22. Toronto: University of Toronto Press, 2009.

——. *For All of Humanity: Mesoamerican and Colonial Medicine in Enlightenment Guatemala*. Tucson: University of Arizona Press, 2015.

——. "Medical *Mestizaje* and the Politics of Pregnancy in Colonial Guatemala, 1660–1730." In *Science in the Spanish and Portuguese Empires, 1500–1800*, edited by Daniela Bleichmar, Paula De Vos, Kristin Huffine, and Kevin Sheehan, 132–46. Stanford, Calif.: Stanford University Press, 2008.

——. "'That Monster of Nature': Gender, Sexuality, and the Medicalization of a 'Hermaphrodite' in Late Colonial Guatemala." *Ethnohistory* 54, no. 1 (2007): 159–76.

——. *Women Who Live Evil Lives: Gender, Religion, and the Politics of Power in Colonial Guatemala*. Austin: University of Texas Press, 2002.

Fields, Sherry. *Pestilence and Headcolds: Encountering Illness in Colonial Mexico*. New York: Columbia University Press, 2009.

Florescano, Enrique. *National Narratives in Mexico: A History*. Translated by Nancy T. Hancock. Norman: University of Oklahoma Press, 2006.

Florescano, Enrique, and Isabel Gil Sánchez. "La época de las reformas borbónicas y el crecimiento económico, 1750–1850." In *Historia general de México*, vol. 2, edited by Daniel Cosío Villegas and Bernardo García Martínez, 183–302. Mexico City: El Colegio de México, 1976.

Foucault, Michel. *The History of Sexuality*, vol 1: *An Introduction*. Translated by Robert Hurley. New York: Pantheon, 1978.

——. "Illegalities and Delinquency." In *The Foucault Reader*, edited by Paul Rabinow, 226–33. New York: Pantheon, 1984.

French, William E. "Prostitutes and Guardian Angels: Women, Work, and the Family in Porfirian Mexico," *Hispanic American Historical Review* 72, no. 4 (1992): 529–53.

García Peña, Ana Lidia. "Madres solteras, pobres y abandonadas: Ciudad de México, Siglo XIX." *Historia Mexicana* 53, no. 3 (2004): 647–92.

García Vázquez, Iskra, Sandra Edith Moncayo Cuagliotti, and Benjamín Sánchez Trocino. "El parto en México, Reflexiones para su atención integral." *Ide@s Concyteg* 7, no. 84 (2012): 811–44.

Garza, James Alex. *The Imagined Underworld: Sex, Crime, and Vice in Porfirian Mexico City*. Lincoln: University of Nebraska Press, 2007.

Gill, Miranda. *Eccentricity and the Cultural Imagination in Nineteenth-Century Paris*. Oxford: Oxford University Press, 2009.

Gonzalbo Aizpuru, Pilar. "La Casa de Niños Expósitos de la cuidad de México: Una fundación del siglo XVIII," *Historia Mexicana* 31, no. 3 (1982): 409–30.

Gonzales, Manuel G. *Mexicanos: A History of Mexicans in the United States*. Bloomington: Indiana University Press, 2009.

González, Ondina E. "Consuming Interests: The Response to Abandoned Children in Colonial Havana." In *Raising an Empire: Children in Early Modern Iberia and Colonial Latin America*, edited by Ondina E González and Bianca Premo, 137–62. Albuquerque: University of New Mexico Press, 2007.

Goodman, David. "Science, Medicine, and Technology in Colonial Spanish America: New Interpretations, New Approaches." In *Science in the Spanish and Portuguese Empires, 1500–1800*, edited by Daniela Bleichmar, Paula De Vos, Kristin Huffine, and Kevin Sheehan, 9–34. Stanford, Calif.: Stanford University Press, 2008.

Gorbach, Frida. *El monstruo, objeto imposible: Un estudio sobre teratología Mexicana, siglo xix*. Mexico City: Itaca, 2008.

Gruzinsky, Serge. *Images at War: Mexico from Columbus to Blade Runner (1492–2019)*. Durham, N.C.: Duke University Press, 2001.

Guedea, Virginia. "La medicina en las gacetas de México." *Mexican Studies/Estudios Mexicanos* 5, no. 2 (1989): 175–99.

Gutiérrez, Ramón A. *When Jesus Came, the Corn Mothers Went Away: Marriage, Sexuality, and Power in New Mexico, 1500–1846*. Stanford, Calif.: Stanford University Press, 1991.

Haffner, Paul. *The Mystery of Mary*. Leominster, Herefordshire: Gracewing, 2004.

Haslip-Viera, Gabriel. *Crime and Punishment in Late Colonial Mexico City, 1692–1810*. Albuquerque: University of New Mexico Press, 1999.

Hernández Sáenz, Luz María. *Learning to Heal: The Medical Profession in Colonial Mexico, 1767–1831*. New York: Peter Lang, 1997.

Herrera-Ruiz, Maribel, Rubén Román-Ramos, Alejandro Zamilpa, Jaime Tortoriello, and J. Enrique Jiménez-Ferrer. "Flavonoids from *Tilia americana* with Anxiolytic Activity in Plus-Maze Test," *Journal of Ethnopharmacology* 118, no. 2 (2008): 312–17.

Hijazi, A. M., and A. S. Salhab. "Effects of Artemisia monosperma Ethanolic Leaves Extract on Implantation, Mid-Term Abortion and Parturition of Pregnant Rats." *Journal of Ethnopharmacology* 128, no. 2 (2010): 446–51.

Högberg, Ulf, Stig Wall, and Göran. Broström. "The Impact of Early Medical Technology on Maternal Mortality in late 19th-Century Sweden." *International Journal of Gynaecological Obstetrics* 24, no.4 (1986): 251–61.

Holler, Jacqueline. "Hybrid Births: Midwifery and Female Embodiment in Colonial Mexico." Paper Presented at the Fourteenth Berkshire Conference on the History of Women, University of Toronto, June 12–15, 2008.

Izquierdo, Joaquín José. *Raudón, cirujano poblano de 1810; aspectos de la cirugía mexicana de principios del siglo XIX en torno de una vida*. Mexico City: Ediciones Ciencia, 1949.

Jackson, Mark. *New-Born Child Murder: Women, Illegitimacy and the Courts in Eighteenth-Century England*. Manchester, England: Manchester University Press, 1996.

——. "The Trial of Harriet Vooght: Continuity and Change in the History of Infanticide." In *Infanticide: Historical Perspectives on Child Murder and Concealment, 1550–2000*, edited by Mark Jackson, 1–17. Aldershot, England: Ashgate, 2002.

Jaffary, Nora E. *False Mystics: Deviant Orthodoxy in Colonial Mexico*. Lincoln: University of Nebraska Press, 2004.

——. "Monstrous Births and Creole Nationalism in Late Colonial Mexico." *The Americas: A Quarterly Review of Inter-American Cultural History* 68, no. 2 (2011): 179–207.

——. "Reconceiving Motherhood: Infanticide and Abortion in Late Colonial Mexico." *Journal of Family History* 37, no. 1 (2012): 3–22.

——. "Sexual Virtue and Social Mobility in Colonial Mexico." In *Gender, Race, and Religion in the Colonization of the Americas*, edited by Nora E. Jaffary, 95–108. Burlington, Vt.: Ashgate, 2007.

Jaffary, Nora E., Edward W. Osowski, and Susie S. Porter, eds. *Mexican History: A Primary Source Reader*. Boulder, CO: Westview Press, 2010.

Johnson, Lyman L., and Sonya Lipsett-Rivera, eds. *The Faces of Honor: Sex, Shame, and Violence in Colonial Latin America*. Albuquerque: University of New Mexico Press, 1998.

Jordanova, Ludmilla. *Sexual Visions: Images of Gender in Science and Medicine between the Eighteenth and Twentieth Centuries*. Hemel Hempstead, England: Harvester Wheatsheaf, 1989.

Jütte, Robert. *Contraception: A History*. Malden, Mass.: Polity, 2008.

Karchmer Krivitsky, Samuel. "La ginecología y la obstetricia." In *Contribuciones Mexicanas al conocimiento médico*, edited by Hugo Arechiga and Juan Somolinos Palencia, 279–301. Mexico City: Fondo de Cultura Económica, 1993.

Kellogg, Susan. *Weaving the Past: A History of Latin America's Indigenous Women from the Prehispanic Period to the Present.* New York: Oxford University Press, 2005.

Klepp, Susan E. *Revolutionary Conceptions: Women, Fertility, and Family Limitation in America, 1760–1820.* Chapel Hill: University of North Carolina Press, 2009.

Knoppers, Laura Lunger, and Joan B. Landes, eds. "Introduction." In *Monstrous Bodies/Political Monstrosities in Early Modern Europe,* 1–22. Ithaca, N.Y.: Cornell University Press, 2004.

———, eds. *Monstrous Bodies/Political Monstrosities in Early Modern Europe.* Ithaca, N.Y.: Cornell University Press, 2004.

Landers, Jane G. "Female Conflict and Its Resolution in Eighteenth-Century St. Augustine." *The Americas* 54, no. 4 (1998): 557–74.

———. "'On Consideration of Her Enormous Crime': Rape and Infanticide in Spanish St. Augustine." In *The Devil's Lane: Sex and Race in the Early South,* edited by Catherine Clinton and Michele Gillespie, 205–17. New York: Oxford University Press, 1997.

Langer, William L. "Infanticide: A Historical Survey." *History of Childhood Quarterly* 1 (1974): 353–66.

Lanning, John Tate. *The Royal Protomedicato: The Regulation of the Medical Profession in the Spanish Empire.* Edited by John Jay TePaske. Durham, N.C.: Duke University Press, 1985.

Laqueur, Thomas. *Making Sex: Body and Gender from the Greeks to Freud.* Cambridge, Mass.: Harvard University Press, 1990.

Lavrin, Asunción. "Introduction: The Scenario, the Actors, and the Issues." In *Sexuality and Marriage in Colonial Latin America,* edited by Asuncíon Lavrin, 1–43. Lincoln: University of Nebraska Press, 1989.

———. "Sexuality in Colonial Mexico: A Church Dilemma." In *Sexuality and Marriage in Colonial Latin America,* edited by Asuncíon Lavrin, 58–72. Lincoln: University of Nebraska Press, 1989.

———. ed. *Sexuality and Marriage in Colonial Latin America.* Lincoln: University of Nebraska Press, 1989.

Leavitt, Judith Walzer. *Brought to Bed: Childbearing in America, 1750–1950.* Oxford: Oxford University Press, 1986.

León-Portilla, Miguel. *Bernardino de Sahagún: First Anthropologist.* Translated by Mauricio J. Mixco. Norman: University of Oklahoma Press, 2002.

Lindemann, Mary. *Medicine and Society in Early Modern Europe.* 2nd ed. Cambridge: Cambridge University Press, 2010.

Lipsett-Rivera, Sonya. *Gender and the Negotiation of Daily Life in Mexico, 1750–1856.* Lincoln: University of Nebraska Press, 2012.

———. "Marriage and Family Relations in Mexico during the Transition from Colony to Nation." In *State and Society in Spanish America during the Age of*

Revolution, edited by Victor M. Uribe-Uran, 121–48. Wilmington, Del.: Scholarly Resources, 2001.

———. "A Slap in the Face of Honor: Social Transgression and Women in Late Colonial Mexico." In *The Faces of Honor: Sex, Shame, and Violence in Colonial Latin America*, edited by Lyman L. Johnson and Sonya Lipsett-Rivera, 179–200. Albuquerque: University of New Mexico Press, 1998.

López-Alonso, Moramay. "Growth with Inequality: Living Standards in Mexico, 1850–1950." *Journal of Latin American Studies* 39 (2007): 81–105.

López Austin, Alfredo. "La sexualidad entre los antiguos nahuas." In *Familia y Sexualidad en Nueva España: Memoria del primer simposio de historia de las mentalidades*, edited by the Seminario de Historia de las Mentalidades, 141–76. Mexico City: Fondo de Cultura Económica, 1982.

Loudon, Irvine. "The Transformation of Maternal Mortality," *British Medical Journal* 305, no. 6868 (1992): 1557–60.

Malvido, Elsa. "El abandono de los hijos: una forma de control del tamaño de la familia y del trabajo indígena: Tula (1683–1730)." *Historia Mexicana* 29, no. 4, 521–61.

Marko, Tamera, and Adam Warren, eds. *Women, Ethnicity, and Medical Authority: Historical Perspectives on Reproductive Health in Latin America*. San Diego: Center for Iberian and Latin American Studies, University of California–San Diego, 2004. http://escholarship.org/uc/item/894485ro, accessed September 23, 2014.

Marland, Hilary, ed. *The Art of Midwifery: Early Modern Midwives in Europe*. London: Routledge, 1993.

———. "Introduction." In *The Art of Midwifery: Early Modern Midwives in Europe*, edited by Hilary Marland, 1–8. London: Routledge, 1993.

Marley, David F. "Introducción." *Gazeta de México (enero a agosto de 1784)*, facsimile ed., i–vi. Mexico City: Rolston-Bain, 1983.

Martínez, Ana Laura, María Eva González-Trujano, Eva Aguirre-Hernández, Julia Moreno, Marco Soto-Hernández, and Francisco J. López-Muñoz. "Antinociceptive activity of *Tilia americana* var. *mexicana* inflorescences and quercetin in the formalin test and in an arthritic pain model in rats." *Neuropharmacology* 56, no. 2 (2009): 564–71.

Martínez, María Elena. *Genealogical Fictions: Limpieza de Sangre, Religion, and Gender in Colonial Mexico*. Stanford, Calif.: Stanford University Press, 2008.

Mazzotti, José Antonio. "El Dorado, Paradise, and Supreme Sanctity in Seventeenth-Century Peru." In *Creole Subjects in the Colonial Americas: Empires, Texts, Identities*, edited by Ralph Bauer and José Antonio Mazzotti, 407–11. Chapel Hill: University of North Carolina Press, 2009.

McCaa, Robert. "The Peopling of Mexico from Origins to Revolution." In *A Population History of North America*, edited by Michael R. Haines and Richard H. Steckel, 241–304. Cambridge: Cambridge University Press, 2000.

———. "The Peopling of Nineteenth-Century Mexico: Critical Scrutiny of a Censured Century." In *Statistical Abstract of Latin America*, vol. 30, part 1, edited by James W. Wilkie, Carlos Alberto Contreras, and Christof Anders Weber, 602–33. Los Angeles: University of California–Los Angeles Latin American Center, 1993.

McClain, Carol Shepherd. "Reinterpreting Women in Healing Roles." In *Women Healers: Cross-Cultural Perspectives*, edited by Carol Shepherd McClain, 1–20. New Brunswick, N.J.: Rutgers University Press, 1995.

McClive, Cathy. "The Hidden Truths of the Belly: The Uncertainties of Pregnancy in Early Modern Europe." In *The Society for the Social History of Medicine* 15, no. 2 (2002), 209–27.

———. *Menstruation and Procreation in Early Modern France.* Farnham, England: Ashgate, 2015.

McGregor, Deborah Kuhn. *From Midwives to Medicine: The Birth of American Gynecology.* New Brunswick, N.J.: Rutgers University Press, 1998.

McLaren, Angus. *A History of Contraception: From Antiquity to the Present Day.* Oxford: Blackwell, 1991.

Milanich, Nara. *Children of Fate: Childhood, Class, and the State in Chile, 1850–1930.* Durham, N.C.: Duke University Press, 2009.

———. "Historical Perspectives on Illegitimacy and Illegitimates in Latin America." In *Minor Omissions: Children in Latin American History and Society*, edited by Tobias Hecht, 72–101. Madison: University of Wisconsin Press, 2002.

Morin, Claude. "Age at Marriage and Female Employment in Colonial Mexico." Paper presented to the conference "Women's Employment, Marriage-Age and Population Change," University of Delhi, Developing Countries Research Center, March 3–5, 1997. https://www.webdepot.umontreal.ca /Usagers/morinc/MonDepotPublic/pub/CIDHInd97.htm, accessed September 23, 2014.

Morris, Zoë Slote, Steven Wooding, and Jonathan Grant. "The Answer Is 17 Years, What Is the Question: Understanding Time Lags in Translational Research." *Journal of the Royal Society of Medicine* 104, no. 12 (2011): 510–20.

Murphy-Lawless, Jo. *Reading Birth and Death: A History of Obstetric Thinking.* Bloomington: Indiana University Press, 1998.

Nari, Marcela. *Políticas de maternidad y maternalismo político.* Buenos Aires: Editorial Biblos, 2004.

Nazzari, Muriel. "An Urgent Need to Conceal: The System of Honor and Shame in Colonial Brazil." In *The Faces of Honor: Sex, Shame, and Violence in Colonial Latin America*, edited by Lyman L. Johnson and Sonya Lipsett-Rivera, 103–26. Albuquerque: University of New Mexico Press, 1998.

Newson, Linda A. "The Demographic Impact of Colonization." In *The Cambridge Economic History of Latin America*, vol 1: *The Colonial Era and the Short Nineteenth Century*, edited by Victor Bulmer-Thomas, John H. Coatsworth, and, Roberto Cortés Conde, 143–84. Cambridge: Cambridge University Press, 2006.

Noonan, John T., Jr. *Contraception: A History of Its Treatment by the Catholic Theologians and Canonists.* Cambridge, Mass.: Belknap Press, 1986.

Numbers, Ronald L. *Medicine in the New World: New Spain, New France, and New England.* Knoxville: University of Tennessee Press, 1987.

Ortiz, Teresa. "From Hegemony to Subordination: Midwives in Early Modern Spain." In *The Art of Midwifery: Early Modern Midwives in Europe*, edited by Hilary Marland, 95–114. London: Routledge, 1993.

Overmyer-Velázquez, Mark. "Portraits of a Lady: Visions of Modernity in Porfirian Oaxaca City," *Mexican Studies/Estudios Mexicanos* 23, no. 1 (2007): 63–100.

———. *Visions of the Emerald City: Modernity, Tradition, and the Formation of Porfirian Oaxaca, Mexico.* Durham, N.C.: Duke University Press, 2006.

Overmyer-Velázquez, Mark, and Yanna Yannakakis. "The Renaissance of Oaxaca City's Historical Archives." *Latin American Research Review* 37, no. 1 (2002): 186–98.

Palmer, Steven. *From Popular Medicine to Medical Populism: Doctors, Healers, and Public Power in Costa Rica, 1800–1940.* Durham, N.C.: Duke University Press, 2003.

Pender, Stephen. " 'No Monsters at the Resurrection': Inside Some Conjoined Twins." In *Monster Theory: Reading Culture*, edited by Jeffrey Jerome Cohen, 143–67. Minneapolis: University of Minnesota Press, 1996.

Penyak, Lee M. "Midwives and Legal Medicine in México, 1740–1846." *Journal of Hispanic Higher Education* 1, no. 3 (2002): 251–66.

———. "Obstetrics and the Emergence of Women in Mexico's Medical Establishment." *The Americas* 60, no. 1 (2003): 59–85.

———. "Safe Harbors and Compulsory Custody: Casa de Depósito in Mexico, 1750–1865." *Hispanic American Historical Review* 79, no. 1 (1999): 83–99.

Pérez Duarte y Noroña, Alicia E. "Los alimentos en la historia del México independiente." In *Memoria del IV Congreso de Historia del Derecho Mexicano*, vol. 2, edited by Beatriz Bernal, 871–93. Mexico City: Instituto de Investigaciones Jurídicas, Universidad Autónoma de México, 1988.

Pérez Salas, María Esther. *Costumbrismo y litografía en México: un nuevo modo de ver.* Mexico City: Universidad Nacional Autónoma de México, 2005.

Piccato, Pablo. *The Tyranny of Opinion: Honor in the Construction of the Mexican Public Sphere.* Durham, N.C.: Duke University Press, 2010.

Pilbean, Pamela M., ed. *Themes in Modern European History: 1780–1830.* London: Routledge, 1995.

Pilcher, Jeffrey. "Tamales or Timbales: Cuisine and the Formation of Mexican National Identity, 1821–1911," *The Americas* 53, no. 2 (1996): 193–216.

Poole, Deborah. "An Image of 'Our Indian': Type Photographs and Racial Sentiments in Oaxaca, 1920–1940." *Hispanic American Historical Review* 84, no. 1 (2004): 37–82.

Powers, Karen Veira. *Women in the Crucible of Conquest: The Gendered Genesis of Spanish American Society, 1500–1600*. Albuquerque: University of New Mexico Press, 2005.

Premo, Bianca. *Children of the Father King: Youth, Authority, and Legal Minority in Colonial Lima*. Chapel Hill: University of North Carolina Press, 2005.

Priego, Natalia. "Symbolism, Solitude, and Modernity: Science and Scientists in Porfirian Mexico," *História, Ciências, Saúde-Manguinhos* 15, no. 2 (2008): 473–85.

Quezada, Noemí. "Creencias tradicionales sobre embarazo y parto." *Anales de Antropología* 14 (1977): 307–26.

———. "Métodos anticonceptivos y abortivos tradicionales." *Anales de antropología* 12, no. 1 (1975): 223–42.

Quiñones Keber, Eloise, ed. *Representing Aztec Ritual: Performance, Text, and Image in the Work of Sahagún*. Boulder: University of Colorado Press, 2002.

Rabell Romero, Cecilia Andrea. "Evaluación del subregistro de defunciones infantiles: Una crítica a los registros parroquiales de San Luis de la Paz, México, 1735–1799." *Revista Mexicana de Sociología* 38, no. 1 (1976): 171–85.

Rabin, Dana. "Bodies of Evidence, States of Mind: Infanticide, Emotion and Sensibility in Eighteenth-Century England." In *Infanticide: Historical Perspectives on Child Murder and Concealment, 1550–2000*, edited by Mark Jackson, 73–92. Aldershot, England: Ashgate, 2002.

Radkau, Verena. "Los médicos (se) crean una imagen: Mujeres y médicos en la prensa Mexicana del siglo XIX." In *Género, familia y mentalidades en América Latina*, edited by Pilar Gonzalbo Aizpuru, 127–59. San Juan: Editorial de la Universidad de Puerto Rico, 1997.

Reina Aoyama, Leticia. *Caminos de luz y sombra: historia indígena de Oaxaca en el siglo XIX*. Mexico City: Centro de Investigaciones y Estudios Superior en Antropología Social, 2004.

Reyes García Márkina, Manuel de los. "*De jure* and *de facto*: The Penal Code of 1871 and Juridical Culture in Mexico City." In *One Law for All? Western Models and Local Practices in (Post-) Imperial Contexts*, edited by Stefan B. Kirmse, 265–86. Frankfurt: Campus, 2012.

Rico Mansard, Luisa Fernanda Francisca. *Exhibir para educar: objetos, colecciones y museos de la ciudad de México (1790–1910)*. Barcelona: Ediciones Pomares, 2004.

Riddle, John M. *Contraception and Abortion from the Ancient World to the Renaissance*. Cambridge, Mass.: Harvard University Press, 1992.

———. *Eve's Herbs: A History of Contraception and Abortion in the West*. Cambridge, Mass.: Harvard University Press, 1999.

Rivera-Garza, Cristina. "The Criminalization of the Syphilitic Body: Prostitutes, Health Crimes, and Society in Mexico, 1867–1930." In *Crime and Punishment in Latin America: Law and Society since Late Colonial Times*, edited by

Ricardo D. Salvatore, Carlos Aguirre, and Joseph M. Gilbert, 147–80. Durham, N.C.: Duke University Press, 2001.

Rodríguez, María de los Ángeles, and Thomas Calvo. "Sobre la práctica del aborto en el Occidente de México: Documentos coloniales (siglo xvi–xvii)." *Trace: Travaux et Recherches dans les Amériques du Centre* 10 (1986): 32–38.

Rodríguez, Martha Eugenia. "Costumbres y tradiciones en torno al embarazo y al parto en el México virreinal." *Anuario de estudios americanos* 57, no. 2 (2000): 501–22.

———. "La medicina científica y su difusión en Nueva España." *Estudios de Historia Novohispana* 12 (1992): 181–93.

Rodríguez-Shadow, María. *La mujer azteca*. Toluca, Mexico: Universidad Autónoma del Estado de México, 2000.

Ruggiero, Kristin. "Honor, Maternity, and the Disciplining of Women: Infanticide in Late Nineteenth-Century Buenos Aires." *Hispanic American Historical Review* 72, no. 3 (1992): 353–73.

———. "Not Guilty: Abortion and Infanticide in Nineteenth-Century Argentina." In *Reconstructing Criminality in Latin America*, edited by Carlos A. Aguirre and Robert Buffington, 149–66. Wilmington, Del.: Scholarly Resources, 2000.

Ruiz Castañeda, María del Carmen. "La tercera gaceta de la Nueva España, Gazeta de México (1784–1809)." *Boletín del Instituto de Investigaciones Bibliográficas* (1971): 137–50.

Schell, Patience A. "Eugenics Policy and Practice in Cuba, Puerto Rico, and Mexico." In *The Oxford Handbook of The History of Eugenics*, edited by Alison Bashford and Philippa Levine, 476–92. Oxford: Oxford University Press, 2010.

———. "Nationalizing Children through Schools and Hygiene: Porfirian and Revolutionary Mexico City." *The Americas* 60, no. 4 (2004): 559–87.

Scheper-Hughes, Nancy. *Death without Weeping: The Violence of Everyday Life in Brazil*. Berkeley: University of California Press, 1992.

Schlegel, Alice. "Status, Property and the Value on Virginity." *American Ethnologist* 18, no. 4 (1991): 719–34.

Seed, Patricia. *To Love, Honor, and Obey in Colonial Mexico: Conflicts over Marriage Choice, 1574–1821*. Stanford, Calif.: Stanford University Press, 1988.

Sesia, Paola M. "'Women Come Here on Their Own When They Need To': Prenatal Care, Authoritative Knowledge, and Maternal Heath in Oaxaca." *Medical Anthropology Quarterly* 10, no. 2 (1996): 121–40.

Sharp, Jane, "Introduction." In *The Midwives Book or The Whole Art of Midwifery Discovered*, edited by Elaine Hobby, xi–xxxi. Oxford: Oxford University Press, 1999.

Shelton, Laura. "'Al parecer de buena conducta': Community Discipline and Judicial Leniency in Infanticide Trials in Mexico's Northern Borderlands, 1850–1910." Paper presented at the Sixteenth Berkshire Conference on the History of Women, University of Toronto, May 22–25, 2014.

———. *For Tranquility and Order: Family and Community on Mexico's Northern Frontier, 1800–1850*. Tucson: University of Arizona Press, 2010.

Shorter, Edward. *A History of Women's Bodies*. New York: Basic, 1982.

Sloan, Kathryn A. "The Penal Code of 1871: From Religious to Civil Control of Everyday Life." In *A Companion to Mexican History and Culture*, edited by William H. Beezley, 302–15. Chichester, England: Wiley-Blackwell, 2011.

———. *Runaway Daughters: Seduction, Elopement, and Honor in Nineteenth-Century Mexico*. Albuquerque: University of New Mexico Press, 2008.

Socolow, Susan Migden. *The Women of Colonial Latin America*. New York: Cambridge University Press, 2000.

———. "Women and Crime: Buenos Aires, 1757–1797." *Journal of Latin American Studies* 12, no. 1 (1980): 39–54.

Soman, Alfred. "Anatomy of an Infanticide Trial: The Case of Marie-Jeanne Bartonnet (1742)." In *Changing Identities in Early Modern France*, edited by Michael Wolfe, 248–72. Durham, N.C.: Duke University Press, 1996.

Speckman Guerra, Elisa. "Disorder and Control: Crime, Justice and Punishment in Porfirian and Revolutionary Society." In *A Companion to Mexican History and Culture*, edited by William H. Beezley, 371–89. Chichester, England: Wiley-Blackwell, 2011.

———. "Justicia, revolución y proceso. Instituciones judiciales en el Distrito Federal (1810–1829)." In *México en tres momentos, 1810–1910–2010: hacia la conmemoración del bicentenario de la Independencia y del centenario de la Revolución Mexicana: retos y perspectivas*, edited by Alicia Mayer, 189–206. Mexico City: Universidad Nacional Autónoma de México, 2007.

———. "Las flores del mal. Mujeres criminales en el Porfiriato." *Historia Mexicana* 47, no. 1 (1997): 183–229.

———. "Los jueces, el honor y la muerte. Un análisis de la justicia (ciudad de México, 1871–1931)." *Historia Mexicana* 54, no. 4 (2006): 1411–66.

———. "Morir a manos de una mujer, homicidas e infanticidas en el porfiriato." In *Disidencia y disidentes en la historia de México*, edited by Felipe Castro and Marcela Terrazas, 295–320. Mexico City: Universidad Nacional Autónoma de México, 2003.

Spinks, Jennifer. "Wondrous Monsters: Representing Conjoined Twins in Early Sixteenth-Century German Broadsheets." *Parergon* 22, no. 2 (2005): 77–112.

Stepan, Nancy Leys. *"The Hour of Eugenics": Race, Gender, and Nation in Latin America*. Ithaca, N.Y.: Cornell University Press, 1991.

Stern, Alexandra Minna. "Responsible Mothers and Normal Children: Eugenics, Nationalism, and Welfare in Post-revolutionary Mexico, 1920–1940." *Journal of Historical Sociology* 12, no. 4 (1999): 369–97.

Stern, Steven J. *The Secret History of Gender: Women, Men, and Power in Late Colonial Mexico*. Chapel Hill: University of North Carolina Press, 1997.

Tanck de Estrada, Dorothy. "Muerte Precoz. Los niños en el siglo xviii." In *Historia de la vida cotidiana en México*, vol. 3: *El siglo xviii: Entre tradición y cambio*, edited by Pilar Gonzablo Aizpuru, 213–46. Mexico City: El Colegio de México, Fondo de Cultura Económica, 2005.

Tavera Alfaro, Xavier. "Documentos para la historia del periodismo Mexicano, siglo xviii." In *Estudios Históricos Americanos. Homenaje a Silvio Zavala*, edited by Julio Le Riverend Brusone, 319–44. Mexico City: El Colegio de México, 1953.

Taylor, William B. *Drinking, Homicide, and Rebellion in Colonial Mexican Villages*. Stanford, Calif.: Stanford University Press, 1979.

Tenorio-Trillo, Mauricio. *Mexico at the World's Fairs: Crafting a Modern Nation*. Berkeley: University of California Press, 1996.

Tortorici, Zeb. "Women at the Margins of the Unnatural: Abortion and Infanticide in New Spain." Paper Presented at the Latin American Studies Association Meeting, Rio de Janeiro, June 11–14, 2009.

Twinam, Ann. "The Church, the State, and the Abandoned: Expósitos in Late Eighteenth-Century Havana." In *Raising an Empire: Children in Early Modern Iberia and Colonial Latin America*, edited by Ondina E. González and Bianca Premo, 163–86. Albuquerque: University of New Mexico Press, 2007.

———. "Honor, Sexuality, and Illegitimacy in Colonial Spanish America." In *Sexuality and Marriage in Colonial Latin America*, edited by Asuncion Lavrin, 118–55. Albuquerque: University of New Mexico Press, 1989.

———. "The Negotiation of Honor: Elites, Sexuality, and Illegitimacy in Eighteenth-Century Spanish America." In *The Faces of Honor: Sex, Shame, and Violence in Colonial Latin America*, edited by Lyman L. Johnson and Sonya Lipsett-Rivera, 68–102. Albuquerque: University of New Mexico Press, 1998.

———. *Public Lives, Private Secrets: Gender, Honor, Sexuality and Illegitimacy in Colonial Spanish America*. Stanford, Calif.: Stanford University Press, 1999.

Ulrich, Laurel Thatcher, *A Midwife's Tale: The Life of Martha Ballard, Based on Her Diary, 1785–1812*. New York: Vintage, 1991.

Uribe Elías, Roberto. *La invención de la mujer: Nacimiento de una escuela médica*. Mexico City: Fondo de Cultura Económica, Benemérita Universidad Autónoma de Puebla, 2002.

———. "Mexican Obstetrical-Gynecological Surgery in the 19th Century." *Cirugía y Cirujanos* 75, no. 2 (2007): 137–42.

Uribe-Uran, Victor M. "Innocent Infants or Abusive Patriarchs? Spousal Homicides, the Punishment of Indians and the Law in Colonial Mexico, 1740s–1820s." *Journal of Latin American Studies* 38 (2006): 793–828.

Van Patten, Nathan. "Obstetrics in Mexico Prior to 1600." *Annals of Medical History* 4, no. 2 (1932): 203–12.

Vela, Estefanía. "Current Abortion Regulation in Mexico." *Documentos de Trabajo del CIDE* 50 (2010): 1–19. http://www.cide.edu/publicaciones/status /dts/DTEJ%2050.pdf, accessed September 7, 2015.

Voekel, Pamela. *Alone before God: The Religious Origins of Modernity in Mexico*. Durham, N.C.: Duke University Press, 2002.

Volo, James M., and Dorothy Deneen Volo. *Family Life in Nineteenth-Century America*. Westport, Conn.: Greenwood, 2007.

Von Sneidern, Maja-Lisa. "Joined at the Hip: A Monster, Colonialism, and the Scriblerian Project." *Eighteenth-Century Studies* 30, no. 3 (1997): 213–31.

Wertz, Richard W., and Dorothy C. Wertz. *Lying-In: A History of Childbirth in America*. New Haven, Conn.: Yale University Press, 1989.

Wilson, Adrian. *The Making of Man-Midwifery: Childbirth in England, 1660–1770*. Cambridge, Mass.: Harvard University Press, 1995.

Wrigley, E. A., R. S. Davies, J. E. Oeppen, and R. S. Schofield *English Population History from Family Reconstitution 1580–1837*. Cambridge: Cambridge University Press, 1997.

Index

Abortifacients, 33–34, 44, 78, 79–80, 81, 82, 84, 91, 94, 96, 100. See also *Cihuapatli*

Abortion, 9, 38, 77–79, 84; attitudes toward, 92–93, 98–100, 210; colonial, 80–83, 91–96; pre-Columbian, 79–80; in the nineteenth century, 83–87, 96–101; prohibitions on, xiii–xiv, 87–91, 92, 94–95, 102–3; surgical, 86. *See also* Abortifacients; Antiabortive remedies

Abrego, Federico, 86–87

Acosta, Elvira, 99–100

Acosta, Pomposa, 99–100

Advertising, 67, 192, 197

Alcaldes. See Judges

Alsivar, Juana Josefa, 116–17

Altamisa, 81, 82, 85, 102, 210, 213

Alzate y Ramírez, José Antonio de, 144, 146, 159, 162

Anatomy, reproductive, 3, 40, 196, 198–200, 206. *See also* Cervix; Hymen; Pelvis; Placenta; Uterus; Womb

Antiabortive remedies, 46, 66

Arnold, Linda, 14, 123, 135

Arrom, Silvia, 53, 83

Astruc, Jean, 48

Axoxoquilitl, 79

Baptisms, 13, 95, 141, 147, 156, 177, 184, 186, 267 (nn. 18, 37)

Barbers, 7, 47

Barrera, María, 86–87

Bartolache, José Ignacio, 46, 59, 61, 144

Baudelocque, Louis, 27, 64

Birth. *See* Childbirth

Bleeding, 44, 47, 84, 190, 268 (n. 59)

Bloodletters. *See* Phlebotomists; Bleeding

Blum, Ann, 37, 127

Bodies, women's, 5, 57–58, 68–69. *See also* Anatomy: reproductive; Menstruation; Nursing; Pregnancy; Sexuality.

Bolaños, Juan Nepomuceno, 163, 167–69

Boticarios, 7, 47, 60, 62, 78, 81, 82

Bourbon Reforms, 145–46, 151, 159; and children, 109, 119; and education, 143–44; and justice, 98; and marriage, 36; and medicine, 58–61, 174, 184

Bravo, Francisco, 45

Breech of marriage. See *Palabra de casamiento*

Buenas Costumbres, 90, 101, 107, 124, 125, 126, 128–32. *See also* Honor: sexual

Buffington, Robert, 132, 135

Buffon, Comte de (Georges-Louis Leclerc), 150, 159, 160, 161

Caesarean births, xiv–xv, 4, 61, 147, 184–87

Calvo, Thomas, 77

Cangiamila, Francisco, 184–87

Casa de Maternidad, 2, 7, 37, 60, 169, 188, 196, 197, 200; abortions and, 79, 85, 86; monstrous births and, 172; puerperal infections at, 200–207

Casa de Niños Expósitos, 108, 116. *See also* Foundlings

Catholic Church, 14, 25, 88, 147, 184, 193. *See also* Catholicism; Inquisition

Catholicism, 20–21, 23–24, 32, 41, 146–47

Censuses, 11–13

Cervix, 61, 67, 68, 69, 85, 172, 190, 199, 214, 246 (n. 120)

Chamomile, 65, 81, 188

Charles III (king of Spain), 147, 158, 177, 184–85

Charles IV (king of Spain), 109, 157

Cházaro, Laura, 196, 199

Chepa, Josefa, 49

Childbirth, 46, 48, 189–90; attitudes towards, 174–78, 196–97, 210–11; in the colonial era, 176–87, *182*; and concealment, 111, 117, 118, 124, 252 (n. 2); instruments used during, 7, 63, 190–207, *191*, 200–207; medicine to alleviate pain of, 56; multiple, 155–56; positions during, 7, 178–79; rates, 11–13, 37, 77, 82–83, 207. *See also* Caesarean births; Forceps; Labor; Monstrous births; Mortality: maternal; Newborns;

Childhood. *See* Children

Children, 91, 105, 108, 109, 112, 116, 118–20, 127, 131, 159. *See also* Foundlings; Mortality: child

Christianity. *See* Catholic Church

Church. *See* Catholic Church

Científicos, 38

Cihuapatli, 80, 81, 85, 86, 102, 179, 189, 207, 210, 213

Civil Code of 1870, 89, 123, 126

Civil Registry, 90, 124, 126

Clavijero, Francisco Javier, 159, 161

Climatology, 156, 159–60, 171

Coitus. *See* Intercourse

Conception, 5, 23–24, 33, 42, 44, 57, 64, 65, 67, 73–74

Consejo Superior de Salubridad, 192, 193, 200, 203

Contraception, 46, 77, 78, 210; colonial 80–83; pre-Columbian, 79–80; nineteenth century, 83–87

Courts, 26, 96–98, 107–8, 114–15, 122, 123–26. *See also* Judges

Creole patriotism, 3, 142, 146, 158, 159–62

Crime, 38, 98, 107–8, 115, 123, 125, 132, 133, 135–37. *See* Abortion; Infanticide; Criminology; Penal code of 1871; Rape

Criminal Code. *See* Penal code of 1871

Criminology, 38, 132, 143

Cuernecillo de centeno. See Ergot

Curadores, 104, 112, 115, 120–22, 128, 129, 131, 194, 212–13

Curanderas, 7, 8, 9, 30, 33, 53, 57, 62, 78

Departamento de Partos Ocultos o Reservados, 37, 60, 110, 119, 130, 169

Depósito, 95, 112, 120, 253 (n. 27)

Díaz, Francisca, 51–52

Disease. *See* Illness

Divorce, 119

Doctors, 6, 10, 42–43, 46–48, 58–59, 63–64, 69–70, *70, 71*, 116, 121, 181–83; and abortion, 86–87, 91; and midwives, 60–61, 69–73; and regulation, 58–63. *See also* Obstetricians; Surgeons

Dolores, María, 113–14, 213

Dore, Elizabeth, 2

Education, female, 21, 119, 192. *See also* Midwifery: licensing of

Embryotomies, 177–78, 187, 200

Enlightenment, 3, 5, 8, 118, 142, 150–51, 159, 162

Erauso, Catalina de, 25

Ergot, 85, 189, 207, 208

Escarcega, Tomasa, 100–101
Escobar, Teresa, 112, 118
Escriche, Joaquín, 89, 91, 124
Escuela de Medicina, 63, 85, 164, 169, 187, 196, 198
Esteyneffer, Juan de, 33, 66, 187, 189
Eugenics, 3, 4, 38, 143, 171, 172, 206

Ferrer Espejo y Cienfuegos, José, 84–85
Fertility, 12, 44, 46, 142, 149, 151, 156, 169, 171, 210
Few, Martha, 8, 9, 148, 211
Flores y Troncoso, Franicsco de Asis, 4, 38–40, 74, 85, 99, 186, 198–99, 212; and midwifery 6–7, 9, 45, 72–73, 188
Forceps, 63, 172, 188, 190, *191*, 192, 199, 200, 201, 202, 214
Foucault, Michel, 97, 235 (n. 4)
Foundlings, 108, 109, 112, 116
Freud, Sigmund, 15

García, Guadalupe, 125–26, 129, 131
García, Mauricia, 128–29
Gazeta de México, 27, 64, 81, 141–47, 150, 151–62, 167, 177, 185–86
Gender, 2–5, 35, 43–44, 90, 92, 105, 114, 120, 148. See also *Buenas Costumbres*; Honor: sexual; Motherhood; Virginity
Guerrero, Julio, 38

Hechicería. See Witchcraft
Hernández, Francisco, 44, 46, 79, 80, 152–53, 162, 187
Hernández, Isabel, 33–34, 44, 52–53, 80, 81, 183
Hernández, Juana, 111–12, 120
Hippocrates, 48, 55
Holy Office. *See* Inquisition
Honor: public, 90, 113–14, 118, 124, 128, 130, 137; sexual, 1–2, 19, 31, 41, 99, 105, 107, 110, 118, 119, 132, 134, 167, 211. *See also* Virginity; *Buenas Costumbres*
Humors, 33, 65, 66. *See also* Bleeding
Hymen, 26, 27–29, 38–41, 199, 207
Hysteria, 33, 68, 82

Illegitimacy, 91, 99, 104, 116, 118, 124, 125, 131, 185; and paternity suits, 126–27; rates of, 12, 31–32, 37, 83
Illiteracy, 48, 52–53, 129, 194. *See also* Literacy
Illness, 44, 47–48, 67, 81, 82, 174–75. *See also* Mortality; Puerperal infection
Incest, 24, 25, 32, 82, 96, 113
Infanticide, 1–2, 55, 57–58, 83, 87–92, 97, 98, 99, 104–37, 175, 185, 193–96, 210–13; attitudes toward, 105, 111, 112, 210; prohibitions on, 109, 124; prosecution of, 105, 108, 122–28
Inquisition, 9, 23, 49, 64, 92, 94, 95; and midwives, 33, 48, 53, 55–56, 57, 69–70, 72, 80, 183, 184
Insanity, 120, 121–22, 213
Intercourse, 26, 35, 39, 45, 64, 65, 66
Intoxication, 120, 137, 213

Judges, 97, 123, 135; and abortion, 88–89, 91, 92–93, 95, 101, 135; and infanticide, 58, 109, 111–24, 128, 129, 133, 195–96; and midwives, 29–30. *See also* Legal system
Judiciary. *See* Judges

Labor, 46
Lamarck, Jean-Baptiste, 170, 171, 206
Lanning, John Tate, 6
Lara, María de la Luz, 113, 117, 118
Legal system: colonial, 87–88, 109; nineteenth-century, 89–90, 98, 123–24. *See also* Judges; Penal Code of 1871; Civil Code of 1870

Legitimacy, 24, 41, 47, 67, 91, 124.
  See also Illegitimacy
Leite, Angela Marìa, 62
León, Nicolás, 6, 7, 47, 55, 64, 73, 86,
  178, 180, 183
Levret, Andrés, 27, 64
Liberalism, 2, 78, 89–90
Licensing, medical, 8, 59–60
Limpieza de sangre, 24, 25, 47, 60, 212
Lipsett-Rivera, Sonya, 32, 35–36, 119
Lister, Joseph, 201–2
Literacy, 48–49, 52–53, 144
Lizardi, Joaquín José Fernández de,
  180–81, *182*
López, Gregorio, 46, 187

Magistrates. *See* Judges
Marriage, 24; banns, 34; impediments
  to, 24–25, 32, 34. *See also* Divorce;
  Palabra de casamiento
Martínez de Castro, Antonio, 89–90
Maternity. *See* Motherhood
Maternity hospitals. *See* Casa de
  Maternidad
Matrimony suits. See *Palabra de
  casamiento*
Mauriceau, François, 5, 27, 64
Maygrier, Jacques Pierre, 63, *70*
McCaa, Robert, 12, 13, 207
Medicine: African, 6; indigenous, 6,
  7–8, 43–46, 53, 77, 80–81, 86,
  178–87, 188; popular, 7, 10. *See also*
  Obstetrics; Pregnancy
Medina, Antonio, 26, 28, 48, 60–61,
  64, 65, 67–68, 80, 179, 189
Menstruation, 27, 46, 57, 64, 65, 69,
  197; and regulators, 33–34, 78,
  79–80, 81, 84, 102, 212; suspension
  of, 33, 65, 68, 82
Mercurio Volante, 46, 59
Mezcal, 188, 189
Midwifery, 4–7, 8–10; licensing of,
  2–3, 48, 54–55, 59–63, 77, 192–96,

245 (n. 81); texts, 26, 27, 28, 48, 59,
  60–61, 63, 64, 65, 67, 80, 85, 101,
  185, 187. *See also* Midwives
Midwives, 28, 30, 33–34, 42, 46,
  47–55, 57, 80–81, 88, 177, 178, 179,
  184, 187–88, 201, 206; and abortion,
  33–34, 44, 78, 84, 85–88, 91, 94;
  and doctors, 9–10, 56, 58, 60–61,
  68–70, 72–73, 176, 178–79, 180–81,
  183; indigenous, 43–46, 54, 79–80,
  86, 178–87, *180*, 206; and infanticide, 55, 110, 193–96; and the
  Inquisition, 49–50, 52–53, 55–56,
  57, 69–72, 80–81, 94; male, 5, 59,
  62, 68; performing medical
  examinations, 26, 28–31, 49, 58, 62,
  112, 116, 125, 133; pre-Columbian,
  43–46, 79–80, 177–80, *180*, 187; and
  superstition, 9, 181, 183–84, 267
  (n. 23); and witchcraft, 49–50, 52,
  53, 55–56, 57, 80–81
Miscarriage, 78, 80, 82–83, 87, 95, 97,
  99, 101, 102, 112, 113, 128, 131, 183,
  210, 214; preventing, 46, 65, 66
Modernization, 127, 132, 134–35, 145,
  162
Monstrous births, 3, 56, 88, 215; in the
  colonial era 143–59; in the nineteenth century, 162–73
Montaña, Luis José, 245 (n. 75)
Montequitl, 20
Montiel, Tomasa, 124, 175
Mortality: infant, 4, 11, 12, 13, 90, 115,
  116, 174–75; child, 116; maternal, 4,
  12–13, 85, 174, 200–207
Motherhood: ideals of, 2, 5, 105,
  118–22, 126, 128, 130, 131, 132–36,
  211–3l; and lineage, 24; and pregnancy, 65–67; practice of, 21, 175

Nationalism, 2–3, 40, 107, 175,
  196–207, 215. *See also* Creole
  patriotism

Newborns, care of, 82, 174–75, 179–81, *180*, 187

Nursing, 67, 120, 122, 124, 155, 157. *See also* Wet nurses.

Obstetricians, 3, 4, 7 42–43, 68–69, *70, 71*, 181–83 *See also* Obstetrics

Obstetrics, 5–6, 27–28, 47–48, 64–68, 84, 184–87, 188–206; Pre-Columbian, 43–46, 177–80, *180;* and nationalism, 196–207; nineteenth century, 39–40, 170, 196–207; and regulation, 60–63, 67, 68. *See also* Midwifery; Rodríguez, Juan María

Orgasm, 64–65

Osorio, María, 130, 133, 259 (n. 106)

Pacheco, Ramón, 37

Pacheco, Romualda, 30–31

Palabra de casamiento, 25, 32, 57, 82, 96, 118

Parteras. See Midwives

Pastor, José Ventura, 27, 64, 69, *71, 72,* 84, 189, *191*

Paternity, 24, 126–27

Pauw, Cornelius de, 159, 160, 161

Pelvis, 7, 40, 198–200

Penal Code of 1871, 36, 78, 86, 89–91, 97, 98–99, 102, 124, 128, 129, 137

Penyak, Lee, 10, 28, 29, 30, 49

Pérez, María de los Santos de, 126, 135, *136*

Peyote, 57, 244 (n. 46)

Pharmacists. See *Boticarios*

Phlebotomists, 7, 47, 112

Physicians. *See* Doctors

Placenta, 46, 61, 164, 172, 186, 189, 200, 201

Porfiriato, 61, 127, 134–35, 193, 199; and crime, 105, 125, 132; intellectual project of, 37–38, 119, 136–37, 205–6

Posada, José Guadalupe, 165, *166*

Positivism, 2, 4, 6, 38, 39

Pregnancy, 5, 42, 44–45; counsel during, 65–67; signs of 57–58, 65, 68, 73–74

Prostitutes, 55, 104, 117, 134

Prostitution, 38, 55, 131. *See also* Prostitutes

Protomedicato, 2, 46, 54, 60–61, 62, 63, 68, 77, 179, 192

Public health, 2–3, 38, 85, 119, 134, 174–75, 184–85, 192, 197, 202–7. *See also* Consejo Superior de Salubridad

Public Sphere, 41, 78, 89–91, 102, 105, 175, 196–98, 210–11; and honor, 32–33, 37, 99, 113–14, 118, 124, 130, 132, 133, 134; and virginity, 34, 41

Puerperal infection, 7, 188, 200–208

Pulque, 81

Quezada, Noemí, 43

Race, 49–52, 54, 198, 199, 206. See also *Limpieza de sangre*

Ramírez, Getrudis, 110, 195

Ramírez, Ramón, 163, 172, 173

Rape, xiii, 10, 26, 28–31, 35, 38, 39, 49, 58, 67

Rapto, 36, 134

Rodríguez, Joseph Manuel, 185

Rodríguez, Juan María, 3, 40, 66, 68, 74, 143, 164, 169–73, 189, 197–99, 202, 206

Romero, Carlota, 63

Romero, Felipa, 55, 110, 184, 193–95

Rougmanac, Carlos, 38

Royal College of Surgery, 7, 60, 61

Royal Pragmatic, 24

Sahagún, Bernardino de, 9, 43–45, 79–80, 81, 87, 177, 178

Saint-Hilaire, Étienne Geoffroy, 168, 170–71

Sánchez, María Francisca Ignacia, 62

Seed, Patricia, 24, 36
Segura, Ignacio, 80, 179, 184, 185
Serrano, Antonio, 62–63, 192
Sexuality, 5, 20, 26, 32, 35, 36, 37, 38,
    39, 128–29, 167. *See also* Orgasm;
    Intercourse
Shelton, Laura, 13, 127, 130
Siete Partidas, 87, 88, 109
Slaves, African, 32, 51–52, 53, 183
Sloan, Kathryn, 36, 134
Sorcery. *See* Witchcraft
Speckman Guerra, Elisa, 88, 90, 105,
    122, 133, 237 (n. 45)
Stepan, Nancy Leys, 3, 4, 206
Sterility, 45, 64, 79, 160
Surgeons, 47, 59, 61, 62
Syphilitics, 38

Temazcales, 7, 45, 46, 80, 214
Tenedoras, 55, 178, 194
Teodora, Ignacia, 121–22
Teratology, 143, 162, 163, 164, 167, 168,
    169, 170–71
Ticitl, 43–46, 65
Tlaquatzin, 80, 81, 247 (n. 9)
Torres, Ignacio, 28, 66, 68
Torres, María de Jesús, 120, 213
Torres, Petra de, 53, 123
Tribunals. *See* Courts
Twinam, Ann, 32, 34, 116
Twins, conjoined, 149, 154, 155,
    157–58, 161, 164, 167, 170

Uterus, 21, 66, 68, 143, 167, 171,
    172–73, 177, 197, 199, 205, 207,
    211

Valdés, Manuel Antonio, 143–45, 150,
    152
Venegas, Juan Manuel, 27, 33,
    64, 81
Ventura, Mariana del Carmen, 104,
    112, 115, 120
Vidart, Pedro, 27, 64, 65, 189
Villalpando, Cristóbal de, 21, 22
Virginity, 2, 24, 25, 31, 32, 34, 35–37;
    biological, 19; and Catholicism,
    20–21; and honor, 41; medical
    examinations to establish, 26,
    28–30, 38–41; pre-Columbian
    attitudes toward, 20; social 19, 20,
    25, 27, 32, 34–35, 41, 132, 211
Virgin Mary, 21, 23, 24, 41, 94
Virtue, public, 1–2

Wet nurses, 117, 157
Witchcraft, 8, 9, 48, 49, 53, 57, 69–70,
    72, 79, 80, 184
Womb, 24, 44, 45, 57, 61, 66, 68, 72,
    82, 94, 101, 147, 168, 177, 183, 189,
    206. *See also* Uterus; Caesarean
    births

Zárate, Josefa de, 53
Zárate, Manuel de, 145, 157

CPSIA information can be obtained at www.ICGtesting.com
Printed in the USA
LVOW11*0131231016

509858LV00010B/27/P